DARK CALORIES

DARK CALORIES

HOW VEGETABLE OILS DESTROY OUR HEALTH
AND HOW WE CAN GET IT BACK

CATHERINE SHANAHAN, MD

First published in the United States in 2024 by Hachette Go,
an imprint of Hachette Books

First published in Great Britain in 2024 by Orion Spring,
an imprint of The Orion Publishing Group Ltd
Carmelite House, 50 Victoria Embankment
London EC4Y 0DZ

An Hachette UK Company

The authorised representative in the EEA is Hachette Ireland,
8 Castlecourt Centre, Dublin 15, D15 XTP3, Ireland (email: info@hbgi.ie)

7 9 10 8 6

A CIP catalogue record for this book is
available from the British Library.

ISBN (Trade Paperback) 978 1 3987 2073 2
ISBN (eBook) 978 1 3987 2074 9
ISBN (Audio) 978 1 3987 2075 6

Cover design by Amanda Kain
Cover photograph by Ratchat / Getty Images
Print book interior design by Sheryl Kober

Printed and bound in Great Britain by Clays Ltd, Elcograf S.p.A.

Every effort has been made to ensure that the information in the book
is accurate. The information in this book may not be applicable in each
individual case so it is advised that professional medical advice is obtained for
specific health matters and before changing any medication or dosage. Neither
the publisher nor author accepts any legal responsibility for any personal
injury or other damage or loss arising from the use of the information in this
book. In addition if you are concerned about your diet or exercise regime and
wish to change them, you should consult a health practitioner first.

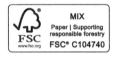

www.orionbooks.co.uk

To everyone whose daily labors strengthen Mother Earth.

CONTENTS

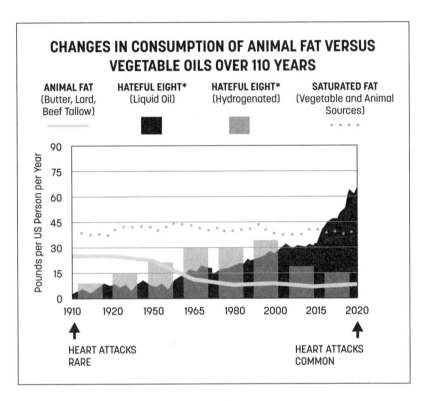

Figure 0-1: This graph showing our historic fat consumption suggests a root cause that doctors don't learn about. In fact, the data goes against everything doctors do learn about nutrition. As you can see, vegetable oil consumption has increased in the past 110 years, while saturated fat and animal fat have not.

I'm showing you that there is no correlation between either saturated fat or animal fat and heart attacks. Nevertheless, doctors learn that there is. The indoctrination with this carefully crafted concept opened the door to flood the American diet with cheaply produced oils that change our body chemistry in ways that breed every disease you can name. That story is what this book is all about.

For sources used to create this figure, see the endnotes for the introduction.

*Corn oil, cottonseed oil, canola oil, soy oil, sunflower oil, safflower oil, grapeseed oil, ricebran oil

INTRODUCTION

Most of us are aware of the dangers of trans fats, sugars, and chemical preservatives added to processed foods like tater tots and Twinkies. But what if I told you that roughly 30 percent of the calories in your diet are likely coming from a substance you probably haven't noticed, with no color, odor, or flavor, and that has effects on our metabolism that medical science knows little about?

Whether you shop at Whole Foods Market or The Dollar Store, the ingredients listed on most of the products in your kitchen right now likely include vegetable oil, or, to be specific, the following phrase: VEGETABLE OIL (CONTAINS ONE OR MORE OF THE FOLLOWING: COTTONSEED, CORN, RAPESEED, SOYBEAN, SUNFLOWER, SAFFLOWER).

Once you start looking, you'll see them *everywhere*, since more than 80 percent of foods with an ingredients label do indeed contain at least one type of vegetable oil.[1]

The reason human health is increasingly in crisis is right there on the label, hidden in plain sight. Yet doctors learn almost nothing about these ingredients.

I was no exception.

When I went to medical school in the early 1990s, I never heard vegetable oils mentioned during lectures on nutrition. They are not part of our initial training or our continuing medical education. There are no medical societies that focus on educating doctors about vegetable oils or their health effects. None of the charitable foundations devoted to researching disease shines any light on the role of vegetable oils in their disease of interest.

I probably would have remained ignorant to this day if I'd stayed healthy. But in 2001, I developed a serious and mysterious medical condition that made it difficult for me to walk, endangering my ability to continue working as a family doctor. The specialists I saw took guesses at what might be going on, but their procedures only made it worse. After exhausting all other angles, I finally went along with something my husband had been saying for years: stop eating so much sugar. He compared my diet to that of an army of ants, and dropped a book with a hopeful-sounding title on my lap, *Spontaneous Healing*. But it turned out that sugar wasn't the big epiphany in that book. Reading it, I ran into the concept of essential fatty acids, which is the term for fats our bodies don't make and that we need to get from our diet, like omega-3.

These days, everyone knows fish oil is a source of omega-3 fats, but back in the 1990s, nobody outside of the researchers who studied essential fats ever talked about them. Essential fatty acids belong to a category of fat called polyunsaturated fats. That makes them different from the types of fats I'd learned were unhealthy, called saturated fats. These polyunsaturated fatty acids have vitamin-like properties, playing roles in fundamental body processes, including blood clotting, reproduction, and fending off infections, among others, so I wondered if they could help me improve my own health. I needed to know more.

Today, I'm a doctor with a specialty in family medicine. But before I went to medical school I'd gone to Cornell University as a PhD student, dreaming of genetically engineering bacteria that could digest plastic. I stayed long enough to learn two important things—truly, both changed my life. One, we were a long way off from designer microbes, which was why I dropped out and went to medical school instead. And two, certain forms of oxygen are highly attracted to closely spaced double bonds. That last bit of knowledge did nothing for me until that pivotal moment in my life when I wanted to learn more about polyunsaturated fatty acids—like those in vegetable oils (more on that in chapter 1).

But I couldn't just crack open ordinary medical textbooks or even look up polyunsaturated fats online. This was 2002, when search engines were rudimentary and online resources like PubMed were limited in scope. Even more frustratingly, I couldn't find the answers in medical journals or at medical conferences, either. I had to look outside the medical system entirely. This was not easy to do in the days when you had to know exactly what you were looking for to find anything online. I was looking for a tiny group of chemical experts who studied polyunsaturated fatty acids, like those in vegetable oils. They are best called lipid scientists, because the only thing they all have in common is that they study lipid science. *Lipid* meaning fat.

Part of the difficulty in finding lipid scientists comes from the fact that they don't all have the same training, background, or titles. Some are toxicologists studying the basic chemistry of toxin formation, for example, while some are industry experts studying how processing, cooking, and extended shelf storage affect toxin formation in these oils. The only thing that unites all lipid scientists is that they have the training and knowledge required to understand the unique chemistry of vegetable oils.

So I bought textbooks. I started with a thousand-page biochemistry textbook and began devouring the science. After months of searching for a book specifically about fats and oils, I found one called *Know Your Fats*, written in 2000 by a stern-appearing lipid scientist named Mary Enig, PhD. The book taught me that vegetable oils were chock-full of "highly unstable polyunsaturated fatty acids," which meant they were prone to forming gummy, sticky residue "in salad bowls and frying pans."[2] What did that mean to anyone eating them? I'd thought that polyunsaturated fats might have been the key to better health, but now I wasn't so sure. *Know Your Fats* didn't have much information other than that, but it was enough to get me very concerned about the healthfulness of these oils. I kept looking.

The investigation took me down a rabbit hole that would unravel everything I thought I knew about diet, health, and chronic disease, and completely change my life. Soon after diving into the biochemistry of fatty acids, my thinking on vegetable oil did a 180. I went from hoping polyunsaturated fatty acids might help me get healthy to wondering if they were the reason I'd gotten sick. According to numerous lipid scientists, these polyunsaturated fats have chemical properties that made them potentially quite dangerous. Yes, we need to eat *some* (as we will see in chapter 2), but today we are eating a lot. In order to better understand how they affect human health, I've had to consider how they are manufactured; how they behave when we cook with them; how our bodies absorb and distribute them through the bloodstream; how they affect our cell membranes, our DNA, our bodies' antioxidants, and various enzymes; where our bodies store these fats; and how they affect the health of each and every major organ and tissue, including our arteries, our brains, our livers, our skin, and so on. What I learned upended my view of what constitutes a healthy diet.

But how did medical science get all of it so wrong? That question took me down another rabbit hole. I learned of an undisclosed conflict of interest between the vegetable oil industry and organized medicine that has existed since shortly after World War II. This alliance has given us all the wrong idea about which fats are good and which ones are bad. It has distorted nutrition science and stalled progress in medicine and health care for over half a century. And it has led to a scenario where the very diet that doctors believe is healthy is in fact making us sick. The entanglements now run deep, extending well beyond just what doctors learn about nutrition. They climb all the way up the ivory towers of our most influential Ivy League institutions, and they are now codified into multiple federal and state laws.

I'm writing this book to expose not just this story but also what has happened to our health because these relationships persist and continue to impair medical science. The entanglements between the vegetable oil industry and leading health authorities originated so long ago that they've now shaped doctors' day-to-day practices. They've molded the nutritional ideology of every medical specialty. This ideology, in turn, impacts health-care guidelines, including how we treat high blood pressure, diabetes, obesity, strokes, cancer, and so on.

After I learned about the harms of vegetable oils and how traditional foods might heal us, I went around the country trying to share this information with other doctors. Unfortunately, I soon realized that the doctors working in the insurance-based system—and I was one of them—no longer have the freedom to do what we think is best for our patients. Many of our day-to-day treatment choices are dictated by practice guidelines handed down to us from on high. On top of that, if we fail to comply, we may even be penalized financially—creating a powerful disincentive to question the status quo. So instead of swimming upstream fighting the entire healthcare industry, I decided to focus on sharing this information directly with the food consumer. With a renewed sense of professional purpose, I began writing my first book, *Deep Nutrition: Why Your Genes Need Traditional Food*, in which I argued that our historical culinary practices represented a great body of nutritional wisdom that enabled us to survive in every corner of the globe.

The Four Pillars of a Human Diet

Before the industrial era, people across the globe ate according to principles that had sustained humanity for thousands of years. Working with the ecology of their particular locale, they extracted maximum nutrition using four simple dietary strategies: (1) Eat fresh food from healthy soil, raw or gently cooked. (2) Preserve and enhance foods using fermentation and sprouting. (3) Extract nutrients that support healthy connective tissue by boiling animal bones, skin, and joint material. (4) Use every part of the animal, including the organs and the fat. Our genes have come to expect the collection of nutrients these strategies deliver, and without them, we can't achieve our health potential. We'll explore the Four Pillars in more depth in chapter 10.

In 2011, my husband cooked up a plan to expand our sphere of influence by several orders of magnitude by connecting with athletes. And why not start with the best? We mailed Gary Vitti, head athletic trainer of the LA Lakers, a copy of *Deep Nutrition*. A week later, Gary called to say, "Everyone who's written a diet book in the past thirty years has sent me a copy. Yours is the first one that changed the way I think about food." Gary was not a person to take chances with a multibillion-dollar franchise, and his endorsement held a lot of sway. The Lakers soon hired me as a staff member to create their PRO Nutrition program, launching a lasting and mutually beneficial relationship between the National Basketball Association and Whole Foods Market. Central to my effort working with them was eliminating vegetable oils from the athletes' diets, because I suspected the oils were slowing down recovery and sapping their energy. We got it out of the food they ate at the Staples Center, during training, on planes, and at every hotel buffet.

The results were incredible, and soon many other NBA teams and players followed suit. This way of eating spread to the multi-championship Golden State Warriors, to the Oklahoma City Thunders, and to other teams, and to individual players such as Kyle Lowry, right after signing his four-year, $46 million contract with the Raptors (he went on to lead them to their first-ever championship victory in 2019). Even college teams followed suit: Villanova had its basketball team, the Wildcats, ditch seed oils in 2015, and they earned their first championship in thirty years in 2016. They won again in 2018. Scores of professional teams and athletes around the world have now adopted these principles.

My work has gone beyond the world of sports as well. I'm delighted to have met many medical influencers who were interested in learning why these oils deserve the title of public health enemy number one, often by diving deep into the science on-air. Everyone I've spoken with has been grateful to have their eyes opened on this important topic, and many of them have since continued to loudly sound the alarm to their audiences.

Dr. Ken Berry, Dr. Paul Saladino, Dr. Mike Eades, Dr. David Perlmutter, Dr. Anthony Gustin, and Dr. Daniel Pompa are among them. One of the best descriptions of the health transformation you get from cutting seed oils comes from Dr. Drew Pinsky, of *Loveline* fame. Speaking on air during one of our conversations, he said, "If you had told me that two weeks into it, I would feel this good, I wouldn't have believed you."

Deep Nutrition was initially published in 2008. It covered just a small sliver of the harms that vegetable oils can do to us, and when I wrote it I wasn't yet sure which was worse, vegetable oils or sugar. Still, it was enough to inspire some forward-thinking entrepreneurs. A few food manufacturers began catering to the small group of consumers seeking vegetable-oil-free products such as mayonnaise, salad dressings, and potato chips. This kind of business has since grown from a handful of boutique producers to major companies that sell their products in places like Costco and Walmart. The first blips and alerts have already started, and vegetable oil is poised to take the same trajectory that sugar has taken toward food-pariah status. But there's enormous pressure to maintain the status quo that has been holding this movement back—and that's why I sincerely hope that you, dear reader, will be able to join and help shape this exciting and urgently needed cultural revolution.

Almost nobody was talking about vegetable oils before *Deep Nutrition*. Since writing it, I've continued to assemble the research into a cohesive body of practical medical insights, amounting to a new paradigm for health and nutrition that I will present to you here. In recent years, I've begun to talk about this paradigm with influencers and other health experts, and I've happily watched the don't-eat-toxic-oil conversation explode on social media as early adopters have proliferated and repeated the information. I've noticed, however, that enthusiasm can seem like fanaticism to doctors, scientists, journalists, and others who only encounter snippets of the argument in a forum unfit for serious scientific discourse. This makes it too easy to dismiss the concept as just another fad. By providing a more complete picture, I hope to make it very clear that the link between vegetable oil and poor health is firmly grounded and can be backed up with hard scientific research. If you've previously heard that seed oils are unhealthy and were intrigued, I'm glad you're here because now you've come to the source of this growing discussion, and you're going to get the full story. I want to take you on a journey of discovery that will change your life for the better and very likely add years, if not decades, to your time here on Earth by revealing the truth about vegetable oils—the dark calories in your diet.

There are three aspects of vegetable oil that I would call dark. First, the truth about vegetable oil has been hidden from medical doctors, and this has negatively impacted the entire field. Second, because people have manipulated our belief systems for profit, and in doing so have sold more vegetable oil, the substance has brought out the worst aspects of human nature. And third, like dark matter in the universe, vegetable oil explains otherwise unexplainable phenomena—and removing it from our diets resolves otherwise unresolvable health conditions.

I want to help you recognize that your life-giving biology is under siege—that these oils will inevitably make you sick (if they haven't already)—and open your eyes to the systems ready to capitalize on your need for medical care. I want to show you this so that you can appreciate what you stand to gain by losing your reliance on these toxic vegetable oils. Then, I'll show you how to get started.

The book is divided into three parts.

In Part One, you'll learn what the scientists who specialize in studying toxin formation in vegetable oils have been trying to tell us. You'll find out how these oils are made, and I'll introduce the basic terms used to describe their toxicity. You'll witness how these toxins pummel our physiology at the cellular and genetic levels, and how that microscopic damage manifests as some of the most terrifying inflammatory, degenerative, and age-related diseases we know.

In Part Two, we'll take a deeper look at a misunderstood nutrient, cholesterol, and at how it came to be a scapegoat for our pressing health issues.

We'll meet the men who managed to scare us into believing that a vital nutrient is bad for our health. We'll discover that, whether by intent or by fortuitous design, by building cholesterol avoidance into the foundation of preventive medicine, an annual physical exam lures healthy people into becoming lifelong patients. We'll see how, just as the processed food industry has commandeered nutrition science, the drug and device industry now controls much of medical science, medical education, and medical research.

Part Three will empower you to take control of your own health and well-being. You'll learn how to identify and avoid vegetable oils at home, at the grocery store, and at restaurants. We'll look at the healthful foods that will put you on the path to healing. The final chapter invites you to detoxify for just two weeks and see how much better you start to feel. My hope is that, once you reacquaint yourself with some healthy, delicious, and easy-to-prepare foods, you'll find living without vegetable oil to be so energizing that you'll want to continue indefinitely.

We doctors will do our best with the information we are taught. But vegetable oils affect our health so profoundly and in so many ways that it represents a whole other world of knowledge that most health professionals are unaware of. The explanations doctors provide may seem sensible enough. But once you see for yourself how vegetable oils can damage every organ in the body and affect people of every age, you might find these ideas making more sense. Many people already have. Around the globe, people are waking up to the idea that vegetable oils have been causing their problems, their families' problems, and their nations' problems this whole time. I want you to be armed with accurate research and knowledge so you can trust your own judgment.

Together, we can put the darkness behind us and create a brighter future for ourselves, our families, and our world.

DARK CALORIES

PART ONE

THE SCIENCE THAT MEDICINE OVERLOOKS

Came from a plant, eat it; was made in a plant, don't.

—MICHAEL POLLAN, AUTHOR AND JOURNALIST

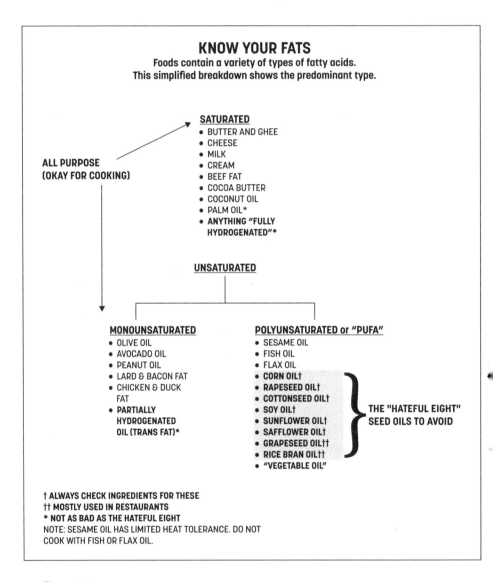

KNOW YOUR FATS

Foods contain a variety of types of fatty acids.
This simplified breakdown shows the predominant type.

**ALL PURPOSE
(OKAY FOR COOKING)**

SATURATED
- BUTTER AND GHEE
- CHEESE
- MILK
- CREAM
- BEEF FAT
- COCOA BUTTER
- COCONUT OIL
- PALM OIL*
- **ANYTHING "FULLY HYDROGENATED"***

UNSATURATED

MONOUNSATURATED
- OLIVE OIL
- AVOCADO OIL
- PEANUT OIL
- LARD & BACON FAT
- CHICKEN & DUCK FAT
- **PARTIALLY HYDROGENATED OIL (TRANS FAT)***

POLYUNSATURATED or "PUFA"
- SESAME OIL
- FISH OIL
- FLAX OIL
- **CORN OIL†**
- **RAPESEED OIL†**
- **COTTONSEED OIL†**
- **SOY OIL†**
- **SUNFLOWER OIL†**
- **SAFFLOWER OIL†**
- **GRAPESEED OIL††**
- **RICE BRAN OIL††**
- **"VEGETABLE OIL"**

} **THE "HATEFUL EIGHT"
SEED OILS TO AVOID**

† ALWAYS CHECK INGREDIENTS FOR THESE
†† MOSTLY USED IN RESTAURANTS
* NOT AS BAD AS THE HATEFUL EIGHT
NOTE: SESAME OIL HAS LIMITED HEAT TOLERANCE. DO NOT
COOK WITH FISH OR FLAX OIL.

Figure 1–1

CHAPTER 1

The Poison in Your Pantry

IN THIS CHAPTER YOU WILL LEARN

- Vegetable oils originated as byproducts of other industries, including soapmaking and confinement animal feeding operations.
- Vegetable oils require a staggering amount of processing to render them "safe" for consumption.
- Vegetable oil is more toxic than other oils and animal fats because of its chemistry.
- Eating a typical five-ounce serving of most restaurant fries (which are nearly always cooked in vegetable oils) equates to the toxicity of smoking twenty to twenty-five cigarettes.

There is a noxious substance in your pantry—and likely your fridge and freezer, too. It has an innocuous and even healthy-sounding name. It is ubiquitous in prepared foods and a staple ingredient in home-cooked meals. Chances are that you and your family are eating it every day. I am referring, of course, to vegetable oil—a substance that all of us eat but too few of us know much about. That's partly because, though most of us grew up with vegetable oil in the kitchen, it is a relatively new food.

A NEWFANGLED FAT

In spite of its healthy-sounding name, vegetable oil doesn't truly come from vegetables like broccoli or carrots. It is sometimes (more accurately) called "seed oil," because it actually comes from seeds. Both terms are used in common parlance, and I use both interchangeably as a blanket term referring to corn oil, rapeseed oil, cottonseed oil, soybean oil, sunflower oil, safflower oil, grapeseed oil, and rice bran oil—members of a group I call the Hateful Eight (see Figure 1–1).

Vegetable oil is an industrial product that didn't exist until a little more than 150 years ago. Before industrial agriculture changed our landscape, many human populations relied on animal fats such as butter, tallow (beef fat), and lard (pork fat). Humanity has been eating animal fats since the Stone Age, and dairy fat for nearly ten thousand years.[1] We've also eaten oils extracted from fatty fruits like olives and coconuts for many thousands of years. But vegetable oils are radically different. To start with, these new fats look different from the old fats—after processing, they are colorless, and they are dyed yellow to hide this. They taste different—they're almost flavorless. And making them requires technologically advanced equipment rather than a simple stone press or butter churn or butcher's knife. Yet despite their lack of flavor and the difficulty of processing them, they are now the largest single source of dietary fats, accounting for more calories in our diets than sugar or flour.

To understand how they became so prevalent, let's take a look at the history of vegetable oil—which began not so very long ago.

Why I Call Them the Hateful Eight

Neither the term "vegetable oil" nor "seed oil" works perfectly to indicate the problematic oils. This is why I created the term "the Hateful Eight," which does. Each member of the Hateful Eight is "hateful" because of its chemistry. Chemistry affects how easily the oil is

---

extracted, what happens during extraction and refining, storage, usage in cooking, the effects of reheating, how it changes in our digestive system, and how it affects our metabolism at low levels versus today's historically high levels of consumption, among other variables. Because not everyone factors all this in, you're bound to run into other people's lists of which oils are good and which to avoid. Just memorize these eight oils and you'll be good to go.

VEGETABLE OIL'S ORIGIN STORY

The story of how vegetable oil became a staple in our diets doesn't begin with hunters in a forest or farmers in a field, like that of other substances we consider food. It begins with chemists in a soap factory.

In the 1890s, facing a shortage of tallow to make soap, the soap and candle company Procter & Gamble turned to a byproduct of the textile industry—cottonseeds. Prior to the mid-1800s, cottonseeds had little commercial value because of their high concentration of an antinutrient called gossypol that causes dangerous spikes in blood potassium levels, organ damage, infertility, and paralysis. However, when the seeds are pressed for oil, and that oil is refined, bleached, and deodorized, the gossypol is largely eliminated (note—unrefined cottonseed oil is still used as an insecticide). Still, cottonseed oil was originally used not as food but as a fuel for lamps. When the petroleum industry emerged and petroleum replaced cottonseed oil as a popular lamp fuel, meatpackers began illegally adding cottonseed oil to animal fats such as tallow and lard to pump up their volume. It was also secretly added to American olive oil.[2] (It's worth pointing out that, if vegetable oils were actually healthier than traditional fats like tallow and lard, this would not have happened—it would be unusual for merchants to adulterate an inferior product with a superior one!) When these practices were exposed, the sale and export of cottonseed oil were depressed, and with a surplus of supply, the oil was once again available on the cheap.

Its low price made cottonseed oil attractive to Procter & Gamble. If the company could figure out how to turn it into soap, cottonseed oil would represent a low-cost source of fat to replace increasingly expensive tallow.

By 1907, with the help of a German chemist, Edwin C. Kayser, the company had succeeded. Kayser contacted P&G's business manager, John Burchenal, about a recently developed method whereby adding hydrogen molecules to oily polyunsaturated fats would solidify them into saturated fats and trans fats (see Figure 1–3). Oil could be converted into solid fat by a process called *hydrogenation*, which is still widely used today. Burchenal welcomed Kayser to the company.[3]

Initially, P&G sold its solidified, hydrogenated cottonseed oil as Ivory soap. But when the company modified the process slightly, the product came out softer, more spreadable—actually, it looked a lot like lard. So why not sell it as a lard substitute? The main challenge would be convincing consumers about the merits of this imitation food. Fortunately for P&G, this was still an era when, owing to the lack of regulatory oversight, advertisers could freely hawk their wares using any claim they might dream up. In 1911, P&G's marketing arm branded the company's newfangled cooking fat as Crisco. Crisco had no flavor—an attribute that P&G's marketing turned into a positive by calling it "clean." The company promoted it to housewives as "a healthier alternative to cooking with animal fats," adding that it could help ensure their children would grow up with "good characters."[4] Indeed, an earlier product, called Cottolene, made from beef suet and cottonseed oil, had been similarly marketed as "healthier, cleaner and more economical" than butter or lard.[5] The scheme worked marvelously well. Crisco quickly superseded Cottolene in popularity.

Even though Americans started consuming the solidified, hydrogenated oil in the early 1900s, our liquid oil consumption didn't change much. Many Americans initially rejected liquid vegetable oil. The 1904 US Department of Agriculture's handbook remarked on an "inexplicable prejudice against the use of vegetable oil."[6] The problem was likely an unpleasant taste or smell from one or more of the process contaminants that could not yet be refined away. (Hydrogenation is more intense and can eliminate those off-flavor contaminants.) Thus our liquid vegetable oil consumption stayed relatively flat until shortly after World War II.

Changes to animal feeding practices dramatically spiked soy production during the postwar era. Americans were now eating more meat, poultry, and dairy products than they had in decades. Farmers had started adding soy meal to feed because it helped fatten up the animals at a faster rate, boosting profits. But animals could not digest soy meal unless it was *defatted*, a process that removed the oil. So, during the 1940s, for the first time in history, the majority of the world's soybeans were crushed to yield separate products: oil and meal. The oil was initially used to make plastics, but by the 1950s major advances in soy oil refining greatly increased its acceptability in cooking and salad oils.[7]

Thus, vegetable oil has a unique history of being released into the food supply as a byproduct of two separate industries, soapmaking and confined animal feeding operations. Having advanced the processing techniques, scientists adapted lessons learned from refining soy and cottonseed to other members of the Hateful Eight. During the ensuing decades, corn, sunflower, safflower, and others made their debut in grocery stores. All eight of these oils are far cheaper to produce than animal fats and don't require refrigeration to reduce spoilage the way lard and butter do, making them immediately attractive to any business producing large amounts of inexpensive, convenient food. What's more, because refining strips away the flavor and most of the nutrition, these oils are chemically very similar, which makes them interchangeable, and this has supply chain advantages. So they caught on.

A seed oil that bears special mention here is canola, a derivative of rapeseed oil. Marketed in the US as canola, this product is generally sold in the UK as rapeseed oil and will be referred to as rapeseed in this edition of the text. Rapeseeds have been cultivated for three thousand years but were unsuitable for human consumption due to erucic acid, a fatty acid that causes liver damage. In 1985, Canadian scientists identified a strain that was naturally low in this harmful compound. Because most seed oils contain mostly omega-6 essential fat and rapeseed is relatively high in omega-3, many people assume that rapeseed oil is healthier than other seed oils. Unfortunately, chemistry says otherwise, as we'll soon see.

Another reason that industrial oilseeds have caught on is their ability to grow in a wider variety of climates than traditionally cultivated plant oils. Coconuts grow only in humid, equatorial tropics. Olives need Mediterranean weather, which only exists in 3 percent of the Earth's landmass. But soy, corn, rapeseed, and sunflowers are highly adaptable and can grow in many climates all over the United States. Over the past one hundred years, a large portion of our arable land has been given over to the cultivation of oilseed crops. Oilseed crops can also be used for animal feed, biodiesel, sweeteners (such as corn syrup), and processed protein powders.

You may think these practicalities have nothing to do with human health, but they do. They determine what we grow in this country and what is promoted to us to eat, and that affects our daily dose.

Procter & Gamble divested Crisco, Jif, and other edible products to other companies, and today no longer sells food. But having pioneered the use of ultra-processed oil as food, their legacy lived on. Next time you make a grocery run, read the ingredient labels: just about everywhere, from the dairy case to the frozen foods section and the snack aisle, you will see seed oils making repeated appearances. This is true of many products with an ingredients list, including salad dressings, canned fish, vegetable preserves such as sun-dried tomatoes, ready-to-eat foods in the deli section, diet drinks, coffee creamers, infant formulas, and nutritional shakes like Boost, Ensure, and Equate. You'll find seed oils in brands promising you they're organic, healthy, GMO-free, and "Whole30 Approved." No matter what kind of grocery store you're in, you'll find seed oils in almost every aisle. No matter where you dine out, you'll find them on the menu. We often hear that fast food is full of saturated fat, but precious few chains use expensive saturated-fat-rich tallow, lard, or butter. And it's not just fast food: vegetable oils now saturate fine dining experiences, and ethnic restaurants also take advantage of them, especially because vegetable oils cost less than healthier alternatives and don't contain the allergens or animal products that many customers want to avoid. These days, vegetable oil is a global industry. It generated more than $115.8 billion in 2020, and that figure is projected to increase to $162 billion by 2027.[8] Candace Rassias is an industry insider who told me that the food service industry as we know it would collapse without vegetable oil. Ventura Foods, the company she worked for, orders shipments by the trainload.[9]

HOW VEGETABLE OIL IS MADE

To keep up with the huge demand, vegetable oil refining takes place inside astoundingly large factories. From the outside, these factories are indistinguishable from oil and gas refineries—like those you see in the opening sequence of *The Sopranos*, as Tony cruises a section of the Jersey Turnpike above the infamously smelly industrial section of the city of Elizabeth.

The process begins as the oilseeds are pumped out of the delivery trucks and into the factory via metal ductwork. They enter a series of large metal cooking and cleaning chambers that heat the seeds to between 400 and 600 degrees Fahrenheit several times, in preparation for oil extraction.

Next, they go into the extraction press itself, where the seeds are crushed through a large metal screw, called an expeller, that squeezes much of the oil from the meal. This first batch of oil emerges as a foamy grayish-yellow liquid with a waxy texture. The crushed meal, containing the solids and residual oil, emerges as dark brown flakes, referred to as the cake. For now, the cake and the oil will go their separate ways. The oil goes straight to the crude oil holding tank, while the cake requires additional treatments to release the valuable oil it still contains.

To release its oil, the cake travels into a solvent treatment chamber to be washed with hexane (a component of gasoline). The solvent removes all but 1 percent of the residual oil from the cake. The cake will be shipped off to a different building for additional treatments required to render it safer for its ultimate use, as an ingredient in animal feed.

The hexane-treated oil, now dark brown, will pass through multiple other chambers to remove most of the hexane and various solids. One important stage collects the waxes as they drain slowly into a grate in the floor. These will be processed into vegetable shortening. Next, the hexane-treated portion is reunited with the expeller-pressed portion in a crude oil tank.

This crude oil is still not safe to eat. When I asked a process manager inside the industry why not, he answered candidly: "Crude vegetable oil contains hydratable and non-hydratable gums, free fatty acids, [partly oxidized] coloring pigments like carotenoids, moisture, [toxic] oxidative components like aldehydes and peroxides, metallic elements, waxes and other impurities."[10] That's a lot to clean up.

Refining the crude oil into a final "edible" oil is complicated. The American Oil Chemists' Society (AOCS) publishes a series of lengthy manuals to educate engineers and chemists on best practices for oilseed production. The flowcharts alone take up quite a few pages. Each flowchart maps out what's involved in each of the major processing steps—degumming, dewaxing, deodorizing...the list goes on. (We'll discuss the deodorizing step again later in this chapter, but for the sake of chocolate lovers, I want to take a moment to try to help you visualize the degumming step in particular. The gum is a dark brown material that emerges from a one-inch diameter steel pipe located about two feet above a cement floor. It plops into a receptacle bowl in gloopy segments, making it look for all the world like a machine having a loose bowel movement. That's where vegetable lecithin, an ingredient used in many brands of chocolate candy, as well as vegan mayonnaise, gets pulled out before undergoing its own set of extensive cleanup operations. Fortunately, the amount used in chocolate is tiny, so even though it faces the same safety challenges as seed oil—we'll see why shortly—it's not much of a dose.) Entire factories may specialize in just one of these major steps. Most flowcharts illustrate between twenty and forty different reaction chambers, each connected by

HOW VEGETABLE OIL IS MADE

STEP 1: OIL EXTRACTION

Oilseeds enter facility.

Heat and pressure used to extract oil creates *lipid oxidation products* (LOPs). Many are highly toxic.

Crude oils are "inedible" and requires extensive processing to clean up stink and mess.

Crude oil exits facility to refinery.

CREATES TOXIC CRUDE OIL

STEPS 2–40: REFINING

Refining is necessary to remove the following "impurities":

- Carcinogenic glicidyls
- Partly oxidized free fatty acids
- Polymerized acylglycerols
- Cyclic fatty acid monomers
- Toxic aldehydes
- **Hexane, if used**
- And too many more to list

Also removed: Minerals and most vitamins
Deodorization: The last refining step creates trans fats. These trans fats are different (more toxic) than the kinds of trans fats created by partial hydrogenation, and labels do not disclose their presence.

UNLESS HEXANE WAS USED TO OPTIMIZE EXTRACTION, SEED OILS CAN BE LABELED ORGANIC.

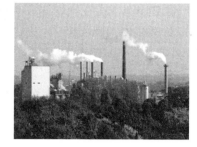

Figure 1–2

what must amount to miles of tubes. I can't imagine that any ingredient requires more intensive processing than vegetable oil.

Vegetable oil is big business, but only a tiny segment of the population eating vegetable oil knows anything about this giant industry. The industry was established by chemists, and it still relies heavily on chemists to oversee many aspects of production, not only for reasons of efficiency, but also to ensure the final product is safe to eat.

WHY VEGETABLE OILS ARE TOXIC: A BRIEF CHEMISTRY LESSON

So why does it take so much processing to make vegetable oils "safe" (or safe enough) to eat? It's because of their chemistry, which determines their stability. And their stability determines how easily they form byproducts during refining, and then during the cooking process, and finally in our bodies.

Fatty acids are the "building blocks" of all dietary fats, including vegetable oils, fruit oils, dairy and animal fats—and our body fat. The three major types of fatty acids are saturated, monounsaturated, and polyunsaturated (often referred to as PUFA). Saturated fats are the most chemically stable. Polyunsaturated fats are the least stable because they are prone to reacting with oxygen—a process called *oxidation*. Monounsaturated fats resist oxygen reactions and are far more stable than PUFAs.

A molecule called glycerol links three fatty acids together to form a *triglyceride*. The blend of fatty acids determines whether the triglyceride fat is liquid or solid. For example, vegetable oils are very high in polyunsaturated fatty acids, which makes them stay liquid even in the fridge. Animal fats are low in polyunsaturates, as are olive and coconut oil, which makes them more solid at cooler temps. (Olive oil should start to solidify in the fridge.)

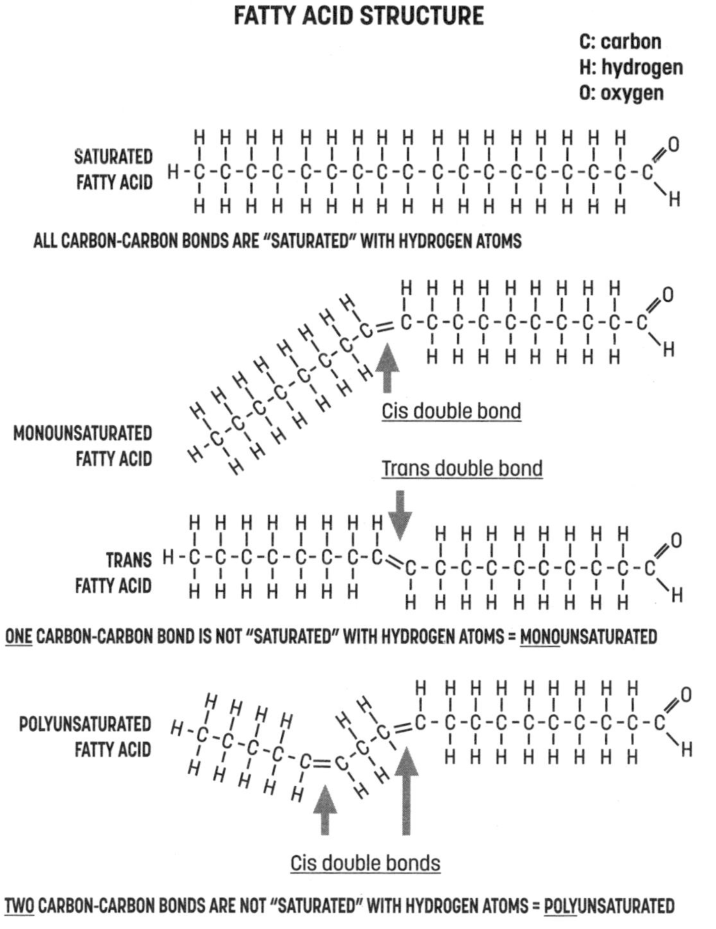

FATTY ACID STRUCTURE

C: carbon
H: hydrogen
O: oxygen

SATURATED FATTY ACID

ALL CARBON-CARBON BONDS ARE "SATURATED" WITH HYDROGEN ATOMS

MONOUNSATURATED FATTY ACID

Cis double bond

Trans double bond

TRANS FATTY ACID

ONE CARBON-CARBON BOND IS NOT "SATURATED" WITH HYDROGEN ATOMS = MONOUNSATURATED

POLYUNSATURATED FATTY ACID

Cis double bonds

TWO CARBON-CARBON BONDS ARE NOT "SATURATED" WITH HYDROGEN ATOMS = POLYUNSATURATED

Saturated fat is "saturated" with hydrogen atoms: Unsaturated fatty acids are "missing" some hydrogens.
Double bonds change the melting point: Each double bond creates a kink that prevents stacking and promotes liquidity.
Cis versus trans: If the missing hydrogens are on the same side, that is cis. If on opposite sides, that is trans. Trans fat is relatively stackable compared to cis fats, and thus partially hydrogenated oils are semisolid.

Figure 1–3

What Is a Double Bond?

The term *double bond* describes how carbon atoms in a fatty acid molecule are connected to each other. They can be connected by single or double bonds. When a fatty acid has no double bonds, it's called a saturated fat, because each one of its carbons is fully saturated with hydrogen.

Hydrogen blocks oxygen, preventing oxidation. So saturated fat is almost completely resistant to oxidation. Monounsaturated fat has one double bond, which makes it somewhat susceptible to oxidation. Polyunsaturated fat has two or more double bonds that are closely spaced together, making it far more susceptible to oxidation than saturated fat. This is why vegetable oil is far more susceptible to oxidation and toxin formation than butter, beef fat, and coconut oil, which contain mostly oxidation-resistant saturated fat.

Oxidation is a familiar term to anyone studying chemistry. Combustion, or burning, is one of the most common oxidation reactions on the planet. Our modern world relies on the oxidation of fossil fuels such as gasoline and coal to power cars, trucks, planes, and trains, and to generate much of our electricity. These oxidation reactions make our lives much easier—even if they create toxins that must be avoided (like those in car exhaust). Consider trees burning in a forest fire: their wood is not toxic until oxidation converts it into the blend of suffocating gases and particulates we call smoke. Similarly, oxidation creates toxins within our foods that weren't there to begin with.

When we talk about toxins in our food, we normally think about one of two things: either natural poisons, like those in many mushrooms or foods contaminated with certain fungi, for example, or man-made toxins like pesticides, heavy metals, and industrial solvents. But the toxins we get from eating vegetable oils are neither naturally occurring poisons nor man-made toxic additives. The toxins in vegetable oils develop as a result of the oxidation of the oil itself. Oil oxidation creates brand-new compounds within the oil that never existed in the seed, and many of these new compounds are mildly to extremely toxic. These toxins are not trivial—many of them are listed in hazmat manuals and require gloves and gas masks to handle, because acute exposure to them is known to "cause damage to essential organs, tissues, and cells."[11] The tendencies of oxygen to convert each major type of fatty acid into toxins is not part of the typical dietitian's curriculum, yet it makes the difference between an oil that's dangerously reactive and an oil that's safely stable. This chemical difference is the most important difference between vegetable oils and traditional fats.

One principle can simplify our understanding of the relative toxicity of various dietary fats: the double-bond principle. The number of double bonds in a fatty acid tells us how easily it oxidizes. The more double bonds, the faster it oxidizes. If the double bonds are closely spaced, as they are in PUFAs, they're double trouble. Since oxidation creates toxins, each *molecule* of PUFA represents a potential source of toxins. Compared to animal fats and the fats in traditional cooking oils, such as olive and coconut oil, vegetable oils contain manyfold more closely spaced double bonds, and thus have the potential to form manyfold more toxic compounds upon exposure to oxygen. Figure 1–4 shows their relative susceptibilities.

This is basic organic chemistry that has vitally important practical implications for nutrition science. These oxidation reactions effectively weaponize the polyunsaturated fatty acids, enabling them to convert bystander nutrients into toxins. This sort of thing can happen whenever we burn our food, generating compounds that tax our kidneys and liver as they work to eliminate them from the body—which is why it's not good to eat heavily charred food. When it comes to fats and oils, however, these toxic transformations can occur at temperatures *lower* than their smoke point. In fact, the much touted benefit of high-smoke-point vegetable oils is actually not a benefit at all, because it's going to make your food less healthy than a low-smoke-point alternative, such as olive oil.

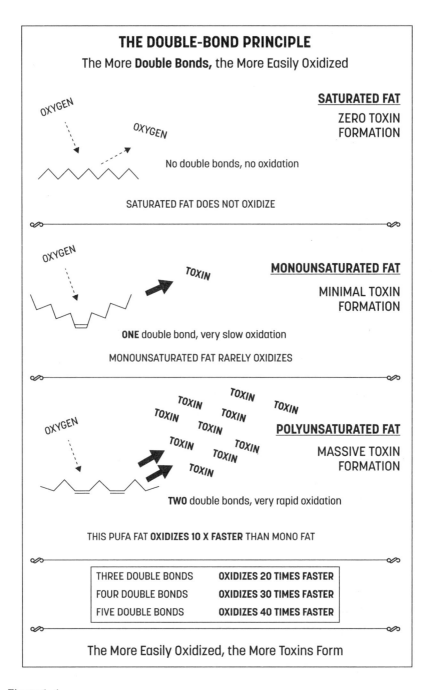

THE DOUBLE-BOND PRINCIPLE
The More **Double Bonds,** the More Easily Oxidized

OXYGEN

OXYGEN

SATURATED FAT
ZERO TOXIN
FORMATION

No double bonds, no oxidation

SATURATED FAT DOES NOT OXIDIZE

OXYGEN

TOXIN

MONOUNSATURATED FAT
MINIMAL TOXIN
FORMATION

ONE double bond, very slow oxidation

MONOUNSATURATED FAT RARELY OXIDIZES

TOXIN
TOXIN   TOXIN   TOXIN
TOXIN   TOXIN
OXYGEN   TOXIN   **POLYUNSATURATED FAT**
TOXIN   TOXIN
TOXIN   TOXIN   MASSIVE TOXIN
TOXIN   FORMATION

TWO double bonds, very rapid oxidation

THIS PUFA FAT **OXIDIZES 10 X FASTER** THAN MONO FAT

THREE DOUBLE BONDS	**OXIDIZES 20 TIMES FASTER**
FOUR DOUBLE BONDS	**OXIDIZES 30 TIMES FASTER**
FIVE DOUBLE BONDS	**OXIDIZES 40 TIMES FASTER**

The More Easily Oxidized, the More Toxins Form

Figure 1–4

Just to be clear, we're not just exposing our bodies to one kind of toxin, but to literally hundreds or even thousands of different types of toxins— some of them too fleeting for scientists to easily study, and that were almost unknown until recently, when they were identified thanks to new technologies. The kind and quantity of toxins that end up in the foods we eat will vary depending on processing, how often they're heated, and what other ingredients they're added to. Heating the oil during manufacture initiates toxin formation. More toxins form in oil that is exposed to light during storage. Still more toxins form when the oil is used to make food, whether in our homes, in restaurants, or in processed-food factories. And even more toxins will form if the food gets heated again, as in leftovers.

The most incredible thing about all these toxins is how fast they multiply. Just one single molecule of some of these toxins can set off a series of reactions that rapidly destroys billions of PUFAs and creates billions of new toxins. The generic term chemists use for all these toxins is *lipid oxidation products*, or LOPs for short. Think of LOPs as lopped off pieces of PUFA.

Toxin development works like a domino effect. One oxidized PUFA can quickly attack its neighbor, turning that PUFA into another LOP that attacks *its* neighbor, and so on. Chemists call this type of domino effect a *chain reaction*. Once a single PUFA "falls" (gets oxidized), the cascading dominoes rapidly oxidize one PUFA molecule after another at a rate of a billion molecules per second, leaving billions of new toxic LOPs in its wake.[12]

Once the chain reaction is started, only two things can stop it. One, simply running out of fuel, like knocking over all the dominoes. Or, two, encountering chemicals that block oxidation reactions, called *antioxidants*. Antioxidants can stop the chain reaction of toxicity, sort of the way adding a twisted domino into the lineup of a long chain will interrupt the flow. The twisted domino diverts the energy off to the side, thus protecting the rest of the dominoes from falling over. Olive oil, peanut oil, and other traditional oils have been selectively bred for thousands of years to yield oils without industrial processing, so they are easier to extract using nondestructive methods that retain antioxidants, making them safer to cook with. Since the processing steps required to make vegetable oils edible remove many naturally occurring antioxidants, cooking with vegetable oils means the toxin-forming oxidation reactions go on for a longer time and do more damage.

Another way to stop these chain reactions is with saturated fat. Saturated fat has zero double bonds and is very oxidation resistant. Think of these fatty acids like dominoes that have been glued down and can't be knocked over. Animal fats, such as butter and tallow, are very high in saturated fat, as is coconut oil and a few other uncommon plant oils, including macadamia nut oil.

Why Seeds Aren't Toxic But Their Oils Are

If vegetable oils like soy and sunflower oil are prone to oxidation, you may be wondering if the seeds are just as bad as vegetable oil. The answer is that all but one of the Hateful Eight oilseeds are perfectly edible. (The exception is, interestingly, the first of the Hateful Eight ever sold as human food, cottonseed, which, as we saw earlier in this chapter, contains toxic gossypol.)

The reason vegetable oils are toxic but their seeds are not has to do with the seed itself, as well as all the intense processing we just covered. Seeds are dormant little plant embryos that can stay dormant for years partly because they contain almost no oxygen. They also contain a variety of antioxidants that block oxidation during germination. The process of making vegetable oil strips away most of the antioxidants while exposing fragile PUFAs to intense oxygen, heat, and chemicals.

If we made processed foods with healthier oils, the fatty acids wouldn't break down, and we wouldn't end up eating quite so many toxins. (Of course, processed foods are still nutritionally impoverished, so I'm not advocating for this.) Vegetable oil is the only food we eat that is so unstable it can't tolerate heat. (Think about that. A cooking oil that can't tolerate heat, that oxygen tends to attack, and that we take into our oxygen-filled bodies.)

Describing all the toxins you expose yourself to from eating foods made with seed oils could fill up volumes of textbooks. Indeed, it has.[13] And yet relatively few people ever read these textbooks or learn about the damning information they contain.

AN ARMY OF OIL EXPERTS AGREE

The squadrons of scientists supporting the edible oil industry work within a silo that few people even know exists. Almost all the science the industry produces is currently buried in technical journals, and these often sit behind firewalls of highly specialized, members-only, professional society publications. Few people involved in health care or medical research read these journals, or, for that matter, even know they exist. Because these journals are so inaccessible, the media rarely pick up stories even when they're damning, as we'll see later on. This prevents most people from ever hearing the truth.

But if seed oil's toxicity is news to you, it's not news to the people in charge of manufacturing these oils. For over 150 years, edible oil scientists have attempted to prevent the fatty acids in vegetable oils from breaking down and forming toxins during their journey from field to fork. Their efforts have consistently failed. It's not that the edible oil scientists don't care about the healthfulness of the products they're in charge of manufacturing. It's that they've been handed an impossible task. Reading through chat groups dedicated to factory managers reveals a daily stream of questions requesting expert help with process problems and challenges in producing relatively toxin-free oils.[14] Reading industry journals reveals a regular stream of scientists reporting on "extremely high levels" of seed-oil-degradation derivatives identified in common commercial products cooked in seed oils.[15] And, for the most part, the rest of the world has remained unaware of these problems.

That said, some people have tried to sound the alarms. One of the most well-respected lipid scientists in the world, Dr. Martin Grootveld, has been trying to warn consumers about toxins in vegetable oils for decades. Dr. Grootveld is a professor of bioanalytical chemistry and chemical pathology, author of over two hundred journal articles, numerous book chapters, and several books, and holder of many prestigious awards and grants. (However, when I asked Dr. Grootveld if he'd ever been invited to present his data at a medical conference, he told me he had not.) He studies oxidation reactions using the best tool for analyzing an array of different molecules all at once: a one- and two-dimensional nuclear magnetic resonance (NMR) spectroscope. This analytical tool identifies molecules by magnetically jiggling the atoms and comparing the jiggling vibrations in the test material against known standards, thus identifying intact and broken (oxidized) molecules by a kind of molecular fingerprint. He has tabulated the myriad toxins that develop in these oils whenever they're heated. His analyses consistently show that heated vegetable oils are loaded with toxic oxidation products, while heated coconut oil and butter contain hardly any toxins at all.[16] Toxins he's identified include acrolein, which inflames lungs when inhaled, and many members of a category of toxin called epoxy-fatty acids, which are involved in the pathogenesis of multiple organ failure and breast cancer and interfere with reproductive functions. Listing just the *categories* of toxins that he's detected in foods fried in vegetable oils would take up half a page.[17]

Remember those early-twentieth-century housewives with their "inexplicable prejudice" against soy oil? They were probably detecting some of the more acrid odors produced by oxidized polyunsaturated fatty acids back in the days before a refining step called deodorization removed them. Deodorization removes a number of volatile compounds, including polycyclic aromatic hydrocarbons like naphthalene (in mothballs) and anthracene (a component of coal tar). However, removing smelly toxins from the bottled oil does not stop oxidation reactions from occurring, and brand-new toxins slowly begin forming again the minute the bottle is exposed to oxygen-rich air. Even light can attack those double bonds and degrade high-PUFA oils. Unfortunately, we can't count on our sense of smell to warn us, since we can only smell those that escape the cooking process as vapors. These volatile compounds tend to be smaller molecules and represent only a tiny portion of the total new compounds formed. Most of the toxins stay behind in our food. (And many volatiles are odorless.)

But the Label Says "Organic"

There are a few issues with the organic labeling of vegetable oils.

The first stems from the two methods used to remove the oil from the seed: mechanical extraction, which makes what is called "expeller-pressed oil," and solvent extraction, which uses hexane. Hexane treatment automatically disqualifies the oil from organic labeling. But the expeller-pressed oil can be labeled organic, even though after extraction it contains the exact same long list of contaminants and toxins as hexane-extracted oil—other than traces of hexane. The second stems from the deodorizing step. This step removes many malodorous and toxic volatiles that form during the earlier steps, but it also unavoidably converts a significant portion of the PUFAs into trans fats. How significant? Testing shows some bottles of expeller-pressed rapeseed oil, for example, contain more than 5 percent trans fats as they leave the factory.[18] But because they weren't purposefully added, these toxins don't count against the organic label. A more honest designation than "organic" would be "hexane-free."

Last, as these intensely processed, mildly contaminated "organic" oils sit on the shelves, they continue to oxidize. After you open them, they oxidize much faster. Toxicologists who perform "real-world" tests on vegetable oils in people's homes and restaurants find that, even before cooking, and whether hexane-free or not, the oils contain significantly higher concentrations of toxins than they did when they were first bottled.[19]

Like all industries, the edible oil industry funds research to improve the quality of its products. Sometimes toxicologists and food scientists will even collaborate on the same grant. The food scientists can try out new ways of making the oil safer, and the toxicologists can test their work.

Perhaps no one has tried harder to make vegetable oils less toxic than Dr. Eric Decker, professor in the Department of Food Science at the University of Massachusetts, Amherst, and one of the most highly cited scientists in agriculture. The focus of his work is preventing oxidation in our food supply, specifically in processed foods, and particularly vegetable oils, which he says are, without doubt, the most oxidation-prone ingredients in our food supply.[20] This matters to the industry partly because oxidation reactions ruin the taste of the foods produced, generating rancid off-flavors, a leading cause of global food waste. The toxicity matters, too, to a degree. During his forty-plus-year career, Dr. Decker has pursued many strategies to protect the fragile PUFA fats from oxidation during refining, cooking, and storage. He's tried adding all types of antioxidants to the oil, including vitamins, proteins, plant-based antioxidants, and synthetic antioxidants. He's tried keeping oxygen away from vegetable oils and foods made with vegetable oils by removing air from bottles and bags and replacing it with inert nitrogen gas. He's tried adding emulsifiers that reduce the oxygen-oil interactions. And he's tried layering a cloud of nitrogen over restaurant deep fryers. He's even tried rearranging the fatty acid molecules within individual triglycerides to see if that would stabilize them. So far, there's no great stand-out solution.

At a 2022 conference attended by oil chemists around the world, Dr. Decker delivered the keynote presentation, called "Why Does Lipid Oxidation in Foods Continue to Be Such a Challenge?"[21] He explained that fully preventing harmful oxidation reactions that create dangerous toxins has proven difficult. Perhaps the most dangerous category of toxins is the *aldehydes*, the family of chemicals that includes the odorous cadaver-preservative formaldehyde and many of the toxins that make cigarette smoke irritating and carcinogenic. Toxic aldehydes that form in frying oil can end up in the food, and this is what keeps scientists like Dr. Decker up at night.

Unfortunately, he is pitting himself against the inevitabilities of physics. Dr. Grootveld told me that the likelihood of ever making vegetable oils safe is about zero: "Thermodynamics dictate that the concentration of polyunsaturated fat is directly related to the amount of toxins that will develop in the oil."[22] It seems then that the only way to protect ourselves from toxins that form in vegetable oil is to avoid vegetable oils, and to use fats composed of more stable fatty acids instead.

There are degrees of toxicity to consider, too. The damage done to polyunsaturates by oxidation follows the same basic principles as burns on your skin: time and temperature. The longer the oil is cooked and the higher the cooking temperature, the more toxins will form. Dr. Decker explains that when it comes to toxin production, "the biggest risk factor is deep frying the oil."[23] Deep frying stresses oils for a long time at high temperatures. Fast-food chains create protocols for employees to reduce toxicity, by, for example, changing the oil once a week, but smaller eateries and chains may not. Dr. Decker warns, "To me, the scary place to go is the diners and the small restaurants. In Germany, they regulate frying oil and test it for toxic volatiles during inspections." If the levels exceed a certain number, that's a violation, and vendors can suffer fines or other consequences. "In the US, we don't even have a number set to define the acceptable level," Dr. Decker explained, and our government authorities don't test for toxins in frying oil during restaurant food safety inspections.

But toxicologists have tested restaurant frying oils. One of the most well-studied type of toxins is called alpha-beta unsaturated aldehydes, now thought to be the most carcinogenic agents in cigarette smoke. In 2019, a paper in the prestigious journal *Nature* reported that a five-ounce serving of french fries cooked in vegetable oil (from a well-known franchise, mind you, not one of those smaller restaurants lacking protective protocols) contains twenty-five times more of these dangerous aldehydes than the World Health Organization's tolerable upper limit for exposure. Dr. Grootveld points out that this amount is equivalent to smoking twenty to twenty-five tobacco cigarettes.[24] (A five-ounce serving has about twenty-five fries, giving us an easy 1:1 correlation between fries and cigarettes for this particular toxic exposure.) These aldehydes are potent mutagenic (DNA-mutating), carcinogenic (cancer-causing), and cytotoxic (cell-killing) agents. Still, they are just one of the many families of toxic compounds present in cooking oils.

Why Banning Trans Fats Has Been a Public Health Flop

In the 1970s, the medical industry directed people to stop using tallow, coconut oil, and butter. Tallow had long been used in the food industry for frying and we needed a replacement. So ingenious food scientists tinkered with the recipe for hydrogenated oils and designed a product—*partially* hydrogenated oils—that could better withstand high-temperature frying for extended periods. These contain trans fats. After doctors woke up to the harms of trans fats, they figured banning them would be a good thing, and successfully lobbied to remove them from the US food supply. The trans-fat ban went into effect in 2018, but large chains had already removed them because

---

of a New York City ban effective in 2007 and a European Union ban in 2008. By January 2020, US food manufacturers could no longer sell products containing partially hydrogenated oils. Currently, they're no longer in the food supply to any appreciable degree. But that leaves restaurants no viable option other than filling their fryers with unstable, regular vegetable oils, as frying in animal fats has fallen out of favor. The trans-fat ban has effectively doubled the consumption of liquid vegetable oil compared to what it was before the ban.

In spite of its mild toxicity, trans fat resists oxidation, making it far less toxic than high-PUFA vegetable oils. This is why food scientists—like Mark Matlock of ADM, a leading global producer of vegetable oils and fats for the food manufacturing industry—warned decades ago that banning trans fats and using liquid vegetable oil in deep fryers would expose us to a variety of toxic oxidation products.[25] By all accounts, using vegetable oils in deep fryers will likely create a larger public health problem than trans fats ever could.

Vegetable oils can contaminate more than just our food. They contaminate the air we breathe, not just in the factories where they are made but in our very environment. After restaurants started making the changeover from trans fats, they dealt with fumes that formed a kind of lacquer on the walls and ceilings that couldn't be cleaned until the industry invented powerful new chemical solvents.[26] The fumes also congeal and harden on workers' uniforms, and they have caused at least two laundromat fires, when the flammable lacquer ignited into flames inside the heat of the dryers.[27] People working over these deep fryers chronically inhale the toxic fumes and are at higher risk of cancer. Indeed, researchers in China have identified an alarming rate of lung cancer in nonsmoking women using vegetable oils during pan frying, deep frying, and stir frying, both in food service settings and their own homes.[28]

Many people know deep frying is not healthy and avoid deep-fried foods. That's why Dr. Grootveld is more concerned about "shallow frying," the industry term for frying food in a pan. (It's different from sautéing, which uses less oil or no oil.) He's published several papers in various prestigious journals warning that you can generate the same "extremely high levels of hazardous aldehydic LOPs" while making popular pan-fried or deep-fried dishes right at home.[29] So it's not just about deep-fried food, and it's not just about restaurants. This could be happening in your kitchen.

I asked Dr. Grootveld if he felt that the food industry knew vegetable oil oxidation presented a potential public health problem (this was before I'd attended Dr. Decker's 2022 conference). Without skipping a beat, he told me, "They're aware of it all right, they just don't want to do anything about it." He then proceeded with a story about a toxicologist who was "obviously employed by the food industry" that he'd caught "sniffing around" his laboratory and who'd asked him to change some of his conclusions in a paper about to be published that would expose a brand-new category of particularly reactive toxins in vegetable oils. When Dr. Grootveld refused, this industry agent "tried to shoot down what we were saying" by publishing an editorial in the same journal. Fortunately, Dr. Grootveld stood his ground, and the journal editors ultimately backed him up. (But it does make one wonder how often other, more easily intimidated scientists have been coerced into hiding the truth.)

THE ONE THING TO KNOW ABOUT OXIDATION

Some of this chemistry we've discussed is complex—and you don't need to memorize any of it to understand the rest of the book. The reason I've included it is to show you that its very complexity is partly why medical science hasn't been able to appreciate the toxicity of vegetable oils. Here's what I do want you to remember: *Vegetable oil's tendency to oxidize has implications for everyday aspects of life that medical science has ignored.* The implications are vast and profound. Indeed, the implications for medical science are so far ranging that I have devoted my career to unraveling them. In the ensuing chapters of this section, we'll be doing that together.

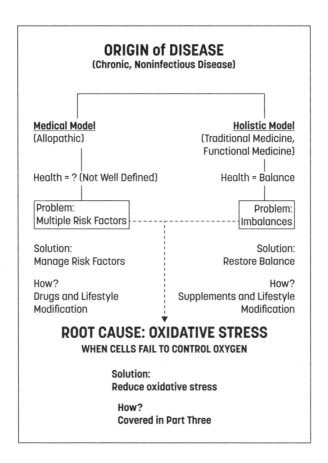

Figure 2–1: All chronic diseases share the same root cause: oxidative stress. The risk factors allopathic doctors talk about, such as sedentism and high blood pressure, either cause or originate in oxidative stress. The imbalances that holistic medicine strives to correct likewise either cause or originate in oxidative stress.

Oxidative stress, in turn, is caused by toxicity and nutrient deficiencies. (Emotional stress, lack of sleep, and lack of physical activity also have toxic effects.) Vegetable oil, being both toxic *and* nutritionally poor, is oxidative stress in a bottle.

CHAPTER 2

The All-You-Can-Eat Buffet of Chronic Disease

IN THIS CHAPTER YOU WILL LEARN

- Vegetable oils promote a cellular chemical imbalance called oxidative stress.
- Oxidative stress can trigger inflammation and/or buildup of cellular debris and garbage.
- These processes are the underlying root cause of every known major disease.
- Our bodies normally prevent this imbalance with an army of antioxidant enzymes that are far more powerful than antioxidants in food.
- A diet full of vegetable oils makes oxidative stress, and chronic disease, inevitable.

To explain the disease we now call epilepsy, ancient Greek physicians invoked a supernatural cause. The symptoms of uncontrollable shaking, frothing at the mouth, and bodily contortions appeared to be a punishment from the gods. Hippocrates, or perhaps one of his students, felt that this explanation could be improved upon, writing in the Hippocratic Corpus that epilepsy "is no more divine or sacred than any other disease but, on the contrary, has specific characteristics and a definite cause."[1] With that assertion, medicine emerged from the shadowy realm of the supernatural to become a science, a discipline rooted in provable realities.

Suggesting that disease is a result of something we can understand may seem basic, but at the time it was revolutionary. The concept seems to me to be a first principle of medicine, a necessary foundation upon which subsequent physicians have since built the entire field. First principles are ideas that we can be absolutely sure are true. Physics is full of first-principle ideas, from Isaac Newton's laws of motion to Euclid's *Elements*. But medicine is underdeveloped this way. Health itself is expressed mainly as an absence of disease, which isn't very useful.

In this chapter, I'd like to elaborate on a concept I think makes for a really good first principle, too: disease starts at the level of the cell. Your body is made up of cells—trillions of them. And all these cells must be in good working order for your organs to be in good working order.

This idea is not entirely novel; it's actually part of medical education. The pathology textbook I bought in medical school begins by discussing "cellular pathology" right on page one. *Pathology* means simply disease. *Cellular pathology* means cellular disease.[2] The idea is also common sense: if you have healthy cells, you're going to be healthy. Likewise, if you have diseased cells, your organs will start to malfunction, and disease related to that dysfunction soon follows.

In spite of this recognition that disease begins in the cell, medical science doesn't go much further with the concept. My medical education did a great job teaching me about how our amazingly intricate cells work and how they cooperate as organs. But after graduation, there is no opportunity to apply those ideas to actually heal our patients. It's as if allopathic medicine got to a point with its basic discoveries and hit a wall, never quite reaching the goal of fixing disease at the root.

That barrier was built by vegetable oil.

In this chapter, we're going to build on what we learned about oxidation in chapter 1 by connecting the dots between oxidation and chronic disease. The gist of it is this: The toxins in seed oils promote a state of cell imbalance called oxidative stress. Over time, oxidative stresses deplete our bodies of antioxidants. Once that happens, our own cells can become a source of additional toxin formation. At that point, we start to develop inflammatory and degenerative diseases. Indeed, oxidation reactions might even explain one of life's deepest mysteries—death.

A RADICAL NEW THEORY

In 1949, Denham Harman, a chemist for Shell Oil Company, started obsessing about death. He couldn't understand why we die. So at the age of thirty-three, and with limited finances, he left job security behind and enrolled in medical school to better understand the human body.

After graduation, Dr. Harman took a part-time clinical position, which left him plenty of time to sit and ponder the aging process.[3] As a chemist, he was accustomed to thinking about chemical reactions, and he was absolutely certain that the mysteries surrounding death itself would come down to a simple cellular process that everyone was just overlooking. During an interview in 2003, he explained that he was on the verge of giving up. "I thought, thought, thought for four months in vain and suddenly the idea came"—free radicals.[4]

Free radicals are destructive molecules that can damage our cells in much the same way that radiation can. Unlike radiation, they form as natural byproducts of reactions involving oxygen, collectively called *oxidation reactions* (like the oxidation reactions we explored in chapter 1). The fact that free radicals can also damage our cellular infrastructure suggested to Dr. Harman that they may very well be the thing that limits our natural life span. He carefully put his thoughts together and exposed them to the world in an article called "Aging: A Theory Based on Free Radical and Radiation Chemistry," published two years later.[5] This theory boldly proposed that our ultimate demise is brought about by oxygen, thanks to the accumulated damage done by those violent free radicals. The idea is that the free-radical byproducts of oxidation reactions slowly destroy our cells one at a time until the tissues and organs depending on them can no longer function and we succumb to infection or injury, develop cancer, or simply die in our sleep.

In the final paragraphs of his article, Dr. Harman makes the provocative suggestion that, if this theory holds, then there may be a "chemical means of prolonging effective life." He was referring to the idea of supplementation with *antioxidants*. Antioxidants were well known to science at the time for their capacity to stop oxidation reactions and prevent free radical damage from spreading within a cell.

Oxidation was a new concept to medicine, a whole new mechanism of disease, different from viruses, bacteria, traumatic injuries, and other things most doctors were familiar with. It did more than just explain why we ultimately die; it also explained why our cells start to malfunction as we age and why we develop degenerative diseases. Being a wholly new concept, the free radical theory was initially ridiculed. But it was rooted in solid science and soon found plenty of supporters. Before long, this three-page paper would launch an entire new branch of science called free radical biology.

By the 1980s, free radicals had increasingly become part of basic medical research into cancer, cardiovascular disease, and strokes. The 1990s saw free radicals linked to Alzheimer's disease and over a hundred other conditions.[6] Dr. Harman's fundamental ideas have since been accepted by most aging experts around the world, as well as by scientists looking for root causes of chronic degenerative diseases such as arthritis, emphysema, and heart and kidney failure, and by toxicologists studying the mechanisms of heavy metal toxicity and other agricultural and industrial pollutants. Dr. Harman put oxidation reactions on the map, which is quite an accomplishment.

Dr. Harman was nominated six times for a Nobel Prize for his work in the field of gerontology, the field of medicine devoted to aging.[7] His ideas now also inspire twenty-first-century biohackers and practitioners of anti-aging medicine. All this stands as testimony to the power of chemistry to lead to major medical breakthroughs, as well as to the benefits of inviting chemists into health and nutrition conversations.

In the decades since this big breakthrough idea, however, the chemical means of prolonging life have continually proven elusive. Dr. Harman himself thought that with a healthy diet, regular exercise, and certain vitamins, particularly vitamins C and E, aging could be slowed by reducing the production of free radicals. He lived a productive life until the ripe old age of ninety-eight, having followed his own advice.[8] But these simple measures do not work to delay the onset of any diseases or extend life beyond 120, as he'd hoped. In fact, his theory has fallen in and out of favor multiple times.

Why the ups and downs?

Over the decades, several generations of investigators have each proposed their set of compounds that might extend our lives or at least stave off degenerative diseases. These scientists have tested antioxidant supplements, including vitamins C and E; phytochemicals such as resveratrol from red wine grapes; algal antioxidants, like astaxanthin (related to vitamin A); NAD+ and other energy metabolites with antioxidant properties; and many more—new ones seem to pop up in the nutrition news every month or so. Other groups of scientists have tested genetic modifications that can make simple organisms like yeasts manufacture more of their own intrinsic antioxidant compounds, most famously compounds called sirtuins.[9] Similarly, scientists have modified worms to produce more of the enzymes that trap free radicals, called antioxidant enzymes, to no effect. Still others have tested calorie restriction, because the process of burning calories generates a great many free radicals. In spite of the fact that calorie restriction could also cause malnutrition, this idea looked particularly promising for a while because it seemed to work in monkeys, which are much more similar to us than yeast. Unfortunately, it came out that calorie-restriction studies were not actually restricting calories below the animals' needs. They were restricting the animals from eating as much as they *wanted*—which usually meant overeating and developing diabetes.[10] In other words, these studies were just showing that overeating is unhealthy—something we already knew. With each new avenue of investigation, the theory has started to shine, only to be dashed when the investigators reached a dead end for one reason or another.

But the idea that free radicals promote diseases that bring about cellular demise, and, ultimately, our death, makes sense. It is also rooted in solid principles of chemistry and cellular biology. So why isn't this field producing the expected results? What are they missing?

They're looking at the problem backward. They're searching for antioxidants that can extend our natural life span, but the problem is we've been consuming more and more vegetable oils, and this depletes our bodies of antioxidants in ways that shorten our life span. This is not something mere supplementation can fully fix.

HOW ANTIOXIDANTS PROTECT OUR CELLS

In chapter 1, we saw that vegetable oils are toxic because of their high PUFA content. However, before we go any further, I need to establish that we do need *some* PUFAs in our diets (we will revisit this—and see how much—in chapter 3). All our essential fatty acids, both omega-6 and omega-3, are polyunsaturates, and we need them for the vitamin-like benefits I mentioned in the introduction. And as with vitamins, without enough of them we can develop deficiency-related conditions, including dermatitis and digestive problems. If a mother doesn't have enough PUFA in her body while her fetus is developing, the baby's vision and intelligence can be limited. Just as every cell in our bodies needs vitamins to function properly, every cell in our bodies needs PUFA for normal function, too.

If you took biology in high school, you may remember that every cell is wrapped in a membrane called (logically enough) the cell membrane. What you may not remember is that our cell membranes are constructed with fat, including a good deal of PUFA. Between 30 and 40 percent of the fatty acids in our cell membranes are polyunsaturated. (The rest is saturated and monounsaturated.)

The PUFA molecules in our cell membranes are chemically identical to the PUFA in vegetable oils, and in fact, the oils we eat are where much of the PUFA in our cells comes from. And just like PUFA in the fryer, oxygen attacks those double bonds, with destructive effects. But unlike in the fryer, the destruction is kept in check. Our bodies protect membrane PUFA with an array of antioxidants, the first and foremost being vitamin E. Vitamin E is the first line of defense; it's the first to "catch" a free radical within the cell membrane. It efficiently blocks oxidation once it starts by taking a hit for the team—the team here being team PUFA.

To do its job, vitamin E nestles down amid a patch of PUFA molecules where it can trap free radicals and expel them from the area. Vitamin E works exactly like that twisted domino I described in chapter 1 to divert the energy of free radicals away from the rest of the PUFA in our cell membranes. Vitamin E gets oxidized itself (taking one for the team), thus protecting its neighboring PUFAs from oxidation. But once vitamin E gets knocked over, it needs to be "stood back up again" (to extend the domino metaphor). And standing up this domino requires a team approach. That's why supplementing with vitamin E can't make up for eating way too much PUFA. Let me show you what I mean.

Antioxidants Work in Teams

Vitamin E is the most famous PUFA-protecting antioxidant, protecting PUFA in our cell membranes and in the lipoproteins that carry cholesterol and other fats in our bloodstream. But vitamin E can't do the job on its own. Antioxidant molecules actually cooperate with each other, working in teams. Team PUFA also includes vitamin C and other compounds discussed below, including glutathione, sulfur, nicotinamide adenine dinucleotide phosphate (NADPH), and a number of others. Some members of the team must come from our diets, and our bodies must make some of them on their own.

To explain this, I have to mix my game metaphors. The team works together to play a molecular game of hot potato, where the potato is a free radical. When vitamin E catches a free radical, it's been oxidized (the domino is knocked down), but it's just a temporary injury to the vitamin E molecule. The oxidation of E causes a kink to form in its tail, flipping the tail outward so that the free radical can't harm any more membrane PUFAs.

Safely shifted out of the membrane, the vitamin E can now pass off its problematic free radical to the other members of the team. The first team member to step forward is the antioxidant vitamin C. Vitamin C takes the high-energy free radical from E, which fixes vitamin E, and its tail straightens out again and flips right back into the membrane where it started, ready to trap any more troublesome radicals (the domino has been stood up again). Now that vitamin C has the free radical, however, it needs to pass it off to another antioxidant compound. In this case, a sulfur-containing molecule called glutathione accepts the free radical. Sulfur gets oxidized during this exchange, and glutathione, in turn, passes its oxidation problem on to another compound, called NADPH.

Each time the various antioxidants pass the free radical along, the free radical's energy state drops a little bit. In this way, the antioxidant team permits the free radical to safely discharge its energy—and the hot potato essentially cools down.[11]

Our bodies support this complex chain of interactions with numerous antioxidant enzymes that play a role in repairing the damage done by free radicals. Each enzyme requires its own set of nutrients and has other requirements for production and operation.

What does all of this have to do with vegetable oils? Vegetable oils promote vastly more free radical reactions than saturated and monounsaturated fats, and supplementing with a few vitamins is not likely to be enough to contain the problem. We know this in part thanks to an underappreciated human clinical trial that was used to determine our vitamin E requirements, called the Elgin Project.

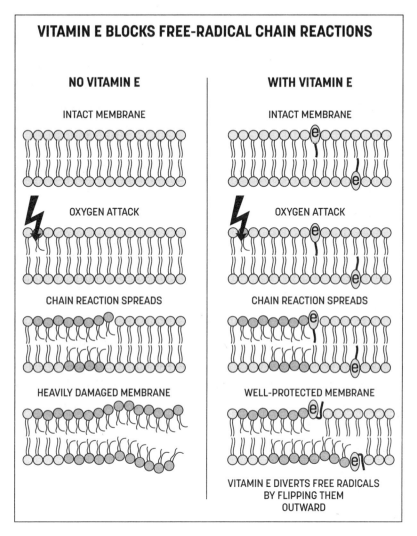

Figure 2-2: This figure shows how having plenty of vitamin E in our cell membranes can limit free radical damage. Cell membranes are constructed of two layers of phospholipids with their "tails" facing each other, as shown. Each phospholipid is made of two PUFA molecules (tails) linked together by a phosphate-containing head group (circle). **Oxygen attack** initiates oxidation reactions that tear through the PUFA, disrupting membrane integrity. Without vitamin E, our membranes would suffer serious damage that might trigger programmed cellular death. **With vitamin E, the damage is contained.** However, the vitamin E is now oxidized and needs a repair job that requires multiple additional nutrients.

This is why supplementing with vitamin E (and not making other dietary changes) has failed to improve health outcomes. **The most important dietary change is to cut out vegetable oils, since that reduces the oxygen attacks.**

PUFA ZAPS OUR ANTIOXIDANTS

In the 1950s and 1960s, researchers at the Elgin State Hospital in Elgin, Illinois, and Chicago's University of Illinois College of Medicine carried out a series of studies on inpatients that tested the impact of PUFA consumption on our vitamin E levels.[12] They knew that Americans were eating wildly different amounts of PUFA depending on whether they used animal fats or plant fats in their cooking. So they wanted to find out if eating more PUFA meant we needed more vitamin E. In short, the answer is yes—*much* more.

Study participants ate either a low-PUFA diet made with lard or a high-PUFA diet made with corn oil. The corn-oil diet contained about 30 percent polyunsaturated fatty acids (by calories), comparable to today's average intake, while the lard diet contained just 4 percent, comparable to many pre-industrial diets. At first, the study confirmed that people eating corn oil do need more E to protect their cell membranes from oxidation than people eating lard—three times more. But after about two years on a high corn-oil diet, something unexpected happened. Suddenly people's blood levels of E started to drop, even though they were getting the same dose of E as they'd been taking all along, and their cell membranes started testing positive for signs of oxidation-related damage.[13] This means that even higher doses of E were no longer enough to prevent corn-oil-induced cellular damage. The fact that it took several years for this problem to occur suggests that after an extended period on a high-PUFA diet, our bodies undergo an important shift. All that PUFA likely exceeded some critical threshold. After that tipping point, the "used" vitamin E (alpha-tocopherol quinone) could no longer get refreshed by its antioxidant teammates, so levels of fresh vitamin E (alpha-tocopherol) dropped.[14]

How did this happen? As the people assigned to the corn-oil diet kept eating corn oil, their body fat changed. The scientists had been testing participants' body fat on a regular basis and discovered that after a few years of eating a high-PUFA diet, their body fat filled up with PUFA. But this aspect of the experiment was almost completely lost to science, and so the effects of long-term PUFA consumption on body fat have been almost completely overlooked—until more recent research brought the question back into the light.

PUFA and Body Fat

Stephan Guyenet, PhD, is a neuroscientist who studies eating behavior—and who has paid attention to vegetable oil. In 2011, it had occurred to him that we've been eating more and more of it, and he wondered what it might be doing to our body fat. In 2015, after reviewing all the available studies reporting on the composition of human body fat from the past fifty years, he published a literature review article covering what he had discovered.

Our body fat is stored under our skin in a layer that doctors call *adipose tissue*. The only way to know what kinds of fatty acids are in someone's body fat is to take a tissue biopsy; you can't get this information from a blood test. A biopsy involves pressing a tiny, cookie-cutter-like instrument into someone's skin, removing the plug of skin and attached fat, packing the sample into dry ice, and rushing it off to a lab for analysis. (This was also how the Elgin Project evaluated participants' PUFA.) These studies get done for a variety of reasons, although not very often. Fortunately, between 1959 and 2008 there were forty-six such studies—enough for Dr. Guyenet to gather meaningful information. The biopsy data showed that the portion of PUFA in human body fat had gradually increased from 9.1 percent of all fatty acids to 21.5 percent during the roughly fifty-year span of time.[15] During that same time, the amount of PUFA in the average American diet had also doubled, increasing from about fifteen pounds per person per year to thirty.[16]

When Dr. Guyenet plotted adipose PUFA against time on a graph, the neat and unusually linear arrangement of the forty-six biopsy data points marching upward year after year—perfectly paralleling the increase in vegetable oil—prompted him to comment that "someone might be suspicious of how I selected the studies." He had included every relevant study available in the English literature and admitted he was "very surprised to see such a consistent trend."[17]

Surprising as it may have been, the lesson was clear: the more vegetable oil people ate, the more their body fat started to look like vegetable oil. Importantly, the process takes years. The Elgin Project scientists determined that the PUFA content of people's body fat slowly increased to match the PUFA content of their diets after about five years.[18]

Excessive PUFA in body fat makes excessive demands on the body's all-important antioxidants. The exact amount of PUFA that's "too much" will vary from person to person, and even within individuals, depending on other elements of the diet. Today's average PUFA intake sits at historically high levels, while our consumption of antioxidant vitamins, minerals, and other necessary cofactors has not risen. Vitamin and mineral deficiencies run rampant within our population, with more than half of Americans over age four lacking adequate potassium, magnesium, choline, and vitamins E and K.[19] Even if we were getting vastly more of all the required nutrients, that doesn't guarantee that our bodies could keep up. It may not be genetically possible.

This high load of PUFA in our adipose tissue causes a fundamental shift in our body chemistry once that tipping point is reached. The process underlying that shift is called *oxidative stress*.

OXIDATIVE STRESS: WHEN YOU BECOME LIKE THE DEEP FRYER

In 2017, a brilliant German chemist named Gerhard Spiteller, who had been investigating the dangers of turning away from stable animal fats and using vegetable oils, died at the age of eighty-five, having gained little recognition for decades of dedicated work. During the last forty years of his life, he'd published nearly one hundred articles on the link between polyunsaturates and diseases related to oxidation and free radical formation. Both free radicals and oxidation reactions can tear through our cell membranes to cause this dangerous state of cellular imbalance. Likewise, oxidative stress can promote free radical formation and oxidation reactions. Oxidation and free radicals are so intimately linked that the free radical theory of aging has at times in its evolution been called the oxidative stress theory of aging.[20] Oxidative stress causes free radicals to form, and free radicals can also promote oxidative stress. Think of free radicals as flying embers that can start fires, and oxidative stress as giant fires that spew hot embers.

Dr. Spiteller may not be a household name, but he is an absolute giant in the field of biochemistry. In the 1950s, he had invented an antibiotic called sulfadimethoxine, a precursor to one of the most widely used antibiotics today, Bactrim, so he had already saved billions of lives. In the 1980s he discovered an antioxidant component of fish oil called furan fatty acid, which appears to be at least as responsible for the benefits of dietary fish as omega-3.[21] Then, in the early 1990s, he started warning the world about the dangers of replacing saturated fats with vegetable oils.[22]

Or at least, he tried to.

As a chemist, he was making his argument using chemistry. But the dizzying array of chemical equations in his papers would be meaningless to most people, so his efforts to communicate were not as successful as they should have been given their importance and potential to positively impact our lives.

Dr. Spiteller's publications show that the very same reactions that occur in deep fryers can also take place inside our cells. This takes us back to the domino effect. Remember, PUFAs have more double bonds than saturated or monounsaturated fats, making PUFAs more susceptible to oxygen attacks and free-radical chain reactions that have a kind of molecular domino effect. Dr. Spiteller determined that if oxygen initiates a single free-radical spark *within our membranes*, the damage can spread like wildfire— or a row of toppling dominoes—just as it does in heated vegetable oils. In other words, oxidative stress can literally fry our biology from the inside out.

In his articles he laid out page after page of chemical equations, mostly stick diagrams of polyunsaturated fatty acid molecules and how they changed and became distorted after interacting with oxygen and free radicals in living tissues. The equations are circular, full of arrows that curve back from the end of one reaction right to where the reaction had started. This is how chemists express the idea of a chain reaction—that domino effect we've been talking about. Dr. Spiteller was trying to tell us that our own cell membranes can deteriorate into toxic compounds. And that those compounds can turn right around and attack more PUFAs, in a loop statement of cellular destruction.

Whenever oxygen kicks off one of these chain-reaction domino effects within a cell membrane, that cell is experiencing oxidative stress.

Oxidative stress is a state of cellular imbalance that disrupts everything the cell is trying to do. It unleashes mutagenic, cytotoxic, carcinogenic toxins and free radicals that can damage proteins and DNA. During episodes of oxidative stress, all semblance of organization is lost. Free radicals fly everywhere, shattering enzymes, mutating genes, and penetrating membranes where they will create more lipid oxidation products. If all this sounds abstract, think of oxidative stress inside your cell as a teeny tiny version of the "biblical" disaster Bill Murray and the Ghostbusters described as "rivers and seas boiling...human sacrifice, cats and dogs living together, mass hysteria." And it's no joke. It's a kind of toxic chaos that portends potential Armageddon for a cell.

Dr. Spiteller wanted to warn us that oxidative stress is contributing to numerous diseases. This is exactly what the free radical biologists have been saying since the 1950s. But there's a big difference between their message on oxidative stress and his. They jumped right to trying to prevent it, throwing antioxidants at the problem before fully understanding it. Dr. Spiteller did the work to understand the *source* of the free radicals, which is the root of the problem. He literally drew the chemical equations showing the connections between oxidized PUFA molecules, free radicals, and the molecules that investigators have found in people suffering from inflammatory and degenerative disease, where they are known as the biomarkers of oxidative stress—things like malondialdehyde, nitrotyrosine, and many more. This is why preventing free radicals and oxidation reactions with antioxidants has proven futile.

It's also why preventing both by avoiding toxic vegetable oils should be a slam dunk.

Antioxidant Supplements Are Mostly Worthless

The world has woken up to the harms of oxidative stress. Thousands of companies selling antioxidant supplements claim to be able to prevent inflammation and related degeneration. Some of the most popular of these supplements include resveratrol, lycopene, zeaxanthin, and megadoses of vitamins. Unfortunately—or fortunately, if you look at it from the point of view of saving money by not buying worthless products—these products are more likely to harm than hurt you. Most of the antioxidant compounds you can buy are made by plants for plants, and serve no function in our bodies. It would be like giving a firefighter a bunch of fruits and vegetables and telling him to go fight fires. It just doesn't help, and if he's carrying a Fukushu kumquat when he needs a firehose, that's going to get him into trouble. Worse, most of these antioxidants can promote oxidation under certain circumstances, so in that case it would be like giving our firefighter a flame thrower.

Rather than taking antioxidant supplements or megadoses of vitamins, I recommend supporting your body's firefighting crew with basic tools, mineral supplements as well as a simple multivitamin. It's important not to overdo the dose because too much of even these nutrients can provoke oxidation. (For more on supplements to support your antioxidant enzymes, see the Resources section.)

Dr. Spiteller devoted his last decades to laying out the evidence that PUFA oxidation contributes to one health problem after another: it is involved in the plaque formation that promotes heart attacks and strokes, the oxidized protein plaques and tangles of Alzheimer's disease, and the inflammation that drives autoimmune disease, diabetes, cancer, and more.[23] He was describing a universal mechanism of pathology that is known to be responsible for myriad diseases—but in a way that no one seemed to notice. It's heartbreaking, it's one of the consequences of silos in science, and it has prevented doctors from understanding patients' pain and suffering. It's particularly heartbreaking because all of us do learn in medical school that oxidative stress promotes inflammation. We just don't learn that vegetable oils are the main reason why our patients experience oxidative stress.

LINKING OXIDATIVE STRESS TO INFLAMMATION

Oxidative stress starts small and often goes undetected, but we can actually feel some forms of oxidative stress as it spreads. Oxidative stress is intimately linked to the body's inflammatory response, and inflammation causes many symptoms including pain, warmth, congestion, and swelling.

Inflammation can make us uncomfortable, but in some ways it's necessary for daily life. Inflammation clots your blood so you don't bleed to death from a paper cut. When you have a cold, inflammation is what gives you a runny, stuffy nose. Inflammation also readies the immune system for battle against infections. After a joint injury, such as an ankle sprain, inflammation helps break down the frayed ends of your damaged ligaments to clear the way for rebuilding and repair. The pain keeps you from walking until your tissues can be rebuilt and made strong again. The redness, swelling, itching, and pain you experience after a mosquito bite or a bee sting are examples of inflammation. These are all functions of the body's acute inflammatory response, which is how the body responds to trauma and infections. So we need inflammation—and we need oxidative stress to get it going.

All inflammatory responses in our bodies start with oxidation of the polyunsaturated fatty acids in our cell membranes. The body's inflammatory response system works like this: Infection or trauma damages cell membranes. The cell membrane damage activates special enzymes that oxidize the PUFAs in those membranes, triggering a cascade of additional reactions that magnify a tiny distress signal into something really loud. We've seen that PUFA oxidation happens so fast that chemists call it a chain reaction. Our bodies take advantage of the speed of this process, which enables the inflammatory reaction to spread quickly and contain the problem. Without membrane PUFA oxidation, there can be no inflammation—and no defense against infection or trauma. In other words, PUFA oxidation is designed by nature to trigger a life-saving inflammatory response system.

But the system can get tipped out of balance. If we experience oxidative stress too often, we experience inflammation too often. This is one of the most important and most harmful consequences of high-PUFA body fat.

In contrast to acute inflammation, which is helpful, *chronic* inflammation is a problem. Chronic inflammation can make us feel chronically unwell, or even confuse the immune system and cause autoimmune diseases such as rheumatoid arthritis or Graves', celiac, and Crohn's diseases. Inflammation is quite the buzzword today—and for good reason: many of us are living with the consequences of chronic inflammation.

If our diets constantly promote PUFA oxidation, we can deplete our bodies of antioxidants. This is what the Elgin Project showed. A diet high in vegetable oils will eventually deplete the body of antioxidants, tipping the system out of balance and promoting inflammatory disease.

These days, inflammatory diseases keep doctors in business. Most of our chronic diseases are inflammatory conditions. Some, such as gout and scarlet fever (an autoimmune disease related to strep throat), were linked to inflammation centuries ago. More recently we've discovered that out-of-control inflammation contributes to all autoimmune diseases, including celiac, Crohn's, thyroiditis, and rheumatoid arthritis. In 1986, a research paper listed over one hundred conditions that had already been linked to oxidative-stress-induced inflammation.[24] It has been implicated in heart disease, insulin resistance, and diabetes (more on those in the next chapter).[25] More recently we've added chronic pain syndromes and long COVID.[26] The menu of inflammatory conditions a doctor learns to diagnose represents a virtual all-you-can-eat buffet of chronic disease.

The inflammation involved in these conditions can be direct and noticeable immediately, or indirect and noticeable only later. Gastritis is an example of the former, and celiac of the latter. Either way, once inflammation starts, our bodies will continue to experience it until the PUFA oxidation completely stops. But, as we know, PUFA oxidation is a chain reaction. That means once it starts, everything happens blazingly fast, and all it takes is one little spark left unquenched before it flares up all over again. Fully quenching each inflammatory fire requires an arsenal of antioxidant equipment. With so many PUFAs in our diets and in our body fat, we can run out of firefighting equipment.

The number and diversity of diseases associated with inflammation has attracted a lot of research attention. But there is still one gigantic piece of the puzzle missing. Nobody can explain why oxidative stress and inflammation have become such a problem recently, particularly over the past thirty or forty years. That missing link is driving billions of dollars' worth of medical research every year.

I have yet to see any of the medical scientists doing the research for inflammatory diseases suggest that the missing link could be vegetable oil, with one important exception, discussed in "The Omega Imbalance Theory of Inflammation" below. But it's one of those ideas that won't go away, because it's solidly rooted in the basic sciences of chemistry and cell biology. One simple explanation can make the link without the need to spend another research dollar: on a vegetable oil diet, inflammation takes so long to quiet down that people's symptoms continue, or worsen, long after the initial infection or injury has resolved.

COMMON INFLAMMATORY DISEASES
CUTTING VEGETABLE OILS IMPROVES ALL OF THESE

AIRWAY INFLAMMATION
- Allergies*
- Asthma*
- Chronic sinusitis*
- Chronic obstructive pulmonary disease (COPD)*

SKIN INFLAMMATION
- Acne*
- Atopic dermatitis*
- Eczema*
- Hidradenitis suppurativa*
- Seborrheic dermatitis*
- Sunburning easily*
- Urticaria (hives)*
- Lichen sclerosis**
- Pemphigus**
- Psoriasis**
- Vitiligo**

BRAIN INFLAMMATION
- Concussion*
- Migraine headache*
- Attention-deficit/hyperactivity disorder (ADHD)**
- Anxiety disorders**
- Bipolar disorder**
- Depression**
- Dysthymia**
- Multiple sclerosis**

OTHER ORGAN INFLAMMATION
- Angioedema*
- Chronic cystitis (bladder)*
- Fatty liver*
- Visceral fat*
- Atherosclerosis and peri-arterial fat*
- Myositis**

GLANDULAR INFLAMMATION
- Chronic prostatitis*
- Polycystic ovarian syndrome (PCOS) and irregular periods*
- Thyroiditis**

GUT INFLAMMATION
- Celiac**
- Collagenous colitis**
- Crohn's**
- Lymphocytic colitis**
- Ulcerative colitis**

JOINT INFLAMMATION
- Lupus**
- Psoriatic arthritis**
- Rheumatoid arthritis**

PAIN SYNDROMES
- Chronic daily headache*
- Premenstrual syndrome and painful periods*
- Neuropathy*
- Fibromyalgia**

FATIGUE SYNDROMES
- Chronic fatigue**
- Long COVID**

METABOLIC SYNDROMES
- Insulin resistance*
- Obesity*
- Type 2 diabetes*
- Cancer**

*These conditions respond quickly to dietary change. They are caused by direct, primary inflammatory responses. They stop progressing and begin the process of resolution within days of improving nutrition, although complete resolution can take much longer.

**These conditions require more patience. These occur after chronic inflammation causes secondary problems. For example, chronic inflammation causes immune system malfunction and autoimmune diseases.

Figure 2–3

Does Fish Oil Reduce Inflammation?

In the 1990s, Artemis Simopoulos, a scientist with the National Institutes of Health, proposed that the root cause of our modern epidemic of inflammatory disease might be related to an aspect of vegetable oil that I haven't talked about much here. There are two types of PUFAs in vegetable oils, called omega-6 and omega-3. In response to infection or trauma, enzymes in our cells transform these two kinds of fatty acids into different sets of chemicals with complementary effects. Omega-6 fatty acids tend to promote inflammation, and omega-3s tend to shut it down. It's likely that in our evolutionary past, our dietary ratio of these two was closely balanced, maybe 1 to 1, or 1 to 2. Today it's more like 1 to 10, or 1 to 20, in favor of the pro-inflammatory omega-6. Since vegetable oils contain much more omega-6 than omega-3, Dr. Simopoulos thought this might be why so many people were suffering from inflammatory diseases. In the late 1990s, before anyone had an opportunity to test the idea in experiments, a journalist proposed writing a book called *The Omega Diet*. The book encouraged people to balance their omega-6 by supplementing with omega-3, and it was wildly popular. Unfortunately, the book ignored the role of oxidative stress.

Since then, scientists have tested the imbalance theory in human clinical experiments and have shown that even a very imbalanced 19-to-1 ratio of omega-6 to omega-3 does not increase the body's inflammatory responses, at least under normal circumstances.[27] Still, it could in theory worsen symptoms during extreme stresses, such as when someone is experiencing serious infections or trauma. In such circumstances, having way more omega-6 than omega-3 could very well promote blood clotting, excessive swelling, and a few other serious problems. But even if vegetable oils were balanced in omega-3 and omega-6, they would still deteriorate into toxins during cooking, and we would still suffer from excessive oxidative stress and inflammation.

This is why fish oil and other omega-3 supplements don't often help. In fact, they often just add fuel to the fire. That's why after decades of trying to prevent asthma attacks, heart attacks, cancer, and other diseases with fish oil, the results are consistently unimpressive. Fish oil may be helpful for rheumatoid arthritis and chronic dry eye, but not much else. Avoiding seed oils will work for everything, and it will work even better.

Inflammatory diseases catch our attention. But oxidative stress doesn't always trip off the inflammatory process in a way that's dramatic enough to trigger symptoms. It can also cause a slow-acting, silent form of cellular damage that can take many years for doctors to identify as a medical problem. A kind of gunk can start building up in our cells to the point that they can no longer function. I believe this is how vegetable oil promotes many of the diseases of aging that we call degenerative diseases.

THE "GARBAGE CATASTROPHE": A THEORY OF AGING AND DISEASE

One drizzly day in the spring of 1906, a German pathologist named Alois Alzheimer peered into a microscope to examine tiny samples of a woman's brain at his hospital in Munich. He discovered "a peculiar substance" filling many of the cells.[28] The woman was a fifty-year-old who had recently died after years of worsening memory, increasing disorientation, and hallucinations. He called these formations "senile plaque," as they were usually seen in much older people. Soon, other pathologists around the world noticed the same tiny blobs in people prematurely affected with dementia. They began calling them Alzheimer's plaques.

While the dreaded dementing disease is now all too familiar, the origin of the "peculiar substance" eluded scientific explanation for nearly one hundred years. Finally, in 2000, researchers settled on their answer: oxidative stress. The cellular garbage forms because oxidation damages bits and pieces of cellular protein in ways that the cell's garbage disposal systems can't clean up. So the oxidized gunk just accumulates within the cell until it forms amyloid plaques big enough to show up under a microscope.

Researchers were confused for so long because amyloid doesn't just result from oxidative stress, it also causes oxidative stress—a common theme we've encountered before. So scientists were stuck in a chicken-or-egg loop statement, unsure if the plaques came first and caused the disease, or the disease developed first and caused the plaques. With the root cause question settled, they were able to explain another mystery of Alzheimer's: Why don't anti-inflammatory therapies help? They soon recognized that these plaques trigger little to no inflammation because the affected brain cells slow down their metabolic activity, seemingly in a desperate attempt to control oxidative stress by going into a kind of cellular hibernation.[29] This adaptation unfortunately slows down the brain's processing speed—and that's when symptoms usually begin. Over time, brain cells shrink or die, the brain atrophies, and those who are affected slowly lose themselves as they succumb to dementia.

Many degenerative disorders follow a similar progression. If you follow sports news, you may have heard about *tau protein*, the marker of traumatic brain injury found in football players who've suffered repeated concussions and severe personality changes. Tau protein is another form of oxidized cellular gunk. Another common disease-related blob is oxidized *alpha-synuclein*, which causes Parkinson's disease and another form of dementia called Lewy body dementia (the second most common dementia after Alzheimer's). Lewy body dementia is harder to diagnose, starts earlier—often as attention deficits—and progresses faster. An example outside the nervous system is *drusen*, blobs that build up in the eye and that can cause a form of blindness known as macular degeneration.

Another common garbage blob is *lipofuscin*. This dark pigment is responsible for age spots on the skin and is associated with all the above disorders of the nervous system, although it's unclear if it plays an active role. It's also found in people with certain forms of kidney disease, some people with high blood pressure, and with a painful bowel disease called brown bowel syndrome.[30]

Chemically, the various oxidized garbage blobs behave like the black, sticky, tar-like gunk on the bottom of an oven that resists easy cleaning. But, unlike us when we clean our ovens, our cells can't use solvents to clear away the buildup—they simply have to live with it. They try to cope by wrapping the sticky, dark material in a protective membrane. Or by scooching the tiny garbage blobs out of the way, so they're unlikely to harm anything else. Over time, however, more and more of them pile up. The diseases related to this sort of debris all develop more or less in proportion to the size of the pileups. Interestingly enough, not everyone with this sort of material in their tissues develops disease, which probably has to do with their genetics.

Genes Versus Diet

Genetics is much less powerful than diet when it comes to determining our susceptibility to disease—which makes me glad I didn't stick it out in Cornell's molecular biology PhD program. Genetics does determine how well your body fights off oxidative stress in various tissue compartments—such as brain versus liver or bone marrow. This means that your genes mostly determine *which* diseases you'll likely get by following an oxidative-stress-inducing diet. Whether you get the disease or not comes down to what you eat.

If the modern diet is an all-you-can-eat buffet of chronic disease, then your genetics tell you what's most likely to end up on your plate.

Scientists encounter oxidized cellular garbage associated with age-related diseases so often that, in 2001, a Swedish pathologist who studies lysosomes (the cell's garbage disposal units) coined a phrase for it: "the garbage catastrophe." He published a paper on the subject called "Garbage Catastrophe Theory of Aging: Imperfect Removal of Oxidative Damage?"[31] He explained that since these damaging accumulations are a result of oxidative stress, then perhaps by manipulating our cellular ability to withstand oxidative stress, future technologies might prevent aging and age-related diseases. Of course, he wouldn't have known that our modern diet powerfully promotes oxidative stress. If he did, he might have considered that *preventing* oxidative stress—by avoiding vegetable oils—might be a more practical strategy.

Bottom line, the fact is that the normal aging process itself is driven by oxygen and by oxidation reactions. Because PUFA accelerates oxidation reactions, high-PUFA vegetable oils accelerate the aging process. Cutting vegetable oil slows it down.

With oxidative stress currently linked to so many conditions, it would seem logical that doctors would be equipped to identify and treat it. Unfortunately, that is not yet the case.

Doctors are taught that a "Western-style diet" contributes to these degenerative diseases, which is true. But the devil is in the details, and we learn that the two most harmful elements in a Western diet are saturated fats and cholesterol (more on this in Part Two). We hear this over and over again in spite of the lack of direct scientific evidence that these two nutrients can promote diseases related to oxidative stress. There is, however, direct experimental evidence that polyunsaturated fats play a causative role in a wide variety of human diseases, but it's not built into a doctor's training. Just to give you one example, let's take a look at the tau deposits of Alzheimer's disease. When scientists try to create tau during animal experiments, they find that saturated fats do not readily promote tau deposits, and cholesterol actually inhibits tau formation.[32] But polyunsaturated fats are a different story. PUFAs are the most effective inducers of tau protein

COMMON DEGENERATIVE DISEASES
CUTTING VEGETABLE OILS SLOWS THESE AGE-RELATED PROBLEMS

BRAIN DEGENERATION
- Alzheimer's*
- Essential tremor*
- Lewy body dementia*
- Parkinson's*

KIDNEY DEGENERATION
- White coat hypertension and essential hypertension*
- Kidney failure*

HEART DEGENERATION
- Heart failure*

JOINT DEGENERATION
- Osteoarthritis**

BONE DEGENERATION
- Osteoporosis**

AIRWAY DEGENERATION
- Emphysema**

BLOOD VESSEL DEGENERATION
- Aneurysm**
- Varicose veins**

*These conditions result mainly from oxidative stress INSIDE the cell.

**These conditions result mainly from oxidative stress OUTSIDE the cell, activating enzymes that break down the collagen supporting our skin, joints, bones, and other connective tissues.

Figure 2–4

assembly, initiating its formation seven times more powerfully than mono-unsaturated fats, and fifty times more powerfully than saturated fats.[33]

As a result of our miseducation on root causes, doctors spend a lot of time focusing on risk factors that we don't truly understand.

WHAT YOUR "RISK FACTORS" REALLY MEAN

When you go to the doctor for a physical exam, he or she will screen you for risk factors that might indicate you're likely to develop a serious disease that might be preventable with medications. But this universal practice has little or no net benefit.[34] Risk factors are not root causes, and in treating our patients' risk factors with drugs, while ignoring the real root causes, we are doing more harm than good.

The risk factors we most commonly screen for include smoking, obesity, sedentary lifestyle, family history of diseases, high blood pressure, diabetes, and cholesterol. Other risk factors that not every doctor will test for include abnormal uric acid; homocysteine; lipoprotein (a), or Lp(a); and high-sensitivity C-reactive protein (hs-CRP, a sign of certain subtypes of immune system–mediated inflammation)—and there are actually many more. All of these risk factors put our patients at higher risk of heart attacks. These same dozen or so risk factors also indicate higher risk for many other diseases, including Alzheimer's, strokes, several cancers, heart failure, liver disease, and a huge array of other degenerative and chronic conditions.

Quite a coincidence that so many different diseases can be associated with the exact same list of risk factors, isn't it? It's not actually a mysterious coincidence, of course. The simple, logical explanation is that most of the risk factors *themselves* have the same root cause: oxidative stress.

But although medical journals inform physicians that these diseases are associated with oxidative stress, it's presented as yet another risk factor. It's not yet clear to medical science that oxidative stress is the one root cause we should all be paying attention to (much less that we need to stop eating vegetable oils in order to control it). As a result, we can't help people very much. Worse, many doctors believe that the drugs we use for managing some of these risk factors are fixing the problem at its root. But the risk factors are not causing the disease. By using drugs to manage the outward signs of oxidative stress, but failing to fix the underlying problem, we allow the oxidative stress to continue unchecked while also exposing people to side effects of drugs.

As evidence that modifying these risk factors does little or nothing for anyone, I submit the story of homocysteine. If you have too much homocysteine in your blood, your diet might be low in one or more B vitamins. In the 1990s, research showed that people with higher homocysteine levels had a higher rate of heart attacks, strokes, and cognitive decline. So doctors started ordering this test and treating high homocysteine with vitamins, which successfully lowered homocysteine levels. We thought we'd solved the problem until further research showed that this did nothing to prevent heart attacks, strokes, or cognitive decline.[35] This has been dubbed "the homocysteine paradox."[36] But it's hardly a paradox. It's simply that the underlying problem behind high homocysteine is oxidative stress. And the fact that vitamin supplementation improves homocysteine levels, but not the more meaningful problem—actual disease—is further evidence for the need to address the root cause of oxidative stress.

The homocysteine story has implications for all of our other so-called risk factors. If we can improve a risk factor without reducing disease, then what are we really accomplishing? Over the years I've been in practice, I've seen time and again that risk factor management often fails to produce the expected outcomes. Yet we continue to manage these same risk factors the same way, burying our heads in the sand. I see this as a direct outgrowth of our ignorance about vegetable oils.

Now that we've learned about oxidative stress, we can understand another insidious way that a diet full of vegetable oils harms us at the cellular level. I've come to understand that these oils can contribute to diseases that we now attribute to lack of willpower, unpleasant personality traits, and random chance. In the next chapter, I want to show you the link between vegetable oil and the biggest challenge that medical science is facing, but that our training does not prepare us to treat. It has to do with how cells generate *energy*. Oxidative stress is not only driving chronic inflammatory and age-related diseases, it's also driving the obesity and diabetes epidemics by changing our cravings and our relationship with food.

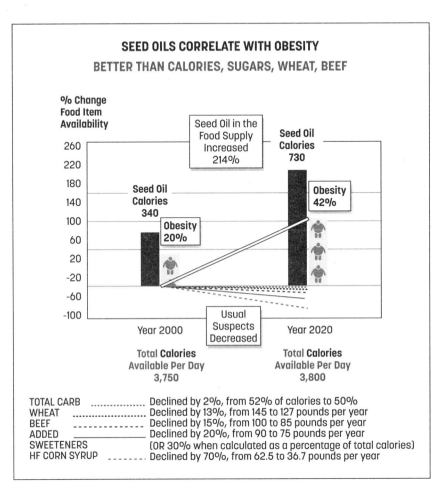

**SEED OILS CORRELATE WITH OBESITY
BETTER THAN CALORIES, SUGARS, WHEAT, BEEF**

% Change
Food Item
Availability

Seed Oil in the Food Supply Increased 214%

Seed Oil Calories 730

Seed Oil Calories 340

Obesity 20%

Obesity 42%

Year 2000

Usual Suspects Decreased

Year 2020

Total **Calories** Available Per Day 3,750

Total **Calories** Available Per Day 3,800

TOTAL CARB	....	Declined by 2%, from 52% of calories to 50%
WHEAT	....	Declined by 13%, from 145 to 127 pounds per year
BEEF	– – – – – – – –	Declined by 15%, from 100 to 85 pounds per year
ADDED SWEETENERS	——————	Declined by 20%, from 90 to 75 pounds per year (OR 30% when calculated as a percentage of total calories)
HF CORN SYRUP	– – – – – –	Declined by 70%, from 62.5 to 36.7 pounds per year

Figure 3–1: The correlation between vegetable oil and obesity is clear enough that we don't need statisticians to find it for us. Nor do we need statisticians to tell us that these other commonly imputed dietary factors do not correlate. Even so, **medical science ignores this data.**

To understand how vegetable oils might make us gain weight, we need to consider how they affect the body's ability to generate energy. **This chapter takes advantage of what we already know to explain one possible mechanism** linking vegetable oil to obesity and metabolic disease.

Note: The 214 percent increase in liquid vegetable oil consumption shown here is related to the trans-fat ban, which increased the consumption of liquid vegetable oil relative to solid (hydrogenated) oil. For sources used to create this figure, see the endnotes for this chapter.

The Metabolic Problem Your Doctor Can't See

IN THIS CHAPTER YOU WILL LEARN

- We often say our metabolism slows down with age, but this can't explain childhood obesity.
- The problem is inflammatory body fat, which slows energy production in our cells.
- When our cells can't get energy from our body fat, this can make us crave sugar, avoid activity, and gain weight.
- The name of this metabolic problem is insulin resistance.

The World Health Organization describes obesity as the largest health threat facing humanity. In late October 2022, many of the world's greatest medical minds gathered in the gilded rooms of London's Royal Society of Medicine to discuss what might be done to stop its spread. There was just one problem: the presenters had contradictory ideas about what causes it in the first place. Some blamed genetics. Some blamed epigenetics. Some blamed inactivity. Some blamed a lack of shared family dinners due to overburdened parents, chaotic schedules, or so much screen time. Also included in the list of contributing factors were pesticides, herbicides, heavy metals, sugar, corn syrup, and, of course, the microbiome. (This is by no means a complete list, by the way.) At the meeting's closing session, the host expressed his exasperation, saying, "There's no consensus whatsoever about what the cause of it is."[1]

In the midst of all this brain power, not one of the speakers invited to share their research at this prestigious event ever mentioned the fact that roughly a third of our calories now come from vegetable oil.

Forget for a minute everything you've heard about nutrition. Just consider this one statistic: industrial vegetable oils now account for up to 80 percent of the average US person's fat calories, and one-third of our total calories. You don't need to be an obesity expert, or even a doctor, to recognize that anything making up such a large portion of our daily calories certainly warrants mention. You don't need computations to find a striking correlation between vegetable oil intake and obesity, and a striking absence of correlation between obesity and other dietary variables, including—remarkably—calories. Unfortunately, doctors, nutritionists, dietitians, and obesity researchers are completely in the dark about the negative health effects of vegetable oil.

I was one of them. In my early years practicing medicine, when my overweight patients told me there must be something wrong with their metabolism, I had doubts. If thyroid and other basic tests came out normal, I'd silently chalk it up to lack of self-control. To all my former patients who came to me for help with losing weight in those early days, I owe you an apology. You were right. You did have a metabolic problem. That problem is *insulin resistance.*

Metabolism Is All About Energy

Metabolism is about so much more than weight. You've probably noticed that when you wake up full of energy you feel good—far better than when you don't. This feeling isn't just in your head; it's also in your cells, and this feeling happens more often the healthier

---

> your metabolism is and the more efficiently it generates energy. Oxidative stress gets in the way of all that. It prevents you from feeling excited to take on the day. It promotes a metabolic derangement that makes us crave sugary and starchy foods to boost our energy. This metabolic shift toward sugar is called insulin resistance.

Insulin resistance is the first step in the development of type 2 diabetes. It is incredibly common, affecting even more of the US population than overweight and obesity, and yet most people don't even know what it is. In this chapter, we're going to see how vegetable oil gradually disrupts our metabolic health by changing the chemistry of our body fat. As our bodies take steps to deal with that chemical change, we develop insulin resistance. It's a four-step process:

1. Vegetable oil gives us high-PUFA body fat with inflammatory properties.
2. When cells try to burn inflammatory body fat, they end up not getting enough energy.
3. To supplement their energy, cells use more of the limited amount of sugar in our bloodstream, causing low-blood-sugar symptoms.
4. As this continues, the body gradually elevates its blood sugar set point and in the process becomes insulin resistant.

STEP 1: INFLAMMATORY BODY FAT

We began to explore this step in chapter 2 when we looked at two key pieces of research, the Elgin Project and Stephan Guyenet's adipose analysis. Both showed that a diet high in vegetable oil builds body fat that is full of oxidation-prone, inflammation-inciting PUFA.

Given the evidence suggesting we have too much adipose PUFA today, but that we definitely need some, before we move on it's important to know how much we need in our diet. For the answer to that we can turn to Chris Knobbe, MD, an emeritus professor of ophthalmology at the University of Texas, Dallas. He became interested in vegetable oil because it may promote blindness from macular degeneration (as a result of the drusen we discussed in chapter 2). He wanted to know exactly how far out of bounds our current total intake of PUFA is in comparison to the days before vegetable oils. And since our body fat PUFA reflects our dietary PUFA, the answer to that question lies in adipose tissue biopsies. He has spent years unearthing data collected from groups of people living all around the world whose dietary and body tissue fatty acids were analyzed while they were still eating a preindustrial-era diet, free of vegetable oils. This information is also helpful because it tells us what our body fat PUFA concentration *should be*.

The kinds of diets Dr. Knobbe studies are called *ancestral diets*, meaning they're representative of the kinds of diets people everywhere used to eat. The specific populations he's studied include groups in Japan, Africa (the Maasai), Papua New Guinea (Tukisenta), New Zealand (Tokelau), Sweden (in the 1950s, when vegetable oil consumption was still limited), and a few more. You might think these far-flung groups of people would eat radically different diets, and when it comes to specific ingredients, this is correct. However, when it comes to nutrients, all human diets are remarkably similar.[2] Dr. Knobbe's exhaustive research puts the historical PUFA content between 1.5 and 3 percent of total fatty acids, the rest—97 percent or so—being saturated and monounsaturated fatty acids. Very few of these cultures have been properly studied, and it's a small sample size, but the results are consistent and significant. *None* of these ancestral cultures exhibited body fat PUFA of over 3 percent.[3] Others have estimated our total PUFA at between 3 and 5 percent.[4] Even though these experts don't fully agree, it's clear that historical PUFA consumption was significantly lower than it is today. And this has had consequences for our body fat.

I think of body fat as a recipe. If the "recipe" for human body fat calls for up to 5 percent PUFA, and in 2008 we already had 21.5 percent (the figure that Dr. Guyenet found in his research), that's a 400 percent overage. If you quadruple a main ingredient in any recipe, you're going to change the dish from one thing to another thing entirely. Since that 2008 data is out of step with our current rate of vegetable oil consumption, today we're likely deviating even further from the human body-fat recipe.

All this is to say that all of us today are in a completely different metabolic state than people were 30, 50, 80, or 150 years ago, when there was far less PUFA in human body fat. This has important implications for our ability to maintain a healthy weight that we need to understand if we want to understand obesity.

When I'm talking about the percentage of PUFA in your body fat I am not talking about your body composition. The term *body composition* typically refers to how much of our body weight is composed of fat on a percentage basis. A healthy body composition for women is between 18 and 24 percent, and for men 8 to 25 percent, although it varies based on age. But this says nothing about how much PUFA we have in that fat. We can have a normal, healthy amount of body fat and still have an abnormally high proportion of PUFA. This was true for participants in the Elgin Project (and another, the LA VA study).[5] In other words, whether you're fat or thin, if you've been eating vegetable oil, your body fat is full of PUFA. The "recipe" overage is the same regardless of a person's weight, and the metabolic consequences of the overage manifest as health problems even among people who are thin.

One rather bizarre-sounding consequence of high-PUFA body fat relates to its melting point. Just as oil has a lower melting point and is therefore liquid at room temperature when butter stays solid, our high-PUFA body fat has a different, flabbier texture than if we followed a low-PUFA diet. A giant of modern nutrition science, Dr. John Yudkin, had already noticed this difference back in the 1980s. He wrote, "The fat in a person who habitually takes a high proportion of dietary fat as vegetable oils...will tend to be rather softer than that of a person whose dietary fat is largely the solid fats of animal origin."[6] I point out this effect of our high-PUFA diet to highlight how our new, modern diet is doing fundamentally strange things to our bodies.

The Properties of Inflammatory Body Fat

When scientists look at the fatty acid composition of people with obesity versus without, they often find partly oxidized PUFAs. In particular, they find the precise set of toxic, partly oxidized compounds that Dr. Gerhard Spiteller and others had predicted. These compounds cause oxidative damage that promotes inflammation.[7] Thin people often exhibit these same compounds, although in lower average concentrations.

Most scientists don't yet identify inflammatory fat by its partly oxidized PUFA content. They identify it by its biological features—what the cells look like, where the fat tends to build up in our bodies, and what the cells can and can't do compared to normal, healthy adipose cells. Inflammatory fat cells are typically smaller than healthy ones. They often build up in and around our liver, pancreas, and other organs, forming what's called *visceral fat*. We can't directly see visceral fat without X-rays or other imaging technology, since it's internal, but it makes our bellies bulge. It also accumulates around our heart, where it dramatically increases heart attack risk.[8]

Importantly, the problem of inflammatory fat is not just localized to our internal organs, it's everywhere. I'll be calling this problematic fat *visceral fat* when referring to its location around internal organs, and *inflammatory fat* when referring to it generally.

Pound for pound, inflammatory fat produces fewer satiety signals, such as leptin, and lack of leptin promotes overeating.[9] It also exudes cellular distress chemicals called *cytokines*. Cytokines normally indicate an infection, and thus attract immune system cells called white blood cells. Inflammatory fat is positively crawling with white blood cells, as if it were infected. But in this case the cytokines are false indicators, which confuses the immune system, contributing to allergies and autoimmune diseases.[10]

Importantly, you can be at a normal weight and still have unhealthy amounts of visceral fat. This is very common: studies have shown that 45 percent of women and nearly 60 percent of men who appeared thin on the outside actually had excessive levels of internal adipose tissue—i.e., they were "fat inside."[11] This thin-outside, fat-inside combination is now called TOFI. Or, simply, skinny fat.

Testing for Inflammatory Body Fat

There are several ways to find out if you have inflammatory body fat. The most direct test is magnetic resonance imaging (MRI), which shows you exactly where fat builds up inside your body, and how much. But this method is expensive, and insurance won't cover it.

You can also step on a specialized bioimpedance scale that measures how fast electrical impulses travel through your body, and many gyms and health clubs have these. They are not very accurate, however.

The best, simplest test is actually the one that tells you if you are insulin resistant or not. As we'll see when we discuss Step 4, insulin resistance is the very earliest sign that high-PUFA body fat is disrupting an individual's metabolic health. It may even pick up the problem before you see visceral fat buildup.

The presence of inflammatory fat is also strongly associated with the absence of normal amounts of muscle. In 2017, human metabolism pioneer Phil Maffetone and his research team proposed their own term to describe this phenomenon of fat replacing normal, healthy muscle and other tissues. This new term is *overfat*. It refers to the presence of excess body fat that can impair health, even for normal weight individuals.[12] Unlike the terms TOFI and skinny fat, overfat applies to all people, regardless of their weight. When Dr. Maffetone's team reviewed the global evidence, they discovered overfat at "an alarmingly high rate of over 90% in adult males and up to 50% in children." The problem was worst in the United States. Most investigators have assumed that our desk-bound, sedentary lifestyle is the sole explanation. However, Dr. Maffetone's article specifically counters this notion, remarking that "the overfat pandemic has not spared physically active people, including professional athletes in various sports and active US military personnel."[13]

The United States may be leading the way in overfat because we led the way in eating soybean oil.[14] Today, every country consumes more of the high-PUFA vegetable oils than ever before.[15] It's entirely possible that this decades-long practice of eating foods that build inflammatory body fat has now essentially changed human body composition on a national, and increasingly global, scale. It's affecting young and old, rich and poor—although the poor are often hit more severely in proportion to their reliance on cheaper foods that are full of vegetable oil.

How to De-PUFA Body Fat

There is no detox formula to clear your body of these toxins, unfortunately. There is just one way to get rid of it: you have to burn it off—just like you have to burn off any unwanted body fat you may have. I have no doubt that we can get our PUFA levels back down to normal, although it takes a while. One study, performed back in 1960, showed that the half-life of PUFA in our body fat ranged between 350 and 750 days, which means it takes that long to clear out just *half* of it.[16] More recent studies pinpoint a similar figure, 580 days on average. Surprisingly, although the time required doesn't vary much with weight, insulin resistance will extend the time it takes.[17] So we're looking at three or four years of avoiding vegetable oils to normalize the amount

---

of PUFAs in our body fat—possibly longer for those who are severely insulin resistant. Fortunately, you will start to feel much better much sooner. Most people notice fewer inflammatory symptoms (such as those we discussed in chapter 2) almost immediately after stopping vegetable oils. We'll explore how to eat to boost your energy and help your body heal in Part Three.

Although we began this chapter by talking about obesity, the problem is not, at the end of the day, a matter of too much body fat; it's a matter of fatty acid chemistry. This is an important distinction, especially with the rise of the healthy-at-any-size movement. When our body fat is full of PUFA, we are, quite tragically, *unhealthy* at any size. I'm not talking about beauty standards. I'm talking about the ability of human body fat to do its primary job, which is to serve as a source of fuel to energize our cells. This takes us to Step 2 on the path to insulin resistance.

STEP 2: INFLAMMATORY BODY FAT FAILS TO ENERGIZE US

We often hear people talking about burning body fat like it's some special state you need to work really hard to achieve. But the truth is, we're all born as fat burners, and we are supposed to easily burn fat between every meal. But when our body fat is inflammatory, it doesn't give our cells the energy they need, and so we can lose this natural ability to easily burn fat.

To understand how inflammatory, high-PUFA body fat might drain our energy, let's start by discussing where, exactly, body fat gets burned.

Every calorie you've ever burned was incinerated inside one of the tiny chambers in your cells called *mitochondria*. Every cell contains mitochondria; some contain thousands. These little chambers are nature's power stations, tirelessly generating energy for your cells day and night. No matter how much or how little physical work you do, your mitochondria are ready to serve your body's energy needs.

Good Calories and Bad

We've all heard that a calorie is a calorie, as if all calories have equal effects on our weight and metabolism. This is wrong. A calorie is a unit of heat energy, not biological energy. The term tells us how much heat is released when a given food combusts in a device called a bomb calorimeter. An apple releases 100 calories of heat energy, as does a tablespoon of butter. However, some nutrients release heat when burned in a calorimeter, but our mitochondria can't use them for energy, such as cholesterol. Burn a lump of cholesterol and you'll get heat. But if we eat too much cholesterol, our liver eliminates it in the form of bile acids which wind up in the toilet.[18] So, as you can see, thermal energy and cellular energy are very different.

That is the essential flaw in the calories in calories out model of weight loss. Our cells produce energy in mitochondria, not heaters. So to understand which calories are good and which are bad, we need to understand how our mitochondria metabolize them. Good calories provide mitochondria with clean energy and turn you into a metabolic rock star. Bad calories detonate inside our mitochondria and make us fat and tired.[19]

Mitochondria don't melt body fat. They literally burn it, using oxygen just like a combustion engine. Scientists first glimpsed the inner workings of mitochondria in the 1950s using an electron microscope, which can magnify objects 300,000 times (light microscopes start getting blurry at a magnification of around 1,200 times). A single mitochondrion is composed of an outer membrane and an inner membrane. The outer membrane is basically a simple envelope enclosing the bean-shaped mitochondrion. The inner membrane is folded into strikingly organized parallel lines that serpentine through the entire structure, making the interior of the mitochondrion look like a miniature marble game. Due to the elegant design of mitochondria, microscopists frequently nominate them as their favorite organelle.

Studding the serpentine inner membrane, we find an incredible protein molecule that can only be seen using an even more high-tech tool called X-ray crystallography and computerized visual reconstruction. This protein looks exactly like the world's smallest turbine, complete with the ability to spin. With that tiny, spinning turbine, mitochondria generate energy for our cells—a kind of cellular energy called adenosine triphosphate (ATP). Cells use ATP to power their tiny biological machines, much as people use electricity to power our household appliances.

Mitochondria are the whole reason we need to breathe. The oxygen our blood delivers to mitochondria pumps the protons that make those turbines spin. When all is working well, it's an elegant process: the faster those tiny turbines spin, the more ATP your mitochondria make, and the more calories you're burning. Three-dimensional reconstructions of mitochondrial proteins in motion are so awe inspiring that some see it as evidence of intelligent design. All of this beauty and complexity can be disrupted, however, when we fail to protect our mitochondrial membranes from oxidative stress.

Your Miraculous Mitochondria

Paleobiologists who study early life on Earth estimate that evolution took a billion years to create mitochondria. The development began during a period known as the great oxygen crisis, starting about two billion years ago. During this time, primitive single-celled plants, called cyanobacteria, dramatically changed the planet by filling our skies with oxygen they produced as a byproduct of their growth. All that oxygen started killing everything, since cell membranes were not yet prepared to protect themselves from free radicals. This led to the largest mass extinction event our planet has ever faced. The only thing that saved us was the development of antioxidants.

That crucial step led to a giant leap forward. With antioxidants protecting their membranes, bacteria could experiment with harnessing oxygen's power to their advantage. The end result of billions of years of such experimentation is our mitochondria, which were originally independently living organisms that got swallowed up by a bigger cell. Mitochondria generated so much energy that life would soon take another major leap forward.

Before mitochondria, all life was limited to slow-growing single cells. The ocean was black and the sky grayish green. After mitochondria, life flourished, the water cleared, the sky turned blue, and the world blossomed into the diversity of plants, animals, and fungi that fills our fossil record with extinct creatures, and fills today's landscapes with vivid color. None of us would exist today without mitochondria, and mitochondria wouldn't exist without antioxidants.

Because mitochondria contain more oxygen than any other part of our cells, they are more dependent on antioxidants than any other part of our cells. What might antioxidant-depleting, inflammatory body fat do to our marvelous mitochondria when they need to burn it?

How PUFAs Damage Our Mitochondria

In 2002, a group of Italian scientists at the Institute for Neurosciences in Padua, Italy, published a study suggesting that forcing mitochondria to burn PUFA might damage the mitochondria and imperil our cells.

They tested the effect of various fatty acids on mitochondrial energy output by feeding isolated cells each type of fatty acid and measuring ATP production.[20] The differences were easy to see, and their report included a graph that I've adapted here. It shows that 100 percent saturated and monounsaturated fats are efficient mitochondrial fuel; 100 percent PUFA, on the other hand, is not. Within minutes of feeding cells PUFAs, energy production drops. In other words, when mitochondria burn PUFA, their power output goes down (see Figure 3–2).

Their experiment suggests that whether it comes in directly from our diet or from our body fat, too much PUFA can do some really, really bad things to both our mitochondria and our cells.

Of course, this experiment tested 100 percent PUFA, and neither foods nor body fat contain 100 percent PUFA. But the study's findings are nevertheless very important: they show that not all fatty acids are equal in the eyes of our mitochondria. Fatty acids with more double bonds—PUFAs—can stall mitochondrial energy output. Not only that, other experiments performed by the same team showed that when burning PUFA mitochondria can start spewing free radicals that spark oxidative stress, which can damage everything in the cell, including the mitochondria.

This study was not the first to show that PUFA makes a poor fuel for our cells. Scientists were making the same observations as early as 1956.[21] And in 1963, a scientist responsible for our understanding of the mitochondrial turbine, Efraim Racker, warned about the same effect in an article titled, somewhat provocatively, "Calories Don't Count—If You Don't Use Them."[22] Dr. Racker was at the time the chief of the Nutrition and Physiology Department at the Public Health Research Institute of the City of New York, and in 1977 President Jimmy Carter awarded him the National Medal of Science. Dr. Racker was not some armchair nutrition expert seeking attention with a provocative title. He was actually referring to a then popular diet book called simply *Calories Don't Count*. Dr. Racker's article pointed out that the book promoted the "increasingly popular polyunsaturated oils used by the processed food industry." And he explained that the book's title was almost accurate, because polyunsaturates actually can shut down mitochondrial energy production—so he corrected it to make it more accurate by adding the phrase "if you don't use them."

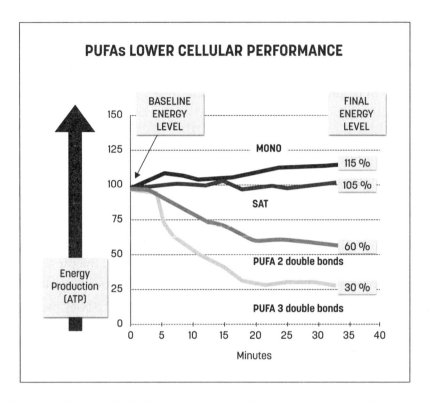

Figure 3–2: This graph holds the key to understanding our modern metabolism. I found the data for it in an obscure scientific journal that reported on an experiment measuring how well each of the four major types of fatty acids supports cellular energy production. It shows that only saturated and monounsaturated fatty acids can do the job— and that the two kinds of PUFAs (omega-3 with three double bonds and omega-6 with two double bonds) can't. This means animal fat and olive oil (among other plant-based oils) help our cells generate energy, and seed oil doesn't.

In addition, the study showed that burning PUFA generates damaging free radicals far faster than burning saturated or monounsaturated fat. The free radicals overwhelm our cells' antioxidant capacity, reducing ATP production and damaging mitochondria, cell membranes, and other vital cell structures.

These findings are true whether the fatty acids came from food or body fat. Think of a lightbulb. The old-fashioned kind produced light but also a lot of heat. A modern LED bulb produces plenty of light with almost no heat, meaning it's a more efficient apparatus. In this case, light is good energy and heat is bad energy.

The same goes for your cells. **ATP production: good energy. Free radicals: bad energy.**

Unfortunately, casual readers may have glanced at the title and thought he was promoting some kind of calorie-free food or fast weight-loss scheme, and just dismissed it. In reality, he was suggesting that vegetable oils were a very poor cellular fuel and would likely harm our mitochondria, with toxic effects. He concluded his article with a solemn warning: "More extensive studies on the toxicity of unsaturated fatty acids may be in order before their indiscriminate use in foods or drugs is condoned."[23]

It's important to point out that the results of the Italian experiment and Dr. Racker's predictions also jibe with the rules of chemistry we've already learned. Chemistry tells us that uncontrolled oxygen-PUFA reactions invariably generate free radicals and oxidative stress. When these reactions occur inside our mitochondria, our mitochondria can't produce energy normally and will start leaking free radicals. This process of leaking free radicals consumes antioxidants, too—which the body can resupply, but it can take a while. Meanwhile, mitochondrial energy output will not be optimal, and the cell will be exposed to damaging oxidative reactions, toxin formation, and the general mayhem previously discussed. All of this is sometimes called *mitochondrial oxidative stress*, and mitochondrial oxidative stress is known to promote a variety of diseases for which medical science currently has no effective cures.[24]

The cell actually has its own defense against this sort of damage, but activating the defensive mechanism comes at a cost. That defense is to take steps to spend less time burning body fat and spend more time burning sugar.[25]

STEP 3: ENERGY STARVED CELLS DEPLETE OUR BLOOD SUGAR SUPPLY

Medical science is finally beginning to recognize that most people who struggle with their weight are struggling because they are not burning their body fat. In a recent medical conference on obesity in New Zealand, the keynote speaker shocked the audience when he presented metabolic test results showing that some people burn almost no body fat, ever.[26] Not at rest. Not during an overnight fast. Not even with light aerobic exercise. And certainly not with more intense activity, since the harder our muscles are working, the more sugar they use relative to fat. Who are these never-fat-burning people? People with ordinary type 2 diabetes, the advanced stage of insulin resistance. These folks are mostly burning sugar, instead.

Think about the problem of high PUFA body fat from the point of view of a cell. Imagine you were managing a cell and needed to keep operations running, but whenever you brought body fat into the cell to use as fuel, energy disruptions slowed things down. You'd want to start looking for an alternative to fueling your mitochondria with fat. Fortunately for you, the bloodstream always contains a small amount of sugar—glucose—which is a much better mitochondrial fuel than PUFA. Unfortunately, our entire bloodstream only contains a teaspoon's worth of glucose.

The teaspoon of glucose in the blood cannot provide for the desperate needs of all the sugar-addicted cells in your body, no longer acting as a cooperative community but thinking only for themselves. Their supply of fuel, normally healthy body fat, has been adulterated by PUFA, causing an increased demand for sugar. The result is hypoglycemia, the medical term for low blood glucose (often referred to as low blood sugar). The healthcare system's callous ignorance of this process is making billions—while allowing millions to needlessly suffer and die.

Human studies have tested a key element of this idea, the part about PUFA increasing our bodies' use of blood glucose between meals. In one study, participants ate either a high- or low-PUFA diet for a week, and then underwent testing to see how much glucose they were burning after an overnight fast. They found that people getting more PUFA were burning relatively more glucose—and relatively less body fat.[27] The fat-burn-suppressing and sugar-slurping effects of polyunsaturates have been surprisingly well documented by a variety of other researchers, too.[28]

Unfortunately, this effect of PUFA is mistaken for a good thing.[29] Researchers have honed in on the glucose-lowering effect of PUFA, interpreting it as increased *insulin sensitivity*. Insulin sensitivity is the opposite of insulin resistance, and increasing insulin sensitivity can reverse the condition even in advanced stages of type 2 diabetes. As a result of this backward interpretation, many articles incorrectly suggest that vegetable oils should reverse insulin resistance and diabetes. The incorrect interpretation comes from a myopic viewpoint that focuses only on one cell at a time, failing to consider that using more sugar might negatively affect the body as a whole, particularly between meals when the supply of blood glucose is most limited.

We need to burn body fat for energy between meals, while exercising, and during a fast. When body fat can't give our cells energy in these circumstances, we're going to feel hypoglycemic. Hypoglycemia is a condition in which your blood glucose is low (and which will become particularly important in the next chapter). When we're hypoglycemic, we might feel hungry. We might feel tired. Uncomfortable blood sugar lows can sometimes occur a few hours after eating, and sometimes wake people up in the middle of the night. This kind of hunger is hard to ignore. When most people get this kind of hunger, they will instinctively eat or drink something to make themselves feel better. To treat the uncomfortable symptoms of hypoglycemia-induced hunger, they may start carrying little snacks to bump up their blood sugar levels to the point where they feel normal again. Some use sugary beverages instead of food. Others use alcohol—which may boost brain energy even faster than sugar.[30] Many people try to prevent their symptoms, taking to eating smaller meals more often.

All these habits tend to make people eat just a few more calories than they used to eat, and more than they burn off. Only a minority of people even realize they're eating more than they used to, and even fewer can boost their activity enough to match that extra intake. And so the vast majority of people caught in this cycle end up gaining weight. It's very important to be able to recognize this kind of hunger in order to learn to prevent it (see chapter 4).

Not only will recurring bouts of hypoglycemia make most people eat more calories than they can burn, they also force a metabolic shift. You see, the body has its own way of raising blood sugar when it senses there's not enough. This takes us to Step 4.

Dr. Cate's Energy Model of Insulin Resistance

Doctors are taught that insulin resistance begins when cells throughout the body become less able to respond to insulin's signal. According to the American Diabetes Association, why this happens is "still a mystery."[31] They claim that weight gain and lack of activity are the most important drivers, as if to say we eat too much and we're too lazy. Exactly backward. Insulin resistance develops first, and it makes us gain weight.

As far back as 1987, metabolic research showed that body weight is not the driving force. As one study put it, "The severity of [insulin resistance] is independent of the degree of obesity."[32] I've been studying the science for more than twenty years, and the model I've developed takes into account the fact that seed oils promote inflammation and don't support energy formation. This floods our bodies with stress hormones like cortisol and glucagon making our liver unable to respond to insulin and forcing it to pump out more sugar. Meanwhile, the pancreas keeps producing more and more insulin to try to get the liver to "hear" the signal.[33–37] All that makes us eat more and move less. Our malfunctioning metabolism makes us gain weight, not the other way around.

STEP 4: FASTING BLOOD SUGAR LEVELS CREEP UPWARD, AND SO DOES FASTING INSULIN; WELCOME TO INSULIN RESISTANCE

In Step 4, the body attempts to adapt to our cells' chronically high demand for sugar by raising our blood glucose levels, keeping them higher than normal between meals and during an overnight fast. This is easily done thanks to our handy, helpful liver.

The liver can respond to distress signals from tissues in need of more energy. The liver can, if asked, elevate our blood glucose well above our normal values to meet a *temporary* need during periods of intense sugar demand, usually due to intense physical activity. When the liver gets these distress signals, it starts releasing more glucose into the bloodstream.

Importantly, this is not supposed to be an ongoing thing. But by this point on the road to insulin resistance, the body doesn't get relief from the intense need for sugar. Cells are now releasing distress signals more and more often, and the liver is releasing glucose more and more often, so that our blood glucose levels often exceed normal values.[38] This is very bad. Too much sugar can stick to our cell membranes, joint tissues, and other critical structures, causing widespread damage.

To be healthy, our bodies must keep blood glucose tightly controlled in a very narrow range, from about 65 to about 85 milligrams per deciliter (mg/dL). Normally, blood glucose only goes higher than that shortly after we've eaten. When blood glucose goes much above 85 or so, the pancreas releases the hormone insulin to bring the sugar back down. Insulin lowers blood glucose by telling fat cells to absorb the sugar. After absorbing sugar, the fat cells will convert it into fat so that it can be stored. Insulin also tells the liver to stop raising blood glucose. But here in Step 4, the liver can no longer stop raising glucose just because insulin says so. Here in Step 4, the liver gets contradictory "more glucose" signals coming in at blood sugar concentrations that would normally be high enough to shut liver glucose production off.

Much of the intense demand for sugar here in Step 4 is coming from the brain. When other cells use up more glucose than normal, our brain cells often run out of energy, making us *feel* like our blood glucose is low even when it is normal. Sometimes we might feel like our blood glucose is too low even when it's high enough to trip the insulin-release switch. And because of that, the liver is often getting instructions to raise the blood glucose level at the same time that it's getting instructions to lower it.[39] Whenever the liver raises glucose hoping to meet the body's needs, the pancreas releases insulin, hoping to bring the level back down. Inflammatory body fat has pitted our organs against one another, forcing them to engage in an ongoing battle to win control over our blood glucose levels. This causes blood glucose swings from high to low and back again and again.

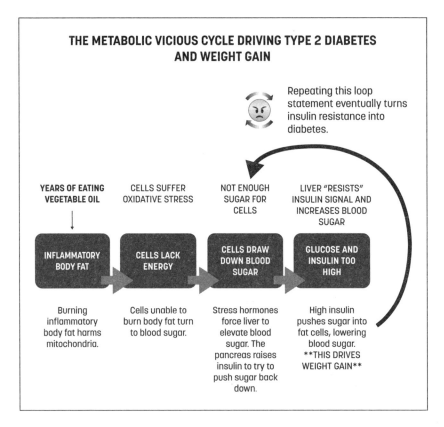

THE METABOLIC VICIOUS CYCLE DRIVING TYPE 2 DIABETES AND WEIGHT GAIN

Repeating this loop statement eventually turns insulin resistance into diabetes.

YEARS OF EATING VEGETABLE OIL	CELLS SUFFER OXIDATIVE STRESS	NOT ENOUGH SUGAR FOR CELLS	LIVER "RESISTS" INSULIN SIGNAL AND INCREASES BLOOD SUGAR
INFLAMMATORY BODY FAT	CELLS LACK ENERGY	CELLS DRAW DOWN BLOOD SUGAR	GLUCOSE AND INSULIN TOO HIGH
Burning inflammatory body fat harms mitochondria.	Cells unable to burn body fat turn to blood sugar.	Stress hormones force liver to elevate blood sugar. The pancreas raises insulin to try to push sugar back down.	High insulin pushes sugar into fat cells, lowering blood sugar. **THIS DRIVES WEIGHT GAIN**

Figure 3–3: Vegetable oils are the root cause of insulin resistance and diabetes, but medical science can't piece the puzzle together like this. Because **doctors do not learn about the link between vegetable oil and oxidative stress (or how it drives insulin resistance),** they are unable to help their patients escape the vicious cycle. They can't even recognize the problem until it has progressed to prediabetes.

If everyone understood the information on this page, **millions would be alive today who are not.** This figure sends a powerful message that invites people to think about their health in a new way. Figure 8–1 in chapter 8 shows how a simple diet change enables us to escape the vicious cycle.

Feel free to print and share this figure and the corresponding figure in chapter 8. For a downloadable PDF of both figures, visit https://drcate.com/darkcaloriesdownloads.

The worse our insulin resistance gets, the higher our blood glucose levels go.[40] At first, the blood sugar levels are only a little high. After a while, blood sugar levels get to the point that our doctors tell us we have

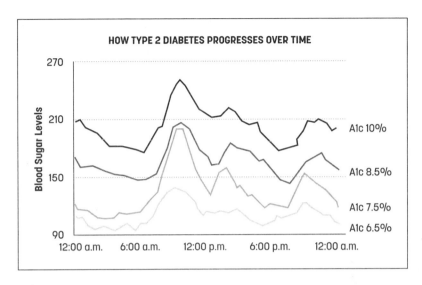

Figure 3–4: These are twenty-four-hour continuous glucose monitor (CGM) tracings from **four groups of people at different stages in their development of diabetes.** Blood sugar is on the left, ranging from 90 to 270. Time of day is on the bottom. The A1c levels (on the right) reflect the groups' average blood sugar. Normal A1c is between 4.8 and 5.5 percent. The group with the worst diabetes has an average A1c of 10 percent.

As you can see, these lines are all similar. **They all go up after eating and come down between meals to a relatively similar degree.** What can we conclude from this? That diabetes is not just a disease of glucose spikes; it is also about the baseline being raised due to an elevated need for sugar between meals. The person with an A1c of 10 percent may not have had a normal between-meal blood sugar in years.

Cutting carbs will reduce the peaks significantly, but may not bring the baseline down. For that you need to get the vegetable oil out of your diet—and your body fat.

For sources used to create this figure, see the endnotes for this chapter.

prediabetes. As our blood glucose levels climb, the lows don't dip quite so low, but we still feel bad during the dips. Prediabetes, or even moderate insulin resistance, can make us feel like our blood sugars are low even when they're normal. If insulin resistance remains unchecked, blood glucose numbers get into the range of full-blown type 2 diabetes. Once we've developed diabetes, we often feel like our blood sugars are low unless they are actually high. As diabetes progresses, not only do our peak blood sugars rise higher and higher, so does our baseline blood sugar. People with more severe diabetes have significantly higher baseline levels, meaning their blood sugars may not have been normal in years (see Figure 3–4).

Insulin resistance is the body's answer to the energy problem caused by having body fat that is too full of PUFA to give our cells the energy they need. But it's not a good solution. The greater availability of sugar somewhat solves the immediate problems, but not very well. In the long run, insulin resistance completely rearranges our metabolism in ways that ultimately cause a whole new set of problems.

Scientists who understand oxidative stress have sorted out exactly how oxidative stress leads to insulin resistance inside a cell.[41] But doctors don't learn about any of that. Instead, doctors learn that insulin resistance is one of those "multifactorial" diseases, caused by abdominal fat, a lack of exercise, too much sugar, stress, old age, inflammation, genetics, and so on. According to the Centers for Disease Control and Prevention (CDC), "it isn't clear exactly what causes insulin resistance."[42] And it won't be, until medical science starts paying attention to scientists who study vegetable oil and the mechanisms of its toxicity.

Since most people think sugar is the main ingredient causing metabolic illness, I'd like to set the record straight.

SUGAR BUILDS NORMAL BODY FAT; VEGETABLE OIL BUILDS INFLAMMATORY BODY FAT

It's a common perception that sugar causes obesity and drives diabetes. Sugar is addictive, so we seek it out even when we're not hungry. And it's fattening, since it's empty calories. Eating sugar spikes blood glucose well above the normal range (even when we don't have diabetes), and blood-glucose spikes can also promote oxidative stress. To avoid sugar-induced oxidative stress, we should only consume a tiny bit at a time—or just avoid it.

All that said, there is reason to be skeptical that sugar is as bad as some people say. Frances Sladek, a professor of cell biology and toxicology at the

University of California at Riverside, has been studying soy oil in our food supply for many years. She knew that our intake of soy oil had increased a thousandfold over the course of the twentieth century. She also knew, as many of us do, that our intake of added sugars had increased. And, along the way, there has been a parallel rise in obesity and type 2 diabetes. Fructose sugar has been considered particularly unhealthy, fattening, and capable of promoting diabetes, based on the parallel rise in high-fructose corn syrup and obesity between 1980 and 2000.

But these are just correlations, which can't prove causation. To test causation, she designed an animal experiment. The experiment had two arms, one to study PUFA versus saturated fat, and the other to study the effect of adding fructose to each of those fatty acids.[43] Mice were given a diet based on either coconut oil or soybean oil. The coconut-oil diet matched the amount of PUFA we were historically eating back in 1900, before there was much in the food supply, and the soy-oil-based diet matched the amount of PUFA we were eating in the year 2000.

The results of her study aligned with everything we've discussed in this chapter. The mice eating soy oil built inflammatory fat—just as we do. The inflammatory body fat ended up in places body fat normally doesn't go—just as ours does. "Fat was everywhere when we opened them up," Dr. Sladek said during an interview.[44] The animals' inflammatory fat was similarly crawling with white blood cells and exuding the same kinds of cytokines found in people. The animals' inflammatory-fat-filled organs also showed signs of dysfunction, particularly their livers, which were filled with huge fatty droplets that caused "ballooning" of the liver cells—the hallmark of fatty liver. When she looked at the animals' mitochondria, she found dysfunction and signs of oxidative stress.

Dr. Sladek's study also linked inflammatory fat to diabetes. Even though the coconut-oil-fed mice got fat, it wasn't inflammatory fat: they developed only mild insulin resistance, and their blood glucose stayed normal. Only the high-PUFA mice developed the extreme insulin resistance and high blood sugars diagnostic of type 2 diabetes.

Adding fructose to coconut oil made the mice slightly fatter than the coconut oil alone did, and it caused slightly more insulin resistance. Even still, their blood sugars were completely normal and all the mice remained diabetes-free.

In a surprise twist, adding fructose to the soybean oil actually seemed to protect against the development of inflammatory fat. The soy-oil-plus-fructose mice developed less visceral fat, less liver disease, less insulin resistance, and less diabetes than the mice that got soy oil without fructose. "This was rather surprising given the considerable attention given to high fructose corn syrup in the diet," she said.[45]

Fructose is the most fattening, oxidative-stress-inducing sugar in our diets, and it failed to promote insulin resistance as efficiently as vegetable oil. So this study suggested that in the which-is-worse contest between sugar and vegetable oil, it's not even a fair fight. Vegetable oil wins hands down.

By solidifying our understanding of the dietary villain hierarchy, we can concentrate our efforts in the right place. Americans' sugar consumption has actually dropped during the past few decades as our rates of obesity have doubled: between 1999 and 2016, the average American cut down on total added sugars by roughly 20 percent (see also Figure 3–1).[46] If sugar were the primary driver of obesity, we should be getting thinner, not fatter.

Cutting out sweet-tasting sugar is immensely more difficult than cutting out flavorless oils. If there's an easier first step to take that's actually more important, I think people deserve to know.

A "METABOLICALLY DIFFERENT" GENERATION

So just how common is insulin resistance? Incredibly common. In 2019, researchers analyzed data from the National Health and Nutrition Examination Survey 2009–2016 (NHANES, a program of the National Center for Health Statistics) and produced a kind of metabolic report card. Judging by respondents' waist circumference, blood glucose levels, blood pressure, triglyceride and cholesterol numbers, and whether they were taking any related medications, the authors concluded that the prevalence of metabolic health in American adults is "alarmingly low."[47] This cluster of symptoms is all part of what is sometimes referred to as the metabolic syndrome, and it is an indirect measure of insulin resistance. More than two hundred million Americans were surveyed, and only a little more than 12 percent of the respondents were considered metabolically healthy.

We do have a better, more direct test for insulin resistance available to us that's not done often enough. This value would give us more accurate insights into our population's health. It's called the homeostatic model assessment of insulin resistance, or HOMA-IR. The test tells you exactly how much insulin your body uses to control your blood sugar. The more insulin it uses, the more insulin resistant you are, and the more likely you are to already have or to later develop type 2 diabetes and all of its complications. The less insulin it uses, the better your insulin sensitivity and the healthier your metabolism.

Getting your HOMA-IR score is relatively easy. You need a fasting morning blood test for blood glucose and a simultaneous insulin level. Plugging those two values into a simple calculator tool (available free online) gives you the final HOMA-IR score. What's not so easy is finding out what number constitutes a normal value. Some experts use a cutoff as low as 1.0, others as high as 3.8.[48] The disagreement comes in part from the fact that these numbers are based on population averages for glucose and insulin, which have been creeping upward over the decades.[49] The experts citing 1.0 are basing their figure on older data than the folks who use 3.8. The 1.0 figure comes from 1985, and 3.8 comes from 2013. In the intervening twenty-eight years, our metabolic health deteriorated. Given this, I think it's wise to use the older value of 1.0 as the cutoff for normal insulin sensitivity.[50]

According to data taken from the 2015–2018 NHANES, *almost nobody in the United States has a HOMA-IR score below 1.3.*[51] This dataset included 6,247 adults aged eighteen to forty-four. Unfortunately, they used a cutoff of 2.5 or less for "normal," so finding the proportion of people with a score of 1.0 or lower required digging into the supplementary data tables, and even there I didn't find a precise answer. All I can gather is that the number of people with values of 1.0 or better was so low that it didn't reach the threshold of even reporting how many people fell into this category. Certainly it would be less than 1 percent. In other words, nearly all Americans over the age of eighteen—more than 99 percent—have insulin resistance.

This is a shocking figure. It's gotten less attention than it deserves because the authors used the wrong cutoff for their "normal" HOMA-IR value. Using a higher cutoff, 2.5 instead of 1.0, puts the prevalence of insulin resistance at just 40 percent, which is what got reported. Why would they use the wrong value? As our metabolic health has deteriorated, our average HOMA-IR has increased. The authors of the NHANES paper chose 2.5 as the cutoff rather than using the previously determined 1.0 value that indicates metabolic health. In effect, they graded us on a curve, drastically underestimating the real prevalence of insulin resistance among American adults.

Insulin resistance is increasingly common in children as well. In 2009, Melinda Sothern, PhD, a public health expert with hundreds of publications and dozens of distinguished scientist awards, presented the keynote lecture at the annual American Diabetes Association meeting. She opened with a warning: "We have a new generation of children who are metabolically different."[52] Her team of investigators had been studying childhood obesity, and they had recently discovered that the "new generation" (born between 1990 and 2001) was developing insulin resistance at higher rates than all previous generations. Those with more severe insulin resistance also had high levels of inflammatory fat in and around their internal organs, and their muscles were marbled with fat.[53] Seemingly unaware of the increased consumption of vegetable oils and their ability to cause insulin resistance, she and her team had not explored the connection, and could not explain why any of this was happening.

She also warned that the younger generation's issues extended beyond obesity and diabetes: insulin resistance also made children less likely to grow normal amounts of muscle or to reach average height.[54] Others have shown that obese children with insulin resistance are very likely to suffer from sleep-disordered breathing. Sleep-disordered breathing, also called sleep apnea, prevents oxygen from getting to our brains. Children with the condition have been shown to experience a variety of learning and intellectual problems that might haunt them for the rest of their lives.[55]

Health problems may be appearing in our younger generations well before insulin resistance develops, although it's hard to say because the HOMA-IR test is so rarely done. We do know that sleep-disordered breathing is becoming increasingly common even in children of normal weight, putting them at risk for the same intellectual complications of inadequate brain oxygen.[56] The newer generations also suffer from a variety of non-obesity-related problems. Every parent knows that rates of life-threatening peanut allergies are up. Autism and learning disorders are increasing.[57] Childhood cancer, while thankfully still rare, has been trending upward since the CDC started tracking it in 1975.[58] Career-ending elbow injuries in children pitching in softball and baseball are also on the rise, as are ligament tears in kids playing soccer.[59] These statistics are just the tip of the iceberg. According to a Blue Cross Blue Shield report published in 2019, "Millennials are seeing their health decline faster than the previous generation as they age," starting around age thirty-five.[60] Intergenerational sperm counts are plummeting, too, having dropped 62.3 percent since 1973.[61] All of this suggests that children born into a vegetable-oil-laden world don't get a fair shot at good health.

A GRAVE NEW WORLD

We are living in a strange time, when our much-celebrated modern, high-tech medicine can't explain what causes insulin resistance, a metabolic abnormality that almost everyone has, and that causes untold amounts of suffering.

Just as the modern diet is profoundly unhealthy compared to the kind of diet humans historically ate, the modern metabolism is profoundly unhealthy, too. The modern diet is nutrient poor and toxin rich. Therefore, the modern metabolism is constantly forced to generate oxidative stress and then adapt to it. The modern metabolism must navigate a delicate balance multiple times a day. It must burn enough body fat to produce energy—but not so much that the oxidative stress starts to damage mitochondria and cells. The adaptation our metabolism most often settles into is to burn less body fat—and more sugar—between meals.

The modern insulin-resistant metabolism is simply not capable of generating energy as nature intended. It's best defined as an inefficient metabolism. It's so inefficient that our daily lives are full of energy disruptions. Generating energy is not supposed to be this much of a challenge.

Life is all about adaptation. Over the course of our own long evolutionary journey, our metabolism and our DNA have adapted to myriad swings in atmospheric sulfur, methane, and oxygen, and to 100-degree changes in average global temperatures, years without sunlight, and more. We've just seen that our metabolism is now adapting to this bizarre new source of energy we've forced upon it by ratcheting our blood sugar levels up higher and higher. As our organs fight over how much sugar should be in our bloodstream, we are subjected to blood sugar swings. Most of us now need higher-than-normal blood sugar levels just to feel okay, and many also now have blood sugar levels so high that we are considered diabetic. What sort of effect might this barrage of altered metabolic states have on our behavior?

In the next chapter, I'm going to show you some of the research in this field that suggests filling our body fat with vegetable oil is changing our relationship with food—and with one another. I'll show you how our modern metabolism subjects our brains to energy shortages that are altering our eating habits, killing our desire for activity, sabotaging our self-control, blunting our ability to plan and to relate to friends and family, and even hijacking our sense of well-being and self-worth.

CHAPTER 4

Fat Bodies, Starving Brains

IN THIS CHAPTER YOU WILL LEARN

- "Hangry" is now common, but it's not normal hunger; it's the first sign of a broken metabolism.
- When we get hangry, it means our brain is starving for energy, and this can make us behave badly.
- Low brain energy is known to impair our self-control and cognitive functions, and can even promote violence and mental illness.
- Many people snack to give their brain the energy that their metabolism can't, which makes them gain weight.
- Because this is not well known, people believe they lack willpower, blame themselves, and give up on trying to eat healthier.

When I first learned what a healthy diet looked like and started focusing on using food to help more of my patients, I noticed one question coming up more often than anything else: *What can I snack on?* When I was working with the LA Lakers, snacking was their top priority too. I used to bluntly warn, "There's no such thing as a healthy snack." For one thing, every time we eat between meals, we take ourselves out of fat-burning mode and put our metabolism into fat-building mode. (Indeed, in randomized controlled trials where people consume equal amounts of calories, those eating more frequently feel hungry more often and gain more weight than people eating less frequently.)[1] But clients would get so blown away by the anti-snacking message, it simply didn't process; the next time I saw them, they'd repeat the question. So I took a different tack. When they asked me about healthy snacks, I'd ask them a question in return: How often did they want one, and why? Often, people said they were hungry just two or three hours after having eaten a solid meal. No wonder the question kept coming up. After all, it's natural to assume that if you're hungry, you should eat.

But is that right? Should you eat every time you're hungry?

Even though hunger is intimately related to the obesity crisis, there's very little research devoted to understanding it. So there's no consensus on basic questions such as, If you get hungry every few hours, do you need to eat every time? Is it bad if you don't? Experts are completely divided on the issue of hunger. Some say that eating every time we're hungry will get in the way of weight loss, and that we need to use willpower and push the hunger down. Others say that by ignoring our hunger we are harming our metabolism and our health. Some suggest we're not actually hungry, we're just addicted, since processed snack foods like chips and cookies are specifically created to be hyperpalatable so we'll keep going back for more.

But, as we'll see in this chapter, we aren't snacking only because we're hungry or bored, or the food is addictive and cheap, or it's so easy to chomp through giant packages. We're snacking because, thanks to seed oils, we have a kind of hunger that is almost entirely new to the human experience.

These days, if you ask people to describe how they feel when they're hungry, you often hear something like, "When I don't eat, I go rampant. I go all over the place." A news crew recently did a man-on-the-street style interview, asking people how they felt when they were hungry, and that was the first response they got.

The other interviewees offered, "When I get hungry, I act hangry. I say things I have to apologize for later." "When my kids don't get their snack, they get very cranky, and they get agitated." (Though the word was used as early as 1918, *hangry* was added to the *Oxford English Dictionary* only in 2018—perhaps indicating how very common a state it has become.)

My patients tell me that being hungry makes them more dependent on fast food and junk, because they need something right away, and cooking takes too long. Some are *afraid* of their hunger, and worry about being caught without food, for example while driving. "Being hangry is the worst thing when I'm driving. If I'm in my car while I'm hangry that could cause an accident." This isn't normal hunger.

Hunger could not have always been such an oppressive, intrusive experience, or I doubt our species would have made it to the present day. Our issues with hunger are a direct outgrowth of the fact that most of today's population is insulin resistant.

In the last chapter, we saw that our high-PUFA body fat doesn't give cells the energy they need, and so our energy-hungry cells slurp up oversized portions of the limited supply of blood sugar. This leaves less sugar for the brain to meet its energy needs. When our brains don't get the energy they need, it's just like the commercial says: "You're not you when you're hungry." But as we will see, the problem goes far beyond moods. Low brain energy has also been implicated in mental health issues.

GOOD HUNGRY, BAD HUNGRY

Normal hunger is about nutrition. The sensations of normal hunger are mostly due to a hunger-stimulating hormone called *ghrelin*, which is tied to our circadian rhythms. (When your cat jumps onto your keyboard at exactly ten minutes till dinner, it's responding to ghrelin.) The stomach releases ghrelin into the bloodstream around our normal mealtimes. Ghrelin travels to our appetite regulation center, located in a brain structure called the hypothalamus. When ghrelin stimulates our appetite center, it registers as hunger that feels nothing like hangry. It's a gentle reminder: "Hey, it's about time to eat—I'm ready when you are," often accompanied by a mild grumbly feeling in the stomach as it releases acid and other digestive juices. If we don't eat, all this shuts down after a few minutes and we no longer feel hungry, especially if we get distracted. Normal hunger can actually be energizing, because the ghrelin helps us burn fat—and if your cat or dog starts acting wild around feeding time, that's from the extra boost of fat burning, which gives them extra energy. It might seem surprising that a hunger hormone energizes us, but nature programs us this way because, for most of life on Earth, hunting or gathering food requires expending a good deal of energy. Today, many people take frequent hunger as a sign of a healthy metabolism. But, as we'll see, more often than not, it's actually the opposite. This new, unhealthy hunger doesn't go away until we feed it, and it actually originates not in the stomach but in the brain. This new hunger is all about satisfying our brain's demand for *energy*.

The brain is both an energy-demanding and a uniquely sugar-dependent organ. It constitutes just 2 percent of our body weight but burns 20 percent of our calories. Unlike other cells of the body, the brain is walled off behind a protective barrier, called the blood-brain barrier, so it doesn't have direct access to big molecules like fat. The brain does have access to sugar, however, since it's a smaller molecule. While our muscles and bones and other vital organs all have direct access to whatever fat may be in our bloodstream, the brain does not. So the brain uses a whopping 25 percent of our blood sugar. Without a steady supply of sugar, the brain cannot properly support the complex activity it's performing for us all day. Just maintaining the electrical grid that keeps the brain alive accounts for a good part of its energy usage. Managing important bodily functions like blood pressure, heart rate, breathing, and body temperature demands a good deal more.

Because the brain is so energy hungry, it contains specialized cells that detect minuscule fluctuations in blood sugar. These glucose-sensing cells are designed to help keep everything on an even keel. You can think of them as a fuel gauge, although they do more than just detect low energy; they can also take steps to fix the problem. One way they adjust blood sugar upward is by regulating your appetite. When your blood sugar starts to drop faster or farther than normal, these cells send an electrochemical impulse to the part of your brain that makes you feel hungry.

These fuel-gauging cells in the brain also detect other sources of brain energy, too, the most famous being *ketones*. If your metabolism is healthy, most of your cells can seamlessly switch over to using body fat when your blood sugar drops. If blood sugar stays low, the liver starts releasing ketones. Ketones quickly get into the brain and are one of the brain's favorite fuels, so all is well—even if you don't eat for hours. But as we just learned in chapter 3, when we are insulin resistant, all our cells have a harder time getting energy from fat, and need to use more sugar. Insulin resistance also disrupts the process of making ketones from body fat, leaving our brain with no good fuel sources.[2] This is why this kind of hunger can feel like an emergency; in insulin resistance, it *is* an emergency. Our tiny cells contain just about twenty seconds of energy reserves.[3] When our mitochondria can't generate enough energy, cells can start to die.

What Is a Ketone?

Ketones are special molecules the liver makes mainly out of body fat. When our insulin levels drop, usually a few hours after a meal, our bodies start breaking down fat stores and releasing fatty acids into the bloodstream. These fatty acids are too big to enter the brain, but most other cells in the body can use them. To convert fatty acids into a kind of fuel the brain can use, the liver chops them up into smaller pieces, called ketones. Our brains can use ketones for energy whenever our blood sugar levels are low. The process of making ketones is called *ketogenesis* (genesis meaning "making").

Unfortunately, insulin blocks this process, and when we're insulin resistant, our insulin levels are often too high to make useful amounts of ketones from body fat unless we are able to exercise heavily or fast for extended periods.

The most important thing to remember from what we learned about insulin resistance in chapter 3 is that it can make you feel like your blood sugar is low *even when it's in the normal range*. Remember, insulin resistance is all about an increased need for blood sugar (see Figure 3–3). As you get more and more insulin resistant, your body needs your blood sugar to get higher and higher all the time, elevating your baseline. When it goes just a little bit lower than what your body thinks it needs, you feel hypoglycemic. And that means you might start feeling hungry while your blood sugar is still in the normal range, or even above the normal range.

Can't Focus?

Some experts believe that no matter how little or how hard you concentrate, your brain needs about the same amount of fuel, accounting for roughly 20 percent of the calories you burn at rest. On the other hand, it's also clear that, when performing any task, the area of the brain responsible for coordinating that task gets more blood delivered to it and uses up more sugar. So other experts suggest that concentration does require more energy. But it's not yet clear how much. What is clear is that we *notice* low blood sugar more when we're trying to concentrate, and the lack of brain energy disrupts our thinking ability. This disrupted thinking ability, or "brain fog," is one of the eleven most common symptoms of hypoglycemia.

So how does this kind of hunger feel? Hypoglycemia can make us ravenously hungry, as if we've been starved for days even though it's often only a little past our normal mealtime. One of my patients calls it zombie eating because it feels like an almost mindless drive to consume anything in front of him. Other symptoms include brain fog, irritability, anxiety, fatigue, shaking, nausea, sweats, weakness, dizziness, headache, and heart

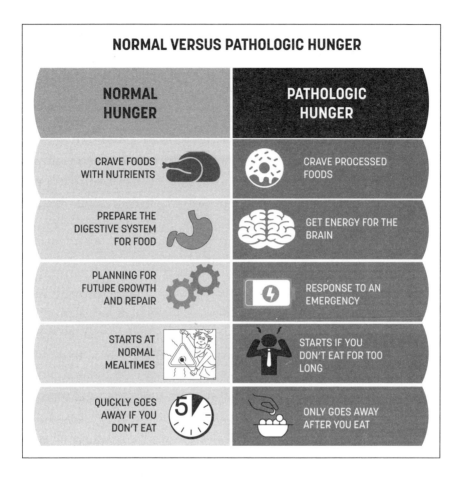

Figure 4–1: Normal hunger and pathologic hunger cause different symptoms and can be distinguished by how they make us feel, what brings them on, and what extinguishes the feelings, as shown here. Pathologic hunger symptoms are due to low blood sugar, and so are identical to hypoglycemia symptoms.

During an episode of pathologic hunger, we experience a metabolic emergency that, if ignored, will harm our health. **No amount of willpower can overcome this metabolically driven hunger**, and it eventually makes most people gain weight, even athletes (especially in the off-season).

Pathologic hunger indicates insulin resistance, and if you've been "hangry," that is a sign of possible insulin resistance. As insulin resistance worsens, we feel these symptoms when our blood sugar levels are normal, or even higher than normal. The long-term treatment for pathologic hunger is to resolve our insulin resistance. In the short term, we can prevent these symptoms. (Part Three shows how to do both.)

palpitations. All eleven of these common hypoglycemia symptoms represent an abnormal kind of hunger that is a reflection of *pathology*, the medical term meaning disease. So I also call this list of eleven common hypoglycemia symptoms the warning signs of *pathologic hunger*. Of course, these symptoms can be due to other processes, so it's important to discuss them with a doctor before jumping to any conclusions (see Figure 4–1).

I teach all my patients to recognize all eleven hypoglycemia symptoms because they are the best way to detect insulin resistance—and to gauge our recovery from it. Importantly, when we're metabolically healthy, we don't get any of these symptoms when we're hungry, because our bodies are perfectly capable of keeping our brains well supplied with fuel for many hours, or even a few days. So simply monitoring for the presence or absence of these symptoms gives us valuable day-to-day feedback on our metabolic activity; it costs nothing, and it can actually provide more helpful information than any sort of technology, including continuous glucometer devices, blood tests, and the $40,000 metabolic cart that athletes use to test their performance. The human brain has been in development for literally billions of years, so its built-in sugar-sensing technology is the most sophisticated, sensitive, and accurate on the planet. We just need to learn to use it.

The symptoms of hypoglycemia fall into two groups. One group is directly related to the fact that the brain is short on energy; the other is related to the hormones the body releases in an attempt to raise our blood sugar back to where the brain wants it to be. Nature intended that these hormones were rarely used for raising blood sugar, and they can have additional negative effects on our moods (see Figure 4–2).

Recognizing Low Brain Energy Symptoms

The two low brain energy symptoms are brain fog (or trouble concentrating) and fatigue. Brain fog is the most common, often making us feel like we are having a senior moment. But of course it's not related to age; it's related to the metabolic need for energy. These symptoms represent a kind

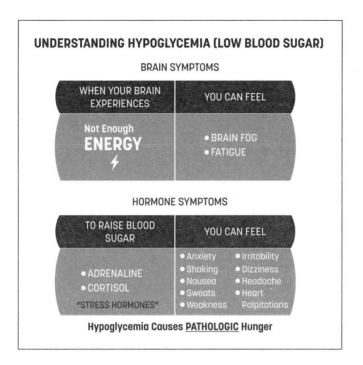

Figure 4–2

of temporary service disruption that, if continued, could actually cause brain cells to die. So, in that sense, you can think of them as a metabolic dashboard indicator that your metabolism needs servicing soon, or permanent damage may occur.

Many people who experience these low brain energy symptoms also feel hungry, so they know what to do: get something to eat. Eating will often end up raising blood sugar enough to solve the immediate problem. The foods that raise blood sugar fastest solve the problem fastest. This is why so many people crave sweet-tasting treats between meals, including soda, juice, sweetened coffee or tea, or candy, donuts, and pastries. However, even though it makes us feel better, it does nothing to solve the underlying insulin resistance.

Hunger is one method our brains use to get our blood sugar back up. Depending on our metabolic health, that food-finding signal might be a friendly little blip on your mental screen or a huge, noisy, blinking pop-up ad that makes it impossible for you to concentrate on anything else.

What if we feel hypoglycemic but can't get anything to eat?

Hunger was plan A. When plan A doesn't fix the problem, the brain cells that detect falling sugar levels will move on to plan B. Plan B is to release the hormones that can raise our blood sugar levels back up again. These are called stress hormones.

Recognizing Stress Hormone Symptoms

Hypoglycemia floods the body with stress hormones, including adrenaline and cortisol. These hormones come from our adrenal glands and are responsible for the many additional, secondary symptoms hypoglycemia can give us. The brain regulates their release by way of the vagus nerve, which travels down the neck, winds around the esophagus and heart, then keeps going down to reach the abdomen, where it regulates the function of all the abdominal organs, including the adrenal glands (which sit on top of the kidneys). This is how the brain boosts adrenaline and cortisol levels. These hormones tell the liver to raise your blood sugar, which solves the brain's energy crisis. But they have a multitude of other effects that are not so beneficial while you're at work on a normal Tuesday.

Adrenaline and cortisol are the classic fight-or-flight hormones. You've probably heard about them in the context of our caveman ancestors running away from lions and fighting off enemies. In the context of a real fight-or-flight scenario, stress hormones are beneficial. They give us an enhanced focus on whatever is right in front of us, a compressed sense of time, and increased muscle strength and coordination. But in the context of pathologic hunger, when it's still an hour before your break, you don't usually experience all that. Instead, you can feel shaking, anxiety, nausea, sweats, irritability, and weakness. Because the vagus nerve also controls the heart rate and blood pressure, its stimulation can cause symptoms related to those functions, which include dizziness, headache, or heart palpitations. Thankfully, most folks just notice one or two symptoms at a time.

The stress hormone symptoms are often more attention-getting and disturbing than the low brain energy symptoms (see Figure 4–2). They can magnify the irritability associated with low brain energy, turning it into a nastier form of hangry than usual. They can also make it easier for minor little things to generate a disproportionate amount of emotional stress.

Stress hormones help give our brain energy by increasing our heart rate, blood pressure, and blood flow. They put more fuels into the bloodstream, helping the liver to dump sugar and the fat cells to release fat. They also instruct the liver to convert the mobilized body fat into ketones.

Let's talk about how well each of these fueling options actually works to solve the brain energy problem when we're insulin resistant.

Fat comes from your body fat, which can't get into your brain—so that doesn't help. Ketones should come from body fat, but insulin blocks ketone formation, and when we're insulin resistant, we may not be able to make enough. That leaves sugar. Only sugar can help rescue us from the internal discomfort caused by pathologic hunger, so the body has to find a way to raise your blood sugar. One way, of course, is making you urgently hungry—that was plan A. The other way is to keep pumping out stress hormones, which can help your liver release stored sugar into the bloodstream while also completely changing our moods—that's plan B.

Your body also has a plan C. Plan C only kicks in after a while as a kind of preventive measure if low brain energy becomes a regular problem. Plan C is to keep stress hormone levels elevated, which dumps more sugar into your bloodstream per minute and supplies your sugar-addicted hungry cells with just a bit more. Studies show that people with insulin resistance may have abnormally high activation of their fight-or-flight system all day and all night.[4] By keeping you in a more or less continual state of heightened fight-or-flight, the brain forces the liver to ignore insulin, and this is how we start to become insulin resistant (as we read in chapter 3). The brain can do this because it directly stimulates the vagus nerve, taking advantage of its stress-hormone-releasing effects. These stress hormones can override the insulin signal coming from the pancreas, which is trying to get blood sugar down to the level where it belongs. The increase of stress hormones represents a metabolic workaround that elevates blood sugar to the point that the brain is happy even though the pancreas is not. And it's a Faustian bargain because of where the sugar actually comes from.

BREAKING DOWN MUSCLE TO FEED OUR CELLS

It would be nice if we could make sugar using body fat, but we can't actually do that very efficiently. When our bodies need to make their own sugar, they have to rely mostly on protein. This process is called gluconeogenesis (*gluc* refers to glucose, *neo* means new, and *genesis* means making). This is how our bodies ensure that we always have some sugar in the bloodstream even if we don't eat food containing any form of sugar. Gluconeogenesis kept our ancestors alive when they lived as hunter-gatherers, sometimes in climates with very little plant growth. They generally had access to plenty of protein-rich game even when they had no access to carb-rich fruits—tubers, nuts, and so on. Gluconeogenesis ensured that they were able to keep their blood sugar levels normal. However, no matter how much protein they ate, they didn't store very much, so they never had much extra protein lying around. This is still the case today. When we eat extra protein, our bodies convert it to fat, very much like what happens when we eat extra sugar. Without a storage form of protein, and with very limited sugar stores, sometimes the only way for our bodies to get sugar is to break down muscle to release proteins that can then be converted to sugar.

Insulin resistance accelerates gluconeogenesis, which accelerates the conversion of protein to sugar. Normally the process of gluconeogenesis produces very little sugar because, normally, we need very little sugar. But when we have insulin resistance and suffer from "sympathetic overactivity" (meaning our stress hormones are abnormally high), the liver accelerates the rate of gluconeogenesis, destructively breaking down more of the body's limited protein supplies all day, every day to feed the sugar monkey on our backs.[5]

In chapter 3, we learned about a consequence of inflammatory fat called overfat, referring to the distortion in body composition skewing toward fat. We also saw that the handy liver can easily raise our blood sugar many times over normal levels by pushing sugar into the bloodstream. These two are related. Insulin resistance keeps us in sympathetic overdrive, which cranks up gluconeogenesis—which breaks down muscle. In other words, when the liver needs to chronically push our blood sugar to higher levels than nature intended, it will make building muscle difficult, and it will make keeping the muscle you have more difficult, too.

This is another reason why I say that hypoglycemia symptoms are really acting like an "engine needs service" light on our metabolic dashboard. They can warn us about the serious problems of metabolic sugar dependence—and insulin resistance. It's important to learn these symptoms so you can tell the difference between pathologic and normal hunger. As we recover from insulin resistance, our pathologic hunger will improve.

Many people have told me they don't experience symptoms of hypoglycemia, however, even though they are severely insulin resistant. Some of these folks who rarely feel hungry turn out to be habitual snackers—just a little bit here and there can spike your blood sugar enough to prevent pathologic hunger. It also blocks your ability to burn body fat, and is not a strategy I recommend. The strategy I recommend is to prevent pathologic hunger by building meals with energizing ingredients that sustain brain energy and function without needing to resort to snacks. (That said, when life gets in the way, there may be times when you still need a snack solution, and I give you the best options in Part Three.) It does seem like some people truly never feel hungry, and in this case it's essential to get a HOMA-IR score, and potentially make use of a special technology called a continuous glucometer device.

Insulin Resistance Makes Us Feel
Low Even When We're High

When we are healthy, we don't feel hypoglycemic until our blood sugar level gets well below the lower end of the normal range, which is 65 milligrams per deciliter (mg/dL). The medical definition of hypoglycemia is actually 50 mg/dL or lower. That number was based on studies done from the 1950s and 1960s showing that people feel and function just fine until their blood sugar dips below 54 mg/dL. As we've seen, most people today are insulin resistant, and when we are insulin resistant, we feel hypoglycemic even when our blood sugar is normal. I've found that mild insulin resistance makes us feel hypoglycemic when our blood sugar level goes under 75 or 80. As folks get more insulin resistant, this threshold goes higher and higher. Patients with prediabetes often tell me they start to feel hypoglycemic when their blood sugar is less than 100. And those with long-standing, uncontrolled type 2 diabetes can even feel hypoglycemic when their blood sugar dips under 200.

Similarly, people with diabetes will often notice that their blood sugar doesn't go down to normal even if they avoid sugar and carbohydrates, which may seem strange: Where is that sugar coming from? Stranger still, people with diabetes can wake up with a high blood sugar level, of, say, 120 (whereas, after an overnight fast, it should be well under 100), and if they check an hour later it will often be even higher, say 140, even though they didn't eat anything. Figure 3–4 shows that for most people blood sugar levels start rising at around 6:00 a.m., which is often *before* breakfast.

None of this makes sense until we understand the process of gluconeogenesis. Gluconeogenesis enables a sugar-dependent metabolism to raise fasting blood sugar higher and higher to meet the body's energy demands. And that's exactly what happens with each passing year: fasting blood sugars creep higher and higher. Once they go over 100, patients are diagnosed with prediabetes. Once they go over 125, they're diagnosed with diabetes. As the need for sugar creeps higher, the blood sugar number where the insulin-resistant person feels hungry and hypoglycemic creeps higher, too.

CONTROLLING HUNGER WITH DRUGS

Pathologic hunger is an unrecognized and powerful driver of weight gain. It overrides the brain's normal appetite control systems, making us feel like we've been starving for days even when it's just been a few hours since breakfast. Normally, the appetite control system receives satiety hormones when we are well fed. Leptin, for example, comes from fat cells and powerfully suppresses hunger. Another satiety hormone, GLP-1, is released by the intestines shortly after we eat, also powerfully suppressing hunger. Scientists recently showed that hypoglycemia completely and powerfully overrides this system to cause "significant increase in food intake" in experimental animals. In one experiment, animals tripled their food intake and generally behaved as if they were desperately hungry (see Figure 4–3).[6] This finding helps to explain why weight loss is such a struggle for even the most motivated among us.

New appetite-suppressing drugs such as Ozempic and Wegovy can override the override, giving people much-needed relief from the discomforting stress signals coming in from all over their bodies. (Such signals may be the chemical explanation for "food noise"—a term for constant hunger and disruptive cravings.) These drugs help people cut calories with much less pain than they could otherwise. But people only need these aids when they're insulin resistant. When we're healthy, we can cut calories painlessly without drugs.

Under normal circumstances, we don't need these drugs because our own GLP-1 and the arsenal of other satiety hormones all work together to

PATHOLOGIC HUNGER OVERRIDES SATIETY
None of our satiety hormones work if our brains are starving for energy.

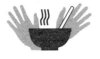

Normal hunger is suppressed by myriad
satiety hormones, most famously leptin and
the GLP-1 receptor antagonists now sold as
weight-loss drugs like Ozempic.

Energy deficiency overrides satiety signals
and creates the most powerful form of hunger.
Quieting this hunger enables you to lose weight
and keep it off without drugs.

Figure 4–3

prevent hunger between meals, particularly when we have plenty of energy stored as fat. These hormones also help us put down our forks after we've eaten enough by making us feel faintly nauseated, thus curbing overeating. Insulin resistance disrupts all this by making us hypoglycemic.

Our appetite-suppressing hormone GLP-1 levels typically spike after a big meal, falling back to normal within a few minutes. Spikes are supposed to make us feel uncomfortably nauseated at the thought of eating more, while normal between-meal levels help to keep us from feeling hungry. This system fails when we are insulin resistant. Enter the GLP-1-mimicking blockbuster weight-loss drugs Ozempic and Wegovy. These drugs continually blast a person's brain with the equivalent of 100 to 1,000 times the level of GLP-1 that normally occurs between meals.[7] For about one-third of the people who take them, they work like a dream to suppress appetite. Although that figure may sound low, it's better than most weight-loss drugs. But naturally, the moment someone stops taking them, the pathologic hunger returns—and for many, sadly, the weight soon follows. The root cause of this form of hunger is not a GLP-1 deficiency, of course. It is the fact that high-PUFA body fat fails to supply our cells with energy. The drops in blood sugar that result cause low brain energy, a metabolic emergency that disrupts our concentration, sets off our fight-or-flight response, and forces us to go seek food. (Fortunately, we don't need to fully reverse our insulin resistance to restore a more normal appetite; all we need to do is to prevent pathologic hunger, one meal at a time—and Part Three shows you how.)

It stands to reason that all these sugar swings, energy deficits, and stress hormones might put us in a less-than-pleasant mood. If this happens once in a while, that can disrupt your day. If it happens every day, it's going to change your life. In fact, new research links hypoglycemia and pathologic hunger to common behavioral problems and even to mental illness.

THE METABOLIC ROOTS OF MENTAL ILLNESS

A research psychologist at the University of Guelph, Dr. Francesco Leri, had always disliked the term "hangry," assuming people just used it as a convenient excuse for bad behavior. But one day he got fed up with hearing about it and decided to tackle this issue directly. Doubtful that blood sugar would ever go low enough to impact mood, Dr. Leri designed a study to prove that the whole idea was wrong. "I was skeptical when people would tell me that they get grouchy if they don't eat," he said in a press release. But his research soon convinced him otherwise. In 2018, the journal *Psychopharmacology* published his experiments suggesting that small but rapid drops in glucose levels could have a lasting negative effect on our emotional states. It was a landmark study because it was the first to show a clear link between the brain's ability to access the energy it needs and mental health.[8]

The experiment tested mice for anxiety using a standardized conditioning procedure that mimicked human anxiety disorders. Conditioning associates an emotional state with something in the environment. For example, ringing a dinner bell at feeding time conditions dogs to start salivating when they hear a bell. Dr. Leri's team conditioned a group of mice by injecting them with a glucose metabolism blocker that gave them a temporary case of low blood sugar, and then stuck each mouse in a new little chamber, to "condition" them to associate that chamber with whatever emotional state they were in. They did the same with a control group, but those mice got an injection of water instead. Once conditioned, the groups were ready for the anxiety test. For the test, both groups of mice were injected with water and then given a choice of two chambers, the conditioning chamber or a new one. The mice who'd experienced hypoglycemia actively avoided the conditioning chamber, indicating that hypoglycemia made them anxious. In contrast, the control group showed no such aversion. In a third phase of the test, both groups of mice got an anti-anxiety medication that also treats depression. With the drug on board, mice who'd previously avoided the chamber no longer did, further solidifying the fact that low blood sugar had created behaviors mimicking human anxiety disorders and depressed moods.

Doctors have long known that people with serious mental illness are more likely to suffer from metabolic syndrome. This line of research suggests that the metabolic issue could be causative. Dr. Thomas Horman, a coauthor on the 2018 paper, said in a press release that "when people think about negative mood states and stress, they think about the psychological factors, not necessarily the metabolic factors."[9] He also included the data in his PhD thesis, where he goes so far as to suggest that our thinking on anxiety and depression is due for a sea change. He noted that low blood sugar triggers stress hormone release and is "a stressor that can cause mood disturbances that may lead to the development of depression or depressive like symptoms." He further suggested that insulin resistance might be a root cause of other "affective disorders," including not just anxiety and depression but also panic disorder, post-traumatic stress disorder (PTSD), obsessive compulsive disorder, phobias, and bipolar disorder.[10]

This concept has implications for all of psychology.

Right now, the bulk of research into the physical origins of mental illness focuses on root causes that those who are affected can do little to mitigate. Historically, the accepted biological roots of psychological problems were limited to thyroid disease, certain vitamin deficiencies, and tumors. In the 1980s, psychiatrists theorized that lower levels of neurotransmitters such as serotonin or dopamine might play a role, and they now frequently use prescriptions that change how the brain processes these chemicals. These drugs sometimes help quite a bit, but sometimes they also cause intolerable side effects, and often they can lead to uncontrollable weight gain. Sometimes, they don't work at all. So if mental health problems stem from metabolic disease, this gives anyone suffering from mental illness a new set of solutions. In chapter 8, we're going to see that research into the use of "metabolic therapy" for psychiatry is starting to take off. If insulin resistance also affects mental health, then knowing how to properly diagnose it is far more important and valuable than we ever realized before.

An abundance of published research linking hunger to bad moods, regrettable decisions, and antisocial behaviors, some violent, already exists. Psychologists at Cambridge University published a review summarizing dozens of human experiments from 2005 through 2021.[11] They found that hungry people are more likely to experience negative emotions (such as anger, irritability, and rage) than people who are not hungry, especially in the context of stressful situations. They wrapped up their article with a conclusion suggesting that ordinary hunger has become a dreaded experience, as "everyday levels of hunger are associated with negative emotionality." If that's the case, people may reorient their lives to prevent the unpleasant, negative emotional states accompanying hunger. They may be too busy thinking about food to be fully engaged in life. But because the psychologists leading this field didn't happen to partner up with metabolic health specialists, they didn't realize they were studying people manifesting the signs of insulin resistance. And so they couldn't possibly have known that their research also suggested that our epidemic of metabolic disease might translate to an epidemic of poor behavior.

LOSING CONTROL

Dr. Roy Baumeister, a leader in the field of self-control and willpower, is one of the most cited and most influential psychologists in the world. He first made a name for himself in the 1970s, after pinpointing the one character trait that would best predict our success in school, at work, and socially. The prevailing idea had been that success depended on a healthy sense of self-esteem. But Dr. Baumeister found that self-esteem can actually get people into trouble—*if* they also lacked self-control. People with high self-esteem but low self-control tended toward violence and antisocial behavior.[12] Shifting gears to focus on self-control, he soon uncovered the real secret to excelling in school, succeeding at work, and enjoying happiness at home. People with more self-control had better mental health, fewer money problems, and less tendency to end up in jail, engage in crime or abuse, become sexually promiscuous, or display prejudicial behavior. They also lived longer.[13] "With self-control, everybody wins," he noted. "It is good for the person who has it, for the people around him, and for society as a whole." Another word for self-control is willpower.

After determining the paramount importance of self-control to health and happiness, he focused next on what makes even the most disciplined people lose self-control from time to time. Here, Dr. Baumeister again broke brand-new ground. His experiments collectively demonstrated that willpower requires brain energy, and that, when people need to exert willpower over and over, their willpower gets weaker and weaker. The idea is now well-known to psychologists as the ego depletion theory. To psychologists, ego is not about thinking highly of yourself. It's the aspect of our psyche that gives us self-control. While the theory is still considered controversial, it seems to be in line with common sense. "It's like a muscle; it needs fuel," said Dr. Baumeister, speaking of willpower.[14] For most of us, that fuel is sugar. And when we're feeling hypoglycemic, we don't have enough.

Dr. Baumeister's studies showed that when we are hungry, we quickly run out of willpower and lose control over our impulses. Over several decades of research, over multitudes of experiments, he found that when we're hungry we are more likely to give in to any kind of temptation. This includes indulgent foods, of course, as well as impulse shopping, sexual encounters, illegal drugs, gambling, alcohol, and more. This is true even in people who normally have good self-control. Feeling hungry depletes our willpower and demolishes our motivation for just about everything other than getting food. Hunger also makes decision-making more difficult. It makes complex planning nearly impossible. It makes us give up when the going gets tough. And his work also showed that it makes us "aggressive."[15]

But Dr. Baumeister wasn't really testing people who were just hungry. Given the 99-percent-plus prevalence of insulin resistance, chances are that many of his subjects were not experiencing normal hunger but pathologic hunger and low brain energy. So everywhere that last paragraph says "hunger," it really should say "low brain energy." Remember, the job of our metabolism is to provide energy to all our cells. Insulin resistance disrupts this all-important metabolic function, thus depleting our willpower and our self-control.

On the other hand, giving people blood-sugar-raising foods vastly improves self-control. In various experiments, Dr. Baumeister and others have found that sugar helps people to "persevere despite frustrating failures," giving them the will—or, literally, the energy—to push themselves harder to complete boring, detailed tasks. Sugar helps people to think better under pressure and to maintain poise while being verbally insulted.[16] Sweet beverages can calm "aggressive individuals" who naturally tend to engage in conflict when provoked, and it "can make strangers less likely to treat each other aggressively."[17]

On the flip side, these findings explain why so many of us seek sugar so often. Sugar can improve our memory and cognition, making us test smarter.[18] It can reduce our impulsivity and increase our attention span, potentially allowing people with attention-deficit/hyperactivity disorder (ADHD) who notice this effect to self-medicate.[19] It can help us work through difficult decisions faster, and plan our days more effectively.[20] It's a cheap, legal, effective, all-purpose performance-enhancing drug. The irony is that we only need it because our modern metabolism has handicapped our performance in so many different ways.

Fatigue, hunger, difficulty concentrating, and low motivational states certainly make it harder to maintain a healthy diet. One of the questions many working parents dread most comes up every day, right around 3:00 p.m.: "So, umm...what are we doing about dinner?" It hits us right about when blood sugar starts to drop, making complex meal planning more onerous. Low brain energy is likely contributing to the fact that 45 percent of Americans between the ages of twenty and thirty-nine rely on fast food every day.[21] It's likely behind the decision made by 62 percent of Americans to replace at least one meal a day with snacks.[22] The cruel irony of these decisions is that we end up eating more of the vegetable oils that steal our brain power away.

When speaking on willpower and self-restraint in the context of dieting, Dr. Baumeister points out that we're in a bit of a bind: "I'm not unmindful of the irony of [needing] sugar to improve self-control."[23] If it takes willpower to avoid sugar, but you need sugar to keep your willpower going, then you're going to need sugar to avoid sugar. Obviously, this is a problem. Dieters are stuck in a metabolic catch-22, where they need the very thing they're trying to avoid in order to avoid it. Dr. Baumeister's research does more to explain our obesity epidemic than anything coming from our obesity experts.

On the job, at school, and at home, low blood sugar spells may be gobbling up productivity. It might be making us feel overwhelmed by tasks we know we should be able to manage. Or it might be distracting us during conversations, so we miss important information. The effects of metabolically driven mood and behavior changes upon individuals and society as a whole run deep and wide. They may even be magnifying our darkest impulses.

HUNGRY FOR VENGEANCE

Criminal psychologists tell us that the leading cause of murder is aggression. Behavioral psychologists tell us that the leading cause of every sort of criminal behavior is poor self-control.

Dr. Brad Bushman is an expert in what drives us to hurt each other. He has been trying to understand our escalating rates of interpersonal violence, particularly domestic violence, which he sees as an existential threat to law and order and the fabric of society.[24] He has published over two hundred peer-reviewed journal articles, testified before Congress, served on presidential committees, and consulted for the FBI. Dr. Bushman's many studies reveal a powerful link between hunger and aggression. And together with a colleague—the self-control expert Dr. Roy Baumeister—he designed a rather creative set of experiments that showed hunger can even cause "greater aggression in married couples."[25] But as we'll see, I think the research actually suggests that our metabolism, not our failure to eat often enough, is driving our bad behavior.

First, Dr. Bushman and several colleagues recruited 107 married couples and studied their sugar levels for twenty-one days. Then, they tested their self-control at the point when their blood sugars were lowest, which was, predictably, just before dinner. To express aggressive impulses (which reflect how much we *want* to physically hurt someone), participants were told, "This doll represents your spouse," and to "insert between 0 and 51 pins in the doll, depending how angry you are with your spouse. You will do this alone, without your spouse being present." They found that people with lower glucose levels consistently stabbed their spousal doppelgänger with more pins than those with higher levels. Those with the lowest levels of blood sugar stuck their voodoo dolls with an average of twice as many pins as those with the highest levels. One individual stuck all 51 pins in their doll every single night—definitely not a happily-ever-after situation.

To see if low blood sugar also made people more likely to *act out* their aggressions, participants returned to the laboratory to play a not-so-friendly game with their spouse. The rules were simple: find out who can press a button faster when prompted by a computer. The winner earned the right to blast the loser with loud noise through headphones. "The noise was a mixture of sounds that most people hate (e.g., fingernails scratching on a chalkboard, dentist drills, ambulance sirens)." The noise levels ranged from normal conversation to approximately the same level as a fire alarm. "The winner could also determine the duration of the loser's suffering by controlling the noise duration," from half a second to ten seconds. What did they find? Once again, lower blood sugar in the evening predicted worse behavior. The lower their glucose levels, the more the test subjects put their spouses through louder and longer bouts of suffering. (In reality, participants competed against a computer, not their spouse, so no eardrums were harmed.) In a TED Talk presentation on the study, Dr. Bushman offered this advice, "Don't talk about anything important with your spouse on an empty stomach."[26] Of course, domestic violence is no joke, and it doesn't all boil down to low blood sugar. Low blood sugar does, however, seem to play a meaningful role.

In an interview about the study, Dr. Bushman explained how low blood sugar translates to such antisocial behaviors. It's straightforward, he said: "Glucose provides the energy the brain needs to exercise self-control." When glucose levels are low, we lose self-control, and any aggressive impulses we have may be expressed.[27] I would add that the surging adrenaline our bodies release during episodes of hypoglycemia can't help, either. He and others in this field tell us that "low blood glucose can be one of many factors that predispose to aggressive behavior." Similar research shows that being hungry makes us every bit as aggressive toward strangers as toward a loved one.

Here's why I think that all this research points to our underlying metabolic problem of insulin resistance. In all these experiments, there is something fascinating, and quite terrifying, that the researchers do not pick up on. People's reportedly "low" blood sugars are actually squarely within normal range, 70 mg/dL or higher. Not even the angriest people with the most aggression had what doctors would consider "clinically meaningful hypoglycemia," a level of 50 mg/dL or lower. It would be one thing if folks were truly on the verge of starving when their behavior deteriorated, but that's not what psychologists are finding. They're showing that people *deemed* to be in good health are regressing to an antisocial behavioral state. But they are *not* actually in good health; we know they're likely to be suffering from undiagnosed insulin resistance, as is 99 percent of the population. And this means we can do something about it besides wring our hands and move on to the next bad news story.

The large and growing body of research linking feeling hungry to behaving badly is giving us clear evidence of a link between disrupted metabolic health and disruptive, childish, and sometimes even violent behavior. Unfortunately, since psychologists are not working with metabolic health experts, they're not making the connections they need to make in order for their research to get the attention it deserves. Right now, the media mostly pigeonhole this sort of stuff into their box of entertaining headlines, along with dogs who can dial 911 and rats dragging various types of fast foods through the subways. That's not where this information belongs, because the implications are deadly serious.

One of the big reasons the world isn't waking up to this connection between insulin resistance and social disruption has to do with the bizarre medical thinking on hypoglycemia itself.

WHY (MOST) DOCTORS DON'T TAKE HYPOGLYCEMIA SERIOUSLY

In our current medical paradigm, most patients experiencing hypoglycemia are not taken seriously unless they're taking insulin and can potentially overdose. Doctors do take the *symptoms* seriously, of course. But once the doctor determines that the brain fog, palpitations, headaches, and so on are not due to other underlying disorders, and are occurring when their patients are hungry, they'll diagnose hypoglycemia, and simply suggest they carry snacks. Unfortunately, snacks don't always help once an anxiety attack or a migraine has already begun. Even worse, many doctors believe that having mild hypoglycemia is healthy.[28] The assumption seems to be that it's a sign of a fast metabolism. Doctors understand that *severe* hypoglycemia can have serious consequences. But they don't typically understand that people with insulin resistance can have severe hypoglycemia *symptoms* even while their blood sugars are normal.

Let's define our terms. A blood sugar below 30 mg/dL is life-threatening hypoglycemia. Between 30 and 50 is severe hypoglycemia. And between 51 and 70 is mild hypoglycemia. Below 50 is where doctors start to take symptoms seriously. Between 51 and 70 is that weird category of "healthy hypoglycemia" that's an unrecognized sign of early insulin resistance— and not at all healthy.

The number 50 was chosen to represent the magical point at which low blood sugar goes from being healthy to problematic based on research showing that blood sugar levels of 50 or less represented an "immediate and long-term danger to the individual."[29] The danger comes from confusion, coordination problems, and slow or disordered mental processing that could make driving or climbing steps and ladders dangerous.

Repeated episodes of low blood sugar can have devastating long-term impacts. Studies on people with type 1 diabetes who use insulin and are therefore subject to frequent episodes of hypoglycemia show that they can permanently lose mental "flexibility," which is essential for getting along with others and solving problems. They may suffer from a tendency to blurt out answers out of turn, termed "rapid responding." They might have trouble with decision-making, lose attention to detail, and experience spatial long-term memory impairments, which makes it hard to remember where they've put things or even recognize where they are.[30] One series of studies showed that recurrent low-blood-sugar episodes can cause significant cognitive impairment and even dementia, which the authors dubbed, sensibly enough, "hypoglycemia-induced brain damage."[31] Given that recurrent severe hypoglycemia can contribute to learning disorders, behavior problems, and even dementia, you'd think there would be at least some concern about the possible harms of recurrent hypoglycemia at milder levels.

Perhaps a more fundamental reason that the medical system treats people with hypoglycemia so poorly may be that the diagnosis itself suffers from a tainted reputation.

At one point in time, ordinary family doctors were listening to their patients, diagnosing them with hypoglycemia, and instructing them about how to modify their diets to prevent it. They didn't go so far as to advise eating fats, but they did suggest using "low-glycemic-index carbohydrates," which is the proper medical term for what I like to call "slow-digesting" carbohydrates. But they were diagnosing so many people with hypoglycemia that it drew suspicion from academics who thought doctors should only diagnose hypoglycemia with lab testing, and not by listening carefully to our patients. They went on an aggressive campaign to shut it all down, calling it a "non-disease," a "pseudo disorder," and most demeaningly, a "psychosomatic illness," suggesting that the symptoms were all in people's heads.[32] Hypoglycemia became a condition of ill repute thanks in large part to these influential articles.

While we've mostly moved past the abject disrespect, we still fail to properly diagnose people with hypoglycemia even if they truly suffer from low blood sugar. The problem is so widespread that a UK nonprofit called the Hypoglycemia Support Foundation specifically focuses on this frustration with the tag line, "Your symptoms may not be in your head."[33]

The problem with relying on labs for the diagnosis of hypoglycemia comes from the fact that blood sugar lows are fleeting and physicians don't typically look for them the way I'm teaching you to do in this chapter (see Figure 4–1). Therefore, unless doctors see a fasting blood sugar below 50 mg/dL printed in black and white on a blood test result, they probably won't take hypoglycemia symptoms seriously no matter how often they happen or how bad they make someone feel. But it's unusual for a fasting blood sugar to go that low unless someone is taking a medication that lowers blood sugar or has a rare disorder. Another problem with standard diagnosis protocols comes from the fact that hypoglycemia mostly happens during the day while people are active, but doctors are taught to test their patients for it first thing in the morning. Even testing later in the day wouldn't necessarily show blood sugar being low, because, as we've been discussing, low blood sugar triggers stress hormones that quickly bring levels back up. Perhaps the biggest barrier to diagnosis is the fact that many people feel hypoglycemic when their blood sugars are normal due to (undiagnosed) insulin resistance.

Due to these diagnostic barriers, securing an official diagnosis of clinical hypoglycemia has been extraordinarily difficult, leaving most people undiagnosed. This is extremely frustrating for the many people who feel their hypoglycemia symptoms are being dismissed. Worse, it's preventing doctors from recognizing the warning signs of a broken, insulin-resistant metabolism. As a result, people are left to fend for themselves, even as hypoglycemia gradually hijacks their eating habits and progresses to more severe forms of metabolic disease. Fortunately, a new technology promises to improve our understanding of hypoglycemia.

CRAZY FOR COCOA PUFFS

After decades of research neglect, small groups of scientists have started to propel the study of hypoglycemia forward. They've taken advantage of a tiny, innovative device called a continuous glucose monitor that adheres to the upper arm and automatically checks blood sugar. It was invented so that people with diabetes wouldn't need to repeatedly stick their fingers. With continuous glucose monitoring (CGM), you don't have to guess when your blood sugar is falling and run to a laboratory hoping that you catch it in the act—it wouldn't stay low that long. You don't even need to poke your finger with a home glucometer. All you need to do is glance at the number on your scanner, and you can even do it after the fact, since the data is stored in the device as well as in the cloud. The device has finally given scientists a tool that can catch those transitory episodes of hypoglycemia, so they can start to understand how it affects our daily lives.

In 2019, a group of doctors decided to use CGM technology to find out if people who claimed to feel hypoglycemic really had low blood sugar.[34] What they learned should put hypoglycemia—and pathologic hunger—on the map. They showed that people with hypoglycemia symptoms frequently had episodes where their glucose dipped below 70 mg/dL, and half of them also had deeper dips, below 50. As we've seen, when blood sugar goes under 50 it causes impaired thinking and a greater risk of accidents. Fortunately, most of these deeper dips lasted less than half an hour.

The authors pointed out that without CGM technology it is unlikely that any of the participants would have received a diagnosis of hypoglycemia at all, since the episodes were brief, and most did not occur in the morning when people usually go to a lab for fasting blood tests. Basically, unless you wear a CGM, you're not going to know if your blood glucose sometimes dips below normal.

It's important to note that participants' fasting glucose levels were actually borderline *high*, with an average of 97 mg/dL among the participants (100 is the cutoff for diagnosing prediabetes). This supports the idea that hypoglycemia symptoms are an early warning sign of insulin resistance.

The other new finding was that, in order to live with hypoglycemia, we basically start obsessing about food and dramatically curtailing our activity. Everyone in the study carried snacks. Some people even ate when they weren't hungry, in hopes of preventing symptoms. Several reported avoiding exercise because it would bring on the symptoms. The authors raised the concern that these adaptive but "obesogenic behaviors" were likely to further jeopardize overall health. I would agree. In fact, my own patients have taught me that insulin resistance can make it hard to consciously control your eating habits. For example, one busy mom in her early thirties told me, "I haven't had anything yet today," but she had brought a half-empty Starbucks venti caramel Frappuccino into the room. Another, a law firm executive in her late fifties, assured me she didn't ever snack—while sucking on a lemon candy. I mention this disconnect between words and actions not to shame anyone but to highlight how a disrupted metabolism can distort our perceptions. If a food makes us feel physically better, then it's only logical to conclude that we needed those calories. And if we *needed* them, then it's hard to fathom how eating them could be contributing to excessive intake. In fact, another study I want to share supports the idea that we can develop eating habits that we're not even aware of.

In 2022, investigators used a real-time brain-scanning technique called functional MRI (fMRI) to map out the areas of the brain that get activated as blood sugar falls. It turns out that, as blood sugar drops, even before it drops below 70 mg/dL, it can activate areas of the brain that drive eating behaviors. Some of these areas operate below the conscious level. As blood sugar falls, it can cause a kind of subconscious hunger that doesn't make you feel hypoglycemic, it just makes you really want food the minute you see it, smell it, or hear someone talk about it. The investigators suggested that these brain pathways could drive "addiction-like" eating behaviors. They warned that telling people to snack to treat their symptoms is dangerously counterproductive and that people could end up snacking "either consciously or subconsciously, to prevent further hypoglycemia."[35] This research tells me that, yes, people can drink Frappuccino and suck on lemon candies without really noticing.

These authors noted that the addiction-like behaviors and unconscious eating were more of a problem for people with worse insulin resistance. They also showed that blood sugar doesn't need to drop below normal to trigger junk food cravings. Half of the study participants started to feel hungry when their blood sugar levels were still as high as 80 mg/dL, ten points above the number now officially considered low, and 30 points above the number considered meaningfully low.[36] Feeling hypoglycemic when we're not highlights what I've been saying about insulin resistance not being a simple problem of *eating* too much sugar: it's a complex problem of progressively *needing* more sugar than the bloodstream is designed to safely carry. As time passes, and a person's blood sugar goes higher and higher, that individual may start to have hypoglycemia symptoms at levels no doctor would consider low, and therefore might suggest the symptoms are just "in your head."

Pathologic hunger is truly the scourge of our time. It's changing our relationships with food. It's potentially damaging our brains. And it's probably disrupting our ability to learn. Of course, the hunger itself is not the root cause. The root cause is the fact that our high-PUFA body fat fails to supply our cells with energy, and that the drops in blood sugar that ensue cause a kind of hunger that I'm calling pathologic. Pathologic hunger is a defining feature of modern metabolism.

If your metabolism is distracting you with fear of hunger—if you're spending even just 10 percent of the time worrying about snacks that you could be spending thinking about life—you're going to be making very different decisions than if you had a healthy metabolism. You might be turning down opportunities for adventure or for meeting new friends. You may not pursue promotions at work. You may miss out on relationships. And you will no doubt blame yourself for your failures—as will other people. Hypoglycemia stays with us for the duration of our metabolic impairments, and it increasingly shapes our day-to-day experience of being human. Still, medical science is barely aware of the problem and offers no real solutions. This is a sad state of affairs, indeed.

In Part One, we've seen that a toxic ingredient has made its way into our food supply in a big way—with most of us none the wiser to its effects.

How did we ever get to this place? How did we, as an intelligent species, get to the point where health-conscious consumers, truth-seeking journalists, and even doctors have overlooked the fundamentals of seed-oil toxicity? And how did our society ever get to the point where practically our entire food system depends on a processed food ingredient that violently assaults our health?

It's been a long time coming. For centuries, America's peculiar form of medicine has suffered from its own chronic disease—a disinterest in nutrition. This state of affairs set the stage for special interests to create an absolutely artificial fear of natural fats that terrorizes us to this day. We're about to learn how a misguided theory of heart disease opened the door for special interests to first hijack the entire science of nutrition, and then to hijack our health. As you'll see, the entanglements between the vegetable-oil industry and the healthcare industry run deep and wide, and they are harder to see because of one word: cholesterol.

PART TWO

DARK HISTORY

The limits of my language mean the limits of my world.

—Ludwig Wittgenstein, Austrian philosopher

CHAPTER 5

The Truth About Cholesterol

IN THIS CHAPTER YOU WILL LEARN

- Doctors have heard that cholesterol causes heart attacks so often, we fail to question the idea.
- Cholesterol is a nutrient, not a toxin.
- More research suggests that lowering cholesterol *increases* the risk of heart attacks than vice versa.
- The fact that vegetable oil lowers cholesterol may be another sign of its toxicity.
- People with lower cholesterol are less healthy and more likely to die than people with high cholesterol.

If you're like most of my patients, you probably believe you eat a relatively decent diet. But do you?

The answer to that question depends on whom you ask. Most of us believe we make the right choices more often than we make bad ones. But in 2022, when a group of dietitians evaluated the eating habits of over nine thousand Americans using their Healthy Eating Index, they gave 70 percent of them an F. The index awarded points for eating fruits, vegetables, whole grains, and protein and for avoiding refined grains, sugar, and cholesterol-elevating saturated fat. Nearly two-thirds—71 percent—of participants had ranked their diets as good, very good, or excellent, while the dietitians ranked only 12 percent of the participants' diets that highly. Fully 94 percent of those who scored an F thought they should have at least gotten a D.[1]

This exuberant overconfidence reflects an interesting human foible: the tendency of people who are unaware of their deficiencies to simply assume that none exist. But we all face this dilemma: no matter how smart we may be, we simply don't know what we don't know. How could we?

Psychologists David Dunning and Justin Kruger have warned that this quirk of human behavior gives experts trained in one field overconfidence in others in which they are not trained—a widely accepted idea which is now called the Dunning-Kruger effect. But their finding implies another possibility that's a bit terrifying: *What if the Dunning-Kruger effect applies to an entire field?* In other words, what if the dietitians grading the healthfulness of people's diets based on their saturated fat content should have been looking at vegetable oil consumption instead? Dietitians, doctors, and other health authorities could all be completely wrong about the healthfulness of common dietary fats. But if they're not looking for evidence that they might be wrong, they would have no way of discovering the error. If our health authorities believe a toxic ingredient is healthy, then how would we *ever* learn the truth?

Answer: We probably wouldn't. At least not for a long, long time.

For a long time, I was one of those doctors. I'd never heard anything negative about vegetable oil during any of my schooling. Not in college, not in medical school, and not during specialty training in family medicine. It's a common perception that doctors don't learn about nutrition, because the topic of food and healthy eating is a brief moment in our long curriculum—but we do actually learn a great deal about the fundamental processes by which our bodies assimilate and utilize nourishment. My experience was unusual because I graduated from one of the few medical schools that offered a nutrition course. I discovered later that a good part of dietitians' curriculum includes those fundamental processes, so we physicians don't need much more education to be caught up with most of what dietitians learn. The problem is, much of our education on nutrition is wrong.

Long before studying nutrition in school, I'd been programmed to accept vegetable oils into my life. It wasn't actually a conscious thought. It was a *feeling*—a feeling of trust and safety. And it was so potent that I still remember the moment it was first injected into me.

I was probably eight or nine. I picked up one of my dad's medical journals lying open to an advertisement for vegetable oils, right at eyeball height on a counter stool in the kitchen. The full-page color picture showed oil that glinted gold like liquid sunlight. And something about the ad copy made me want to run to our refrigerator to check if we had margarine or butter sitting in the door. Margarine. I felt relieved. From that day forward for the next three decades I never questioned the idea that butter was bad for me and plant oils were liquid sunlight, somehow capable of ensuring that my blood would keep flowing. I trusted that they were safe. I saw similar ads again and again, in *Time*, *Newsweek*, and on TV.

Years later, in my high school health classes, I learned that saturated fats are unhealthy because they raise cholesterol. But as with my thinking on vegetable oils, this training had also begun well before high school. Ever since I'd learned to read, I'd eaten my breakfast Grape-Nuts staring at the cereal box, reading the back, the front, the side, as if it were the most fascinating stuff. So many cereals I'd grown up eating claimed to be healthy because they lowered cholesterol. I don't remember ever questioning the idea that cholesterol clogged arteries. After all, something has to cause heart attacks, and cholesterol happens to have a clogged-up, choking sound right in its name—*khhugh*-lesterol. I had this image in my mind of cholesterol building up in my arteries like grease building up in a pipe, slowly choking them off.

I've since come to understand that the vegetable-oil-is-healthy campaign is inextricably wedded to the cholesterol-is-bad concept. Once consumers believe cholesterol causes heart attacks, then publicizing the fact that vegetable oils lower cholesterol makes them the antidote to heart attacks—which makes consumers want to buy them. The combination of package marketing, a plausible-sounding scientific explanation, and the dramatic use of clogged pipe imagery convinced millions of families just like mine that cholesterol was a killer and vegetable oil was heart healthy. We avoided saturated-fat-rich foods like butter and beef because of cholesterol. We bought skim milk because of cholesterol. And we bought margarine and products containing vegetable oil instead of animal fats because of cholesterol.

I've also come to understand that the image of cholesterol clogging arteries is a carefully crafted product of the mid-twentieth century. The origin of this image is a vitally important piece of American history, and we're going to learn more about it later. The reality is that there is a lot more to the story of what causes heart attacks than that simple picture of grease in a pipe. It's a different story altogether. But before we get there, we need to look at the nutrient that's been framed as a public health enemy, cholesterol.

WHAT IS CHOLESTEROL?

The world is seemingly more afraid of cholesterol than of heart attacks. When we cut out seed oils, our cholesterol very often goes up. If we start eating more butter, cheese, and other saturated-fat-rich foods, it can go up quite high, since saturated fat raises blood cholesterol levels. This scares most people quite a bit.

In my first few years of sharing what I'd learned about vegetable oils with patients, after I'd reassured folks that cholesterol was actually nothing to worry about, because it didn't cause heart attacks, I'd often get a puzzling objection: "But high cholesterol runs in my family." It flummoxed me because I initially didn't understand the mistaken belief behind the statement. Eventually, I realized that the concern reflects a common belief that cholesterol is a toxic byproduct that doesn't belong in the bloodstream. So of course my reassurances fell on deaf ears: it would be as if

I'd just told them not to worry about cancerous cells in their body. Now I know that to effectively alleviate worry, I have to tell folks the good things they never get to hear about cholesterol so they can understand why high blood levels might actually be a good thing.

Cholesterol is neither a toxin nor a byproduct. It is a nutrient that every cell in your body requires for basic functions. To the naked eye it appears as a waxy, fat-like substance. At the molecular level, it's bulky and flat, and its unique shape and charge properties make it capable of keeping our cell membranes just flexible enough to avoid solidifying—which would be immediately fatal—but not so fluid that we melt—also fatal. The body goes through a great deal of trouble to make cholesterol because it's so essential. Most cells can make their own if they have to. But cholesterol can come from our diet, too, particularly from foods like eggs, butter, liver, and shellfish. Most of the cholesterol in our blood is made in the liver and our intestinal cells. These cells need cholesterol to manufacture little fat-delivery vehicles called *lipoproteins* that they release into the bloodstream. These lipoproteins contain the cholesterol your doctor measures on blood tests. They work like tiny amphibious vehicles that ferry fat and fat-soluble vitamins through your arteries along a delivery route, making stops at cells that need the vitamins, essential fats, and other nutrients they're carrying—including cholesterol. What do they do with the cholesterol?

Cholesterol is the body's equivalent of duct tape. It's one of the most versatile nutrients our cells have and they use it for solving all sorts of problems. And it's more than just a problem-solver; it's also a building block:

- It enables cell division. The rapidly dividing cells in our intestinal tract, skin, and bone marrow need it more than most other kinds of cells in our bodies.
- It enables cell transport and communication. Cells need cholesterol to create structures called "lipid rafts" that are essential to responding to hormones and to moving large molecules

into the cell, out of the cell, and from place to place within the cell.

- It's the precursor for vitamin D, which forms when ultraviolet light rays strike cholesterol in the skin. Vitamin D helps our bodies absorb calcium.
- It provides waterproofing for our skin and other boundary layers within our bodies.
- It helps our brains and nerve cells conduct electricity. The brain is 15 percent cholesterol by dry weight, a higher proportion than any other organ in our bodies.
- It's the precursor to numerous hormones, called steroid hormones. These include the well-known sex hormones testosterone, estrogen, and cortisol—which give us energy. And there are dozens more, including the supplements many people buy for health and performance enhancement, such as DHEA and adrenal extracts.

Doctors know all this, but the prevailing wisdom holds that too much of a good thing can be a problem. This "too much of a good thing" idea makes no sense, however, when you realize that the levels cardiologists now consider "safe" for people at high risk (70 milligrams per deciliter [mg/dL] or lower) are almost unachievable without drugs. What's more, if cholesterol levels truly needed to be that low for us to be healthy, then healthy people would have lower cholesterol than unhealthy people. But as we're going to explore, it seems that healthier people tend to have higher cholesterol levels.

Still, I wouldn't blame you for doubting this contrarian viewpoint. After all, I'm saying that our country's 1,077,115 physicians are getting it wrong. The sad fact is that doctors can't apply what they learn to draw logical conclusions about cholesterol when they are continually bombarded by messaging about how dangerous it is. Let me give you just one example of how healthcare professionals can be misled.

Large epidemiological studies and meta-analyses have conclusively confirmed the lack of correlation between dietary cholesterol (the cholesterol you take in when you eat cholesterol-containing foods, typically meat and dairy) and blood cholesterol (the level of cholesterol circulating in your blood).[2] The evidence is abundant enough that the government committee that sets the official US Dietary Guidelines revised their report in 2015 to state that "cholesterol is not a nutrient of concern for overconsumption." In spite of this, standard nutrition advice still warns people away from most foods high in cholesterol. Why? Because standard nutrition advice still holds that high levels of blood cholesterol clog arteries and cause heart attacks, and the word association (dietary vs. blood cholesterol) confuses even professionals.

Good Cholesterol, Bad Cholesterol

You've probably heard the terms "good cholesterol" and "bad cholesterol." These terms refer to two subtypes of lipoproteins, those tiny amphibious vehicles that carry fats throughout our circulatory system. One subtype, called low-density lipoprotein (LDL), is said to be the "bad" cholesterol. Another subtype, high-density lipoprotein (HDL), is said to be the "good" cholesterol. These terms are imprecise, at best, since there is only one molecule called cholesterol, and that molecule is the same in all our lipoproteins. Where did they come from? Way back in 1958, a doctor at Cleveland Clinic named Angelo M. Scanu coined the term "good cholesterol" when he observed that people with high HDL tended to have lower heart attack risk.[3] He hypothesized that HDL might clean up the cholesterol that LDL seemed to deposit in our arteries. At some point, people started calling LDL "bad cholesterol" based on these ideas. But by the 1990s, accumulating evidence suggested that LDL does not, in fact, deposit cholesterol in our arteries—*unless it's oxidized.*[4] What's more, we've also discovered that HDL can harm our arteries, too, when it's oxidized.[5] It seems time to abandon these imprecise, outdated terms and focus on the real "bad player": oxidation.

So, we've seen that *dietary* cholesterol isn't something to worry about, but because doctors are confusing dietary cholesterol with blood cholesterol, they still tell people to limit eggs, shellfish, and other high-cholesterol foods—even though there's no evidence that this does anything beneficial.

What about *blood* cholesterol? As unusual as it may sound, blood cholesterol is not a bad thing, either. Because cholesterol is a potent antioxidant, we need it flowing through our arteries to help protect them against oxidative damage. Of course, we're all told that having high blood cholesterol is bad. So let's take a closer look.

DOES CHOLESTEROL CAUSE HEART ATTACKS?

If having higher cholesterol really did cause heart attacks, then people hospitalized for a heart attack would have had high cholesterol levels before their attack. Their levels should be, on average, above the normal range. Likewise, if low cholesterol were protective, people hospitalized for a heart attack would not have had low cholesterol beforehand. But when a very large study asked the simple question, "What is the cholesterol level that people admitted to the hospital with a heart attack have?" that was not what they saw.

In 2009, a multi-center study of 136,905 people hospitalized with heart attacks found that only 25 percent had LDL ("bad" cholesterol) levels that would be considered high at the time they entered the hospital (130 mg/dL or higher).[6] Slightly more people, 35 percent, reported having been previously told they'd had some kind of high cholesterol at least once in their lives. In other words, normal and low cholesterol was a far better predictor of heart attack than high cholesterol.

The Truth Is in the Fine Print

You can catch a glimpse of the lack of foundational support for the cholesterol theory in a surprising place: the Mazola corn oil bottle. The fine print under its "Heart Healthy" label directs you to a side panel with some interesting legalese (you can also find this on the Mazola website). It says, "Very limited and preliminary scientific evidence suggests that eating about 1 tablespoon (16 grams) of corn oil daily may reduce the risk of heart disease due to the unsaturated fat content in corn oil." That sentence is followed by another one that states, contradictorily, that the "FDA [Federal Drug Administration] concludes that there is little scientific evidence supporting this claim."

You might think this would get cardiologists scratching their heads about the utility of treating high cholesterol. But instead of questioning cholesterol's validity as a risk factor, the medical community responded to this information by doubling down on cholesterol-phobia. Here's what they actually said: "These findings may provide further support for recent guideline revisions with even lower LDL goals."[7] In other words, the problem is not that the whole idea is wrong, it's that cholesterol is even more dangerous than we thought. This viewpoint fails to explain the study's observations.

Our guidelines keep moving the goalposts on what's considered a safe level of cholesterol. The authors of the article quoted above were referring to guideline revisions that had taken place in 2004, when doctors were given a new, lower set of cholesterol values to work with. Prior to 2004, a total cholesterol level of 240 mg/dL was considered normal. After 2004, the number was cut to 199 mg/dL. The LDL cutoff was lowered, too, from 130 down to 100 mg/dL. This was hardly the first time the definition of high cholesterol had changed. In 1970, the cutoff for normal total cholesterol was 310 mg/dL. During my career, I've seen that cutoff lowered from 260, to 240, and now 199 mg/dL. Likewise, normal LDL has been ratcheted down from 180 to 100 mg/dL. For a person with multiple risk factors, LDL now needs to be under 70 mg/dL, and some lipidologists (the cholesterol specialists) are still calling for that number to be reduced to "well below 40."[8]

What is going on here? Why do our guidelines keep pushing LDL levels down?

Our guidelines keep changing because the experts writing them don't know what they don't know. These specialists are not listening to the specialists who study the link between oxidative stress and heart attacks. The two groups do not communicate, and as we'll see, the disconnect is not an accident; it's being actively maintained. The lipid scientists have been saying that vegetable oil causes oxidative stress, and that lower cholesterol levels may be an indication of greater vegetable-oil-induced oxidative stress. This explains why, in a population eating more vegetable oils than ever, *lower* cholesterol correlates with heart attacks. But because doctors are working with only partial information, they can't interpret data correctly. Unfortunately, patients are stuck seeing doctors who truly don't know what causes heart attacks—but think that they do.

I've yet to see any guideline acknowledge an important statistic: the cholesterol levels of our *entire* population have been going *down* over time. In 1960, the average adult cholesterol level was 222 mg/dL. In 2000, the average cholesterol level was 203 mg/dL. Today it is 189 mg/dL.[9] If high cholesterol were truly associated with worsening health, one might expect our average cholesterol figures to have gone *up* in tandem with our increasing rates of obesity and diabetes. But that's not what's happened.

THE PERILS OF LOW CHOLESTEROL

The end goal of any public health recommendation is not lowering cholesterol. It's helping you live longer. Dying with lower cholesterol levels is not the goal. Not one human clinical trial has shown that lowering cholesterol produces a beneficial effect. At least not any trial that reported its data truthfully, as I want to show you here.

Vegetable oils do indeed lower cholesterol. This has been proven time and again. It's not controversial at all. And this effect is so predictable, in the 1960s a physiologist named Ancel Keys actually worked out an equation that accurately predicted how much a person's cholesterol levels would drop given a specific dose of PUFA.[10] But the promised benefits of this dietary change rested entirely on the assumption that lowering cholesterol prevented heart attacks, something that Dr. Keys called the diet-heart hypothesis.

During the past seventy years, only one large, randomized, controlled, double-blinded clinical trial in humans has ever directly tested the assumption, and that didn't quite go as planned.

What's a Randomized, Controlled, Double-Blinded Study?

The purpose of this sort of clinical nutrition trial is to compare the effectiveness of a new diet against the standard diet, called the control, in preventing a given health outcome, such as heart attack or death. In this sort of study, you gather together two large groups of people who you think are similar on every variable you can imagine—age, weight, lifestyle, social class. You let one group eat their normal (control) diet and give the other group something you think is healthier, and then follow them for years and see what happens. It's best if the diets are identical in every way except for a single variable, so you can pin any observed effects on that variable. Being randomized and

---

double-blinded means that neither the participants nor the researchers themselves know who is receiving the experimental treatment
and who is not. This helps to reduce the likelihood of any bias on the
researchers' part affecting the results. It also reduces the chance
of the participants' expectations or the placebo effect skewing the
outcome.

In the 1960s and early 1970s, Dr. Keys worked with several cardiologists to design a study called the Minnesota Coronary Experiment, funded
by the American Heart Association. This study was huge, having enrolled
nearly fifteen thousand people. To this day, it stands as one of the most
rigorous diet trials ever conducted. It was so large and so meticulously
controlled that it is unlikely to ever be bested.

When the study results started rolling in, the data surprised everyone. It turned out that lowering cholesterol with vegetable oils did not have
the expected benefits. In fact, a preliminary analysis provided reason to
believe it had some serious harms, including raising cancer risk.[11]

So what did the research team do? Dr. Keys and his collaborators gathered up the data, slides, and other evidence, packed it into a bunch of file
boxes, and kept the boxes in a basement.

Decades later, a savvy scientist working for the National Institutes
of Health (NIH), Chris Ramsden, MD, noticed that a grant had been
approved for a one-of-a-kind experiment to test the diet-heart hypothesis
back in the 1960s, but he couldn't find where the final data had ever been
properly published. After some clever detective work, his team managed
to locate the basement where the files lay hidden, stashed away by one of
the study authors who'd recently passed away; his family hadn't yet gotten
around to selling his home in Minnesota. Some of the data was missing,
but there was more than enough to draw some very important conclusions.

The belated analysis of the remaining original, half-century-old data
showed something shocking. It looked like swapping out saturated fat for

polyunsaturated fat *increased* mortality, even as it also reduced cholesterol. In fact, for every 30 points that eating seed oils lowered a person's
total cholesterol, that person's chance of dying increased by 22 percent.[12] In
other words, the people whose cholesterol dropped the most had the worst
possible health outcome—death. Keep in mind, the study was intended
specifically to demonstrate the validity of the cholesterol theory of heart
disease. Its double-blind randomized design represents the gold standard
of clinical trials. In other words, as much as anything in medicine can ever
be proven, this study proves the cholesterol theory wrong. Dead wrong,
quite literally.

Dr. Ramsden's group published these findings in the *British Medical
Journal* in 2016.[13] Their report specifically emphasized that lowering cholesterol could be dangerous. But the medical world barely responded to
this paradigm-shifting news.

Part of the lackluster response may be related to the fact that busy
medical professionals can't possibly keep up with all the articles being
pushed across our desks every day. Just as TV viewers don't always want
to hear all the details of the news from investigative journalists, prefer-
ring to get the bare-bones bottom line from their favorite trusted anchors,
doctors rely on celebrated medical authorities. When it comes to nutrition
science, we want to hear from physicians who do nutrition research, and
we want to know what we're supposed to do about the newsworthy item.
Is this a better approach? Will we need to change our practices? Or can we
spare ourselves the trouble of even thinking about it?

After Dr. Ramsden's publication of the forty-year-old missing evidence, the medical media turned to one of their favorite sources, Walter
Willett, MD, to summarize Dr. Ramsden's research in a clear, concise way.
As a tenured professor of epidemiology and nutrition at Harvard's School
of Public Health, he would appear to be more than qualified to translate
the findings and put them into their proper perspective. Here's what he
said about the importance of this long-overdue data analysis: "This is an
interesting historical footnote that has no relevance to current dietary

recommendations that emphasize replacing saturated fat with polyunsaturated fat."[14]

I'd like to frame up Dr. Willett's frame-up so that busy readers like yourself can decide if you want to take Harvard's nutrition advice to heart in the future. Thousands of doctors around the world look at their patients' cholesterol numbers every day and advise dietary changes that emphasize replacing saturated fats with polyunsaturated fats based on a theory that would have been seriously undermined (or quite possibly entirely dismissed) had this evidence seen the light of day when it should have.

Consider also that Dr. Ramsden's study—far from being a "historical footnote that has no relevance"—is *not* the only one to find that lowering cholesterol might have negative consequences that doctors and their patients ought to be made aware of. An alarming number of studies now reveal that people with lower cholesterol are more likely to develop scary diseases or die. You have to dig to find them, but here are a few examples of what's out there.

Let's start with cancer. A 2012 article showed the results of three large trials where people were given either cholesterol-lowering drugs called statins or placebos.[15] These trials all showed that people on the statin drugs developed 20 to 25 percent more cancers than people on the placebo. The authors also reported that many articles had found an association between low cholesterol and cancers of the colon, lung, and prostate, as well as dying from any kind of cancer. A 2007 *BMJ* article found "a disturbing, highly significant" risk of newly diagnosed cancer in people with the *lowest* LDL levels.[16]

A 2011 study in Japan suggested that the problem extends to cardiovascular disease, exactly the disease that lowering cholesterol is supposed to prevent. The title of the article makes it clear: "Low Cholesterol Is Associated with Mortality from Stroke, Heart Disease, and Cancer."[17] Mortality means death, in case that wasn't obvious.

Dr. Ramsden had actually published another study that reevaluated lost evidence from another trial also performed in the 1960s and 1970s that was never properly reported.[18] That study was a clinical trial, too—a very large and well-designed one, although not double-blinded like the other study was. It compared a high-PUFA diet to a typical diet of the day, which used animal fat and margarines containing saturated fat (and some trans fat, from the margarine). This study showed that people who ate animal fat and margarines had 13 percent higher total cholesterol than the people on the high-PUFA diet (266.5 versus 243.9 mg/dL). They also had a whopping 60 percent fewer heart attacks (16.3 percent versus 10.1 percent) and fewer overall deaths (17.6 percent versus 11.8 percent).

A potpourri of studies link low cholesterol to a variety of other conditions. In 2016, a study in China showed that every 40-point uptick in total or LDL cholesterol imparted incrementally stronger protection against dementia.[19] Low cholesterol has also been linked to a life-threatening form of infection called sepsis, where the body is overwhelmed by bacteria in the bloodstream and organs start to shut down. And it's been linked to death or near death from COVID-19.[20] Cholesterol has been called "a gatekeeper of male fertility."[21] And it's not just men: many women with premature ovarian failure have very low cholesterol.[22] Inflammatory conditions and autoimmune diseases, including psoriasis, rheumatoid arthritis, and lupus, have also been linked to low cholesterol.[23] And, by the way, we treat those diseases with steroid drugs, which are related to cortisol, a hormone our bodies make from cholesterol. In fact, it's entirely possible that if you have any condition that's been treated with steroids, you might be able to improve that condition by *raising* your cholesterol.

A 2012 publication from Denmark found that people with total cholesterol levels above 200 mg/dL were *less* likely to die during the study's eight-year duration than people with lower numbers.[24] A 2012 Brazilian study on adults aged sixty to eighty-five showed that people with total cholesterol of 170 or less were 50 percent *more* likely to die than people with total cholesterol of 200 or more during the twelve-year study period.[25] Here in the United States, a 2021 publication in *Nature* showed that pushing your LDL down below 80, whether by diet or drugs, doubles your risk of dying in the next eight years compared to people with higher numbers.[26] This particular article concluded, "Further studies are warranted to determine the causal relationship between LDL-C [LDL cholesterol] level and all-cause mortality." In other words, it is time to start looking at why low cholesterol might be killing people. This is just a sampling of the reports clearly linking low cholesterol to death and disease of various kinds. Individually, any one of these studies would call to question our decades-old dietary advice. As a group, these articles should be paradigm shifting, and they should impact most of medical practice. Yet that's not what has happened. In fact, sometimes the authors of studies on PUFAs and the dangers of low cholesterol are subject to undue attack.

THE "WRONG" KIND OF SCIENCE

Dr. Glen D. Lawrence is a professor in the Department of Chemistry and Biochemistry at Long Island University in Brooklyn. His laboratory specializes in polyunsaturated fatty acid metabolism. In 2021, he published an article warning that one way PUFAs lower cholesterol is by disrupting the proper distribution of fats and cholesterol, and in so doing, building inflammatory "atherosclerotic deposits surrounding the arteries."[27] In other words, vegetable oils lower our blood cholesterol levels by depositing oxidized material in and around your arterial walls, where it can cause heart attacks. Dr. Lawrence also pointed out that this idea is not new; many other scientists in a variety of fields have suggested the exact same thing, dating back to the early 1950s.

Dr. Lawrence's description of how cholesterol-lowering PUFAs damage arteries is based on solid science. Yet academics from the University of California, Los Angeles, and other institutions wrote letters to the editor complaining about it. They accused Dr. Lawrence of fearmongering and being out of touch with "reputable researchers."[28] Instead of arguing against his points, the authors primarily argued that he was looking at the wrong kind of evidence. Dr. Lawrence cited mostly animal and in vitro (meaning "test tube," lab-based) studies that his detractors felt should be ignored because they were lower down on "the hierarchy of evidence" as shown by a pyramid-shaped diagram. The two bottom layers of the pyramid were the "in vitro" and animal studies. At the top of the pyramid sits a kind of study called a "meta-analysis of randomized controlled clinical trials," labeled as the "gold standard."[29]

What Animal Studies Can Tell Us

Human clinical trials are limited to what's ethical, thankfully. We can't, for example, test out the most effective diet that would give people heart attacks. For that, we use animal studies (for better or for worse). When researchers try to uncover the answer, they've found it exceedingly difficult to give animals heart attacks at all. In fact, I was unable to find a single animal study where the outcome was heart attack. Instead, the studies report on diets that can give animals atherosclerosis.[30] And even this has proven rather difficult to do using animal fats. Rabbits need to be repeatedly injected with snake venom, or have their arteries burned with electrocautery, or stretched by inserting balloons and inflating them. Mice and rats need to be genetically modified and "subjected to photochemical injury." Scientists agree that "pig models are probably the best way to recreate human plaque," but you have to inject them with a poison called streptozotocin first, which gives them type 1 diabetes.[31]

Even with all these genetic modifications and other health disturbances, in order to give rats atherosclerosis using animal fats, scientists had to formulate a chow with five times more fat than normal rodent chow, and *thousands* of times more cholesterol (by weight). The resulting "atherogenic rodent diet" contains so many additional

---

unfortified calories that, unless the animals eat themselves over-weight, they won't get adequate protein. The daily cholesterol ration in this formula equates to a human equivalent of 22,500 mg, the amount in 92 sticks of butter. Obviously this is not a realistic human diet.[32]

The most efficient way for scientists to give animals atheroscle-rosis is by feeding them either oxidized vegetable oils or oxidized cholesterol.[33] Importantly, the cholesterol in foods such as burgers and chicken does not oxidize to any measurable degree with normal cooking practices.[34] (However, if beef tallow is continually heated for days, as in deep frying, the cholesterol would likely oxidize over time.) This suggests that oxidized fats and oils are key dietary ingredients to avoid if you want to limit plaque buildup and avoid heart attacks.

But labeling the meta-analysis as the "gold standard" is terrifically misleading. These sorts of studies are generally used when individual studies are inconclusive or conflicting in order to discern which way most of the evidence points. Unfortunately, they are often regarded as gospel and beyond reproach so that a single meta-analysis may dramatically change our treatment protocols.

Trusting a meta-analysis more than every other form of evidence is dangerous because it represents the ultimate form of condensed information—a summary of summaries, if you will. That leaves a lot of wiggle room to make the results come out the way we want them to. This is called confirmation bias.

The meta-analysis can be manipulated to produce a variety of different results depending on what studies are included and what studies are excluded. For example, if some studies show that it's more likely to rain in July than in December, and other studies show the opposite, a meta-analysis that included only studies from India, where the monsoon season occurs in summer, may show rain is more likely to occur in July. However, a meta-analysis that included only studies from California, where the monsoon season occurs in winter, would show the opposite. Neither would help someone living in, say, New York predict the weather.

(I think if individual studies are conflicting, we need to consider that there may be some problems with the foundational idea; a key concept may be missing. In the aforementioned example, the missing concept relates to geography and its effect on local climate. In the medical world, the missing concept is often related to vegetable oil and its susceptibility to oxidation.)

When I spoke to one scientist (who asked me not to use her name) about data manipulation, she told me, "I basically watched [one investigator] do everything he could short of inventing and revising the data himself to find a good outcome." Not because he was paid to do so, mind you. Simply because "he was so sure his interventions were going to work" that he lost his scientist's impartiality. This is called an intellectual conflict of interest, and it's quite dangerous since most people are not aware of their own biases.

Since we've all grown up with the ideology that cholesterol is bad, most investigators have this bias. All too often, authors of meta-analyses simply exclude studies that don't support their idea—it's at their discretion, as long as they explain why they made the choices they made. What's more, the authors can also make claims about a study's conclusions that aren't entirely accurate, but the only way to know would be to check the references, and doctors may not have access to the full text (thanks to most journals being behind paywalls), and certainly most doctors lack the time or inclination to fact-check sources in addition to their day-to-day workload.

Another problem with dismissing the foundational types of science that are listed at the bottom of this "hierarchy of evidence" is that most medical knowledge is built on exactly this sort of evidence. If we were to dismiss the base of this pyramid, then we would have to dismiss all of the basic physiology that informs us about how the human body works.

Without basic in vitro science, we would not have discovered cholesterol in the first place. We wouldn't have the germ theory of disease. We'd still be in the dark ages of our understanding of the human body and biology itself.

The pyramid-shaped hierarchy of evidence inaccurately suggests that one type of study is *superior* to all the rest. The reality is, there is a logical progression to building and testing scientific ideas. Each type of evidence has a use, each has its own set of advantages and disadvantages, and all types should be considered. In fact, if the statistical correlations between a nutrient and a disease aren't held up by the foundational mechanistic studies, they probably represent correlations only, and should at least be examined for possible flaws and biases if not dismissed. In other words, basic science belongs at the foundation of the pyramid for *support*. Not because it's lower in quality. If your pyramid of evidence lacks a base, then your idea has not been properly developed.

In fact, the pyramid of evidence for the idea that high cholesterol is harmful rests on a dubious base. That's thanks to the work of the physiologist I mentioned in this chapter and will discuss again in the next, Dr. Ancel Keys. His work, more than anyone else's, is cited as the foundational evidence upon which the cholesterol theory of heart disease rests. His story takes us back to the post–World War II era, at a time when the food supply was dramatically shifting, and when medical science started losing interest in nutrition in favor of pharmaceutical interventions.

CHAPTER 6

Ancel Keys and the Dark Side of the American Heart Association

---

IN THIS CHAPTER YOU WILL LEARN

- The American Heart Association started promoting vegetable oil after receiving money from the vegetable oil industry in 1948.
- Much of this money was used to support one man's attempts to link heart attacks to high cholesterol.
- To make the cholesterol theory look better, this man suppressed data showing that smoking caused heart attacks.
- The AHA now publishes fourteen journals that continue to miseducate doctors about the cause of heart disease.

Back when I first started learning about vegetable oil, I realized I should probably learn more about the history of nutrition science. During my college, medical school, and specialty education years, I'd learned about all kinds of important figures in medical history and details of their discoveries. I'd learned about the "barber surgeons" of the Middle Ages, who provided grooming services, dental extractions, minor surgeries, and sometimes amputations. I'd learned about the history of anesthesia, starting with whiskey, progressing to chloroform, and then to the safer drugs we use today. So it struck me as odd that I'd never been presented with the how-did-we-get-here history of nutrition science. The one thing I'd learned was that a man named Ancel Keys had linked cholesterol to heart attacks in the 1950s and 1960s with his diet-heart hypothesis. A closer look at Dr. Keys and his work provides that how-did-we-get-here story of nutrition science—and what it says about our current nutrition paradigm is troubling.

THE FLAWED FATHER OF THE DIET-HEART HYPOTHESIS

Ancel Keys is a controversial figure in science. On one hand, Dr. Keys is celebrated as the man who discovered the cause of heart attacks, and every medical student learns his name. On the other hand, his methods have been considered substandard since the beginning—although doctors are generally unaware of this aspect of medical history.

The controversy around Dr. Keys's methods begins with the first paper he wrote in support of his diet-heart hypothesis, in 1953, called "Atherosclerosis: A Problem in Newer Public Health."[1] Doctors had recognized coronary artery disease since the Middle Ages, but it was exceedingly rare. As recently as the 1910s, cardiologists could go their entire careers without ever seeing a heart attack. In his paper, Dr. Keys provides his viewpoint that dietary fat consumption drives heart disease by elevating cholesterol in the bloodstream. It was a bold declaration, but men were being struck down in their forties and fifties by deadly heart attacks, and the country was absolutely gripped with fear over this new epidemic. If Dr. Keys had been right, it would have made him a true hero for warning the world at a time when most doctors had almost no experience with the condition. Other investigators were still examining other causes, including smoking, high blood pressure, high blood sugar (aka diabetes), and stress. But Dr. Keys had honed in on cholesterol—and seemed blind to the existence of other factors.

Dr. Keys's 1953 paper boldly asserts that "it is a fact that" people with heart disease "tend to have blood serum characterized by high cholesterol."

But the evidence he offers in support of this "fact" is flimsy, at best. Fifteen of the sixteen tables and figures he provides to back up a link between cholesterol and heart disease only provide irrelevant information, including cholesterol values for healthy men in several major cities, changes in cholesterol levels after eating nothing but rice and fruit for three weeks, changes in cholesterol levels in response to dietary cholesterol in rabbits, chickens, and a few other species—none of which could be used to support his point.

Only one dataset shows any kind of correlation between diet and heart disease at all. Still, it says nothing about cholesterol. This figure is a simple graph with six data points sitting along a line. The graph plotted how much fat people ate in a given country versus the per capita rate of heart attacks in that country. According to the graph, people in Japan ate the least fat of all the six countries he discussed, and also had the fewest heart attacks per capita. People in the United States ate the most fat and sat at the top of the line, outnumbering the per capita heart attack deaths by fifteen to one. The four countries in between sat neatly on the line linking the two extremes. Although the data was skimpy, at least the dietary fat–heart disease correlation looked solid.

The trouble was, he cheated.

Dr. Keys had left out the sixteen other countries that didn't fit along the neat line. This fact was made public by the authors of a 1957 paper that presented a similar graph with all twenty-two countries showing points scattered all over the place with no indication of any such neat perfect line. They concluded by specifically calling out Dr. Keys's blunder, writing, "It is immediately obvious that the inclusion of all the countries greatly reduces the apparent association."[2]

Dr. Keys's written responses to the critics who called out this deception have been described as "sarcastic" where professionalism was called for. Rather than welcoming dialogue around alternative viewpoints, which is generally considered a necessary part of the scientific process, he "did not like challenge from friends or foes."[3] Even his friends described him as a bully. His critics called him "arrogant, blunt and dismissive," and were suspicious of the fact that he never encouraged active debate.[4]

His fraudulent paper has come to be known as the Six Countries Study, even though that's not its actual title, because this story is so often told.

What's less well known about Dr. Keys is that this wasn't the only time he pulled a trick like that. His most famous and influential work was called the Seven Countries Study. This study began in the 1950s and continued for several decades, eventually leading to hundreds of publications. But when you read the study's reports, published periodically between 1970 and 1993, you find lots of unimportant information on irrelevant topics—things like what railroad company employees in Europe did differently from people living in Japan, and musings on the day-to-day activities of people collecting the data in Eastern versus Western Finland. The reports do not adhere to any standard of data collection or presentation. There appears to have been no standardized method of determining what people were eating. There are no figures summarizing the big picture that would support the conclusion that saturated fat led to elevated cholesterol and that cholesterol was causing heart attacks. There's isn't even a simple summary of how many people participated in the nutrition surveys, and there is no single chart that details the total number of heart attacks. This is basic data, and it's entirely missing. Yet the Seven Countries Study has become a cornerstone of medicine; it is still cited today as the proof that high cholesterol causes heart attacks.

Others have reviewed the data from the Seven Countries Study and found it to be full of holes. In 2014, a journalist who had spent ten years researching the history of our current dietary guidelines dug up some disturbing information. When interviewing doctors and scientists who'd worked during the 1970s and 1980s, contemporary with Dr. Keys, she discovered that in those early days many experts had tried to point out flaws with the cholesterol theory. But those who didn't join forces with the anti-saturated-fat campaigners would be disinvited from committees, unable to get grants, and sometimes forced into early retirement.[5] In 2015, a group of scientists who had reviewed the history of saturated fat research up to 1983—when the second official Dietary Guidelines for Americans was published—wrote an article disturbingly titled "Evidence from Randomised Controlled Trials Did Not Support the Introduction of Dietary Fat Guidelines in 1977 and 1983."[6] The scientists showed how, by citing the Seven Countries Study, the dietary guidelines committee was able to position the cholesterol theory as if it had been clinically proven, but that was not actually true.

To come to these contrarian conclusions, in some cases all it took was checking the references. I did this myself when a cholesterol management guideline I was supposed to follow called the ATP-III was released. Whenever the report made a claim that reducing cholesterol was beneficial, it cited a reference. So I checked the references. I found the ATP-III repeatedly referring to scientific articles that kept the real data out of the publication, showing only data that had been adjusted by statisticians, making it impossible to validate the claims of the study. Another trick I noticed was shifting the goalposts. For example, the title and conclusions may claim that saturated fat causes heart attacks, but when you read the study, you see they actually found that saturated fat elevates cholesterol, and then refer to other studies supposedly linking high cholesterol to heart attacks. When you track down those studies, you find deception there, too—such as missing data. Going from article to article, I started to feel like I was Charlie Brown, and the cholesterol theory of heart disease was Lucy, enticing me into kicking that football time and again, and time and again pulling the football away at the last minute, proving me the fool.

Thanks to the body of nonsensical data the Seven Countries Study contains, lowering cholesterol has since become a "surrogate endpoint" standing in for preventing heart attacks. This means that if a study shows that a specific diet—such as one low in fat—lowers your cholesterol, then the authors can claim it will also prevent heart attacks. Likewise, it means that if a diet is known to elevate cholesterol—such as the Atkins diet—then the authors get to claim it will cause heart attacks. Dr. Keys's thoughts still loom large on the nutrition research landscape.

Dr. Keys's force of personality, his bravado and bluster, may have prevented anyone from calling him out, or calling his bluff. This enabled him to grossly misrepresent a very important data point at a pivotal time in the early 1960s: how many cases he had.

A Man on a Mission

For all his flaws, Ancel Keys does deserve credit for one idea: the idea that diet does matter. Dr. Keys clearly believed that our propensity for disease is not entirely set in stone from the moment of our birth. He was operating from a belief that may have seemed to him like a minority viewpoint, the notion that we do have control over our fate— at least when it comes to heart disease. Perhaps it was knowing that to be true that drove him to such extremes. He also was among the first to point out that the US Public Health Service's scope was too limited. The same notorious 1953 paper that misrepresented data had also challenged public health officials to look beyond infectious and occupational diseases. He called for a sweeping campaign to "prevent or decrease the incidence of *all* forms of illness and disability" (emphasis in original), particularly cardiovascular disease.[7] For that, Dr. Keys deserves credit. Of course, since the Public Health Service was a potential source of research funds for him, this was a somewhat self-serving announcement. Still, there were clearly some positives to his campaigning.

But there is a potential moral pitfall you can end up in once you accept that dietary choices can cause illness. That is to blame the victim, and Dr. Keys was certainly guilty of that. A famous *Time* magazine article on Dr. Keys quotes him saying, "Puritans in New

---

England" believed that obesity was "a sin," and expressing this view that "Maybe if the idea got around again that obesity is immoral, the fat man would start to think." He lamented the "weak will" of people who chose "indulgent fatty foods" because they "want to eat themselves to death." He also called obesity itself "disgusting."[8] Given this attitude, he may have blamed people for their own heart attacks long before he ever collected a shred of evidence.

4,820 MISSING CASES

On January 13, 1961, *Time* magazine awarded Ancel Keys the title of Man of the Year. In the era before TV talk shows and the internet, a cover story in *Time* was the ultimate social proof.

The article opens with the implication that the case against saturated fat was already closed. "Americans eat too much fat…. [T]he calorie-heavy U.S. diet is 40% fat, and most of that is saturated fat—the insidious kind, says Dr. Keys, that increases blood cholesterol, damages arteries, and leads to coronary disease." It also paints Dr. Keys as decisive compared to other researchers who were bogged down with details. "[T]hey variously blame hypertension, stress, smoking and physical inactivity, while Keys gives these causes only minor roles."[9]

The article implies that Dr. Keys already had overwhelming evidence, reporting that in support of his idea, "Keys's chief weapon has been the sheer weight of solid statistics." One man, identified only as a Philadelphia physician, is quoted saying: "Every time you question this man Keys, he says, 'I've got 5,000 cases. How many do you have?'"

Indeed, many people cite Dr. Keys's own claims more than they cite verifiable published data. Publicationwise, Dr. Keys *had* amassed an impressive 190 scientific papers under his belt. But most of his articles on heart disease were comments on work *done by others*, peppered with his own prosaic musings about the importance of doing more research. Only three of the investigations into the role of cholesterol in heart attacks represented his own original, clinical work. It appears that by 1961 he'd evaluated the diet and cholesterol levels of just 180 heart attack cases, 72 of them from the Twin Cities and 108 from Naples, Italy.[10] By inflating this number, he successfully passed himself off as the singularly most knowledgeable person on the subject in the world. In 1961, the global effort to gather the data necessary to study the issue had only just begun, so by convincing the world he had so many cases, he gave the distinct impression that other scientists who might disagree with his cholesterol theory could not claim to have more expertise than him on the subject.

In fact, he never did reach 5,000 cases. By the Seven Countries Study's final analysis in 1985, the total case count tallied just 2,289.[11] So it appears that Dr. Keys shut down everyone who tried to question him with a fabricated number—and no one ever called his bluff. His ability to command authority must have intimidated scientists not accustomed to bullying. Perhaps most importantly, though, he'd curated close relationships with influential people, so that, by the time he'd started throwing out grossly inflated claims, he was well protected by his friends in high places.

THE AMERICAN HEART ASSOCIATION BACKS DR. KEYS, SUPPRESSES SMOKING DATA

Dr. Keys didn't work alone. He was aligned with a team of prominent physicians around the world, including Dr. Paul Dudley White, one of the founders of the American Heart Association (AHA) and its former president (who was also President Dwight D. Eisenhower's personal physician), and Dr. Irvine Heinly Page, the acting president of the American Heart Association and the first chair of research at the Cleveland Clinic.

Harvard Medical had accepted Dr. Keys into their inner circle and endorsed his ideas, boosting their acceptance among physicians. Dr. Keys served as a key adviser and spokesperson for the AHA on issues related to diet, lifestyle, and heart disease prevention. The AHA also spent a great deal of effort and money educating the public about Dr. Keys's ideas. Together with Irvine Heinly Page and Jeremiah Stamler (a cardiology researcher then with the Chicago Board of Health, who would be credited with introducing the term *risk factors* into the field), in 1956 Dr. Keys helped to launch the AHA's new "Prudent Diet" in a television campaign. The diet replaced butter, lard, beef, and eggs with vegetable oil, margarine, chicken, and cold cereal.[12] With the weight of prominent physicians behind it, the arguments for the diet were persuasive and it became popular. Millions abandoned traditional recipes in favor of a way of eating that looks like today's modern diet: low fat, low cholesterol, full of processed foods, and saturated with vegetable oil.

The AHA claims to be an evidence-based organization, but in 1956, when it launched its Prudent Diet, the first Seven Countries Study interim report was not yet published. It turns out that the AHA had received an infusion of cash from the vegetable oil industry, as we will see later in this chapter. This undisclosed conflict of interest gave it a financial incentive to promote vegetable oils as part of the Prudent Diet before there was data to back it up.

The AHA also failed to disclose the increasingly convincing link between smoking and heart attacks. In 1956, the AHA issued its first statement on smoking and heart disease, saying, "Much greater knowledge is needed before conclusions can be drawn concerning possible relationships between tobacco smoking and increased death rates from coronary heart disease."[13] In other words, there's not enough data for us to even consider issuing a warning about smoking.

This was false. Two years prior, the *British Medical Journal* had published a landmark study by the epidemiologist and medical doctor Richard Doll that strongly linked smoking and heart disease.[14] Dr. Doll, who had been conducting research on the health effects of smoking for over a decade, had amassed about 230 heart attack cases among the nearly 5,000 people he'd been following. He had found a particularly strong correlation between smoking and heart disease, almost as strong as the association between smoking and lung cancer. Based largely on this data and related work, the British government took a stand against smoking in a 1957 report called "Smoking and Health." The document offered physicians and health officials a one-stop, comprehensive review of the scientific evidence on the harmful effects of smoking, including its association with lung cancer, *heart disease*, and other illnesses. It was the first publication of its kind to recommend that smokers consider quitting, or at least cutting back.

However, during this time, the American Heart Association stayed laser focused on Dr. Keys and his talking points, funding research to attempt to prove the diet-heart hypothesis and ignoring everyone with different ideas. By 1961, the AHA had issued its first definitive dietary guidance to "reduce intake of total fat, saturated fat, and cholesterol" and "increase intake of polyunsaturated fat."[15] Echoing the Prudent Diet, it advised swapping out butter, eggs, red meat, and cheese for margarine, cereal, chicken, and fat-free cottage cheese and skim milk. Supporting the rationale behind this recommendation was a four-page report written by none other than Ancel Keys, along with other members of the AHA.[16] The report contains Dr. Keys's opinions but no supporting data. There is not a single footnote showing readers where to look for the evidence supporting this sweeping dietary recommendation.

To be clear, when the AHA endorsed the cholesterol theory of heart disease, it had no data to support its validity. Instead of data, it offered innuendo. This suggests the strong possibility that when they funded Dr. Keys's trips to seven countries around the world, the results were a foregone conclusion, and that Dr. Keys went through the motions for the sole purpose of making the endeavor look valid. That could explain why he didn't bother to create protocols for systematically collecting and presenting information.

In addition to these irregularities, Dr. Keys and the AHA also failed to warn the public that smoking might be an important factor driving heart attacks, going so far as to downplay the connection between smoking and heart disease even though they certainly knew about it. According to a short book called *The Seven Countries Study: A Scientific Adventure*, by the first five-year analysis in 1963, Dr. Keys knew that smoking twenty-five or more cigarettes daily increased heart attack fatalities by 400 percent, making smoking the most powerful predictor of death by heart attack by far.[17] But he did not include this link between smoking and heart attacks in his 1963 publications. Nor did he do so in the ensuing years.

Dr. Keys suppressed data from another study, too. Also in 1963, he reported on a separate project, a fifteen-year evaluation of heart disease risk factors among Minnesota "Business and Professional Men."[18] His report makes no mention of smoking. But, according to a film made about the project, he was paid to collect smoking data.[19]

It was one thing for Dr. Keys to push his anti-saturated-fat agenda, but for the entire AHA to downplay the smoking risk seems extraordinary. There was no obvious risk to the AHA for recommending against smoking. It seems not to have had any financial ties to the tobacco industry. Yet the AHA failed to issue any further statements on the harms of cigarette smoking until 1985, decades after the 1954 warning from the American Cancer Society and a 1964 US Surgeon General's report that echoed the cancer connection, adding chronic bronchitis to the list of consequences. What would the AHA possibly have to gain by staying mum on cigarettes?

To answer that question, let's take a moment to consider the cuckoo bird. This is the famous bird of Europe whose distinctive voice is imitated by cuckoo clocks. It is less well known for its peculiar parenting style, what's called *brood parasitism*. Female cuckoo birds lay their large eggs in the nests of smaller birds. The baby cuckoo hatches first, and within minutes, the blind, featherless newborn presses its back into the nearest egg, straightens its tiny legs, and heaves the egg up and over the edge of the nest. The baby bird repeats the process until there are no other eggs. The "host" mother then devotes all her time—and food—to rearing just the one baby, the cuckoo.

The nest parasite strategy works for birds, and for scientific theories. Cholesterol was Ancel Keys's egg, and smoking was not. Dr. Keys probably recognized that for his cholesterol theory to dominate the public discourse the way he desired, he would need to kill the other possible candidates for the cause of heart disease in the cradle, so to speak.

THE SMOKING GUN THAT THREATENED THE AMERICAN HEART ASSOCIATION

The AHA wasn't the only organization dedicated to understanding the cause of heart disease. It had competition. And smoking posed a threat to the AHA's desire to dominate the conversation. Aside from the fact that smoking as a cause of heart attacks was a competing theory, there is something unique about this particular risk factor that made it more of a threat to Dr. Keys's status as a global authority and to the AHA's status as the leading medical organization. It's a bit complex, but it takes us back to vegetable oil.

Smoking doesn't elevate blood cholesterol. Nor does it make people gain weight. It doesn't cause diabetes either. If smoking causes heart disease, it must work by a completely novel mechanism that had nothing to do with everything Ancel Keys cared about.

That mechanism is something we've talked about before in this book: *oxidation.* Autopsies of heart attack victims dating back to the 1910s revealed oxidized cholesterol in arterial plaques. As far back as the 1920s, scientists recognized that injecting unoxidized cholesterol into the arteries of lab animals did not give them arterial plaques. *Only* oxidized cholesterol could generate arterial plaques.[20]

Dr. Keys had a talent for biochemistry, so he could very well have recognized how this oxidation scenario threatened his idea. Cigarette smoke by its very nature could be presumed to exert toxicity through some kind of oxidative process, and by the 1950s, intense investigation into what elements in smoke caused this oxidation had already been underway for some time.[21] If oxidation was the mechanism behind heart disease, too, this would present Dr. Keys's ideas with a fatal mechanistic flaw. Remember, saturated fat is almost oxidation proof. Polyunsaturated fatty acids, however, are extremely prone to oxidation, and once PUFA oxidation starts, it can spread until it oxidizes any nearby cholesterol. The oxidized cholesterol stays put in arterial plaques, making it look like a guilty party to anyone without the necessary biochemistry expertise, while the PUFA—having been oxidized—no longer exists.

Given his background in biochemistry, Dr. Keys would certainly have known all of this. If cigarettes could be linked to heart attacks, then so could oxidation, and researchers with biochemistry expertise would recognize that blaming saturated fat makes little mechanistic sense—and his theory could easily be disproven. His entire argument rested on correlational data, which, without a plausible mechanism, would be dismantled.

And there was one more serious threat posed by the cigarette link: the correlation over time between per capita smoking rates and the rise of heart attacks. Cigarette smoking had been on the rise since the turn of the century, in almost exact parallel with the rise of deadly heart attacks, as shown in Figure 6–1. While he could have argued that correlation is not causation, his own arguments were entirely correlational. So if the world had been made aware of the very strong association between smoking and heart disease, that, too, could have snuffed the life out of his theory.

Smoking and heart attack deaths would decline in tandem during the second half of the twentieth century. The AHA has claimed that its anti-saturated-fat campaign is partly responsible, but that, too, is unsupported. As shown in Figure 6–1, the amount of saturated fat Americans ate hovered at a fairly constant level throughout the entire twentieth century. It didn't go up as heart attacks increased, and it didn't go down as they declined.

We often hear the phrase "Correlation is not causation." But without correlation there can be no causation. And saturated fat intake simply does not correlate with heart attack deaths. This graph I'm showing you here is

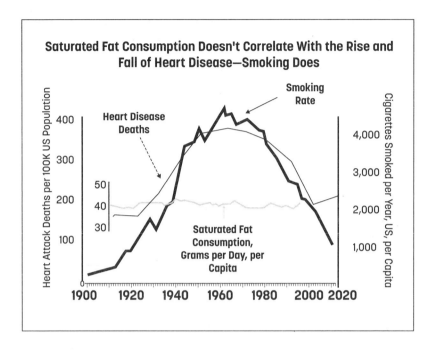

Figure 6-1: If confronted with this figure, our health authorities would have to admit they've been lying to us for decades. (Assuming they admit the data is accurate.)

Vegetable oils and smoking are a deadly combination. Fortunately, when smoking peaked, our vegetable oil consumption was still relatively low. Unfortunately, now that smoking rates have dropped, our vegetable oil consumption has exploded, nearly doubling between 2010 and 2020. (Refer to Figure 0-1 for vegetable oil data.)

Where do we see the effect of vegetable oils? **The kink on the right side of the heart disease death rates is probably driven by vegetable oils.** Remember, vegetable oils manifest many of their health effects by building up in our body fat. But it takes about five years for our body fat PUFA to match our dietary PUFA, and our dietary PUFA is still increasing. If consumption levels out and stays constant (at roughly 77 grams per day), then the full effects of this level of intake will start to manifest five years from now.

For sources used to create this figure, see the endnotes for this chapter.

based on readily available data. If the AHA was truly dedicated to preventing heart attacks, it could have shown this to the world twenty years ago.

To understand why the AHA made the choices it made, we need to understand the impact and motivations of the organization as a whole.

THE AHA BATTLES WITH ITSELF OVER FUNDING STREAMS

Today, the American Heart Association has a billion-dollar-a-year budget, and—thanks to heavy-hitting connections at places like Harvard Medical—its ideology powerfully influences the government's food policy (even though it's not a government agency, as its name might imply).

The US government document that encodes our official nutrition guidelines is called the Dietary Guidelines for Americans (DGA). The committee of people who write the guidelines often includes members who currently or previously played important roles in the AHA. And because other institutions and organizations defer to the AHA for their nutrition ideas, the AHA and its nutrition ideology have more influence on the DGA than any other organization or group of individuals.

The DGA, in turn, dictates what foods are made available in institutions and programs that receive government funding—for example, the taxpayer-funded Supplemental Nutrition Assistance Program (SNAP) that serves an average of 41.5 million people per month. The DGA influences the menu served to the 33 million people admitted to hospitals each year, the 1.3 million nursing home residents, and the 2.1 million people in prisons around the United States. It also dictates what 41 million schoolchildren get served for breakfast, lunch, and snacks, as well as what colleges and universities can serve their 17 million students. Dietitians and physicians generally abide by these guidelines, too, along with every other kind of licensed healthcare professional, from massage therapists to athletic trainers to dentists to nurses and so on. The US Department of Agriculture also abides by the DGA when deciding, for example, which crops get subsidized and which don't. These policies, in turn, determine what farmers grow and how much it costs, and therefore largely determine what's available on most grocery store shelves, most restaurant menus, and mostly everywhere else. All of this gives the AHA substantial, if indirect, influence over the foods many of us eat every day, even if we do not realize it.

Who Funds the AHA?

The story of how the American Heart Association came to dominate nutrition thought begins with the very first industry to fund the AHA. As we'll learn, the AHA was effectively launched with a large sum of money that came straight from the vegetable oil industry. The AHA used this money to support Ancel Keys's cholesterol theory—and to convince the public to start eating vegetable oils. The AHA continues to receive money from industries selling vegetable oil, and the AHA's practice guidelines continue to support the vegetable oil industry today.

Today, our massive processed food industry depends heavily on vegetable oils, as do the companies that grow most of our foods. The AHA's top corporate donors now include heavy hitters from Big Ag and Big Food, including Conagra, Monsanto (before the company closed in 2018), LibertyLink, Kellogg's, Quaker, Tyson, FritoLay, Campbell, and Subway.[22] The AHA's website states that 80 percent of their $1 billion plus annual revenue comes from non-corporate sources. Nevertheless, in 2021, drug and device companies donated just over $40 million, and "other" corporations donated more than $140 million.[23] The AHA uses this money in part to support scientists interested in exploring the benefits of vegetable oils, the harms of cholesterol, and new ways to use drugs that lower cholesterol—and to publish and publicize their findings. The money also goes to lobbyists who influence public health policy at the state and national levels.[24]

The AHA also publishes or copublishes fourteen medical journals on various subjects related to cardiovascular disease treatment, research, and practice standards. The total volume amounts to thousands of articles per year. This makes it easy for the organization to keep the anti-cholesterol message top of mind. Notably, other medical and scientific publication outlets have printed dozens of articles that have called the diet-heart theory to question.[25] The AHA, however, appears to have published none. Funding research through donated money is a cornerstone of the organization, and a mechanism for controlling what doctors learn. The AHA has donated $5 billion to research since 1949 ($461.7 million during the 2021–2022 fiscal year).[26] As a result, it has tremendous influence on health and nutrition research. It gets to decide which topics will be investigated and which studies will be published in its journals—and which studies won't, which, in some cases, means they won't be published at all.

Because of its long history, wide-ranging influence, and extensive publications, the AHA has become the organization that other organizations turn to for guidance on nutrition. This includes other nonprofits, such as the American Diabetes Association and the American Cancer Society, as well as medical organizations like the American Medical Association and the American College of Physicians.

The fact that other organizations unquestioningly accept the AHA's ideology hinders basic, necessary nutrition and toxicology research. During my interview with Dr. Eric Decker, a food scientist I introduced in chapter 1, he pointed out that nutrition leadership is hung up on cholesterol while it should be focusing on oxidation. "My biggest frustration with all these nutrition groups is they don't know how food is made or how food changes during processing," he said. According to Dr. Decker, even experts at the National Institutes of Health don't understand the relevant oxidation science. He explained that whenever he has submitted grant proposals to the NIH to test the health effects of oxidized oil, "the grants would get killed." The criticism of his applications was always the same: "These compounds [the toxins he and others have detected] aren't there in concentrations enough that they're a problem" to human health. Since the NIH's decision-makers don't believe the toxins are present in meaningful amounts, they don't believe it's worth pursuing the research. So Dr. Decker and a tiny handful of toxicologists know about the toxins. But doctors and other scientists do not.

That makes it hard for the food industry to keep the food supply safe. It also makes it hard for toxicologists to do their research. According to Dr. Frances Sladek, whom we met in chapter 3, her biggest challenge is the *perception* that vegetable oils are the healthy fats and saturated fats are unhealthy. Because of that perception, she told me during an interview, the people who need to approve her grants believe the science is already settled. She told me that this perception, more than the financial aspect, is the reason why she's met "huge resistance" and has to fight "an uphill battle trying to get this stuff funded and published."[27] It makes her work all the more valuable, and, in my mind, it makes anyone daring to pursue the truth a scientific hero.

So here we are today, where we have toxicologists and experts in food safety who disagree with the AHA's position on the safety of polyunsaturated fats, and, because the AHA's vast influence gives it control over nutrition thought, these professionals have trouble getting necessary work funded. Meanwhile, the AHA continues to actively promote seed oils, and it continues to support those, like Dr. Walter Willett, who dismiss or discredit experts like Dr. Chris Ramsden who are producing evidence to the contrary. In other words, the AHA is effectively blocking progress in medical science, and, perhaps most egregiously, it is promoting a diet that's actively harming our cardiovascular health. In the beginning, however, the association's culture was very different.

When the AHA was founded in 1924, it was supported only with annual dues from a small collection of doctors concerned about the growing problem of heart disease. Heart attacks skyrocketed after World War I, and the organization felt the pressure of knowing there was so much to learn but such little funding to do the necessary research. In 1942, AHA executive director H. M. "Jack" Marvin, a New Haven, Connecticut, cardiologist, made an ambitious proposal to solve the AHA's "chronic fiscal problems." Lack of funds stood in the way of two of the organization's highest-priority goals: sponsoring research and establishing public health and lay education programs. Without fundraising, the organization would be limited to utilizing the small pool of government funds to achieve its goals. And that pool had just grown a little too crowded for the AHA's tastes.

In 1946, a newly founded organization calling itself the American College of Cardiologists (ACC) threatened the AHA's access to the limited supply of funds. Collaboration with this new organization might have been another option, but apparently that was not on the table.

By 1946, the AHA had grown large enough that it was divided into two camps with polar opposite visions. One group, the expansionists, saw a need "to embark upon a broad expansion of activities and to employ a firm of specialists to outline a fund-raising campaign." The other, the contractionists, wanted to keep "the emphasis upon the small, strictly scientific, professional and clinical aspects of the Association" and didn't see a need to solicit outside funding.

That year, several members of the expansionist group wrote a letter to the AHA's president calling for "a dramatic restructuring of the organization." They lamented the "many other organizations espousing the cause of heart disease."[28] The existence of these other organizations threatened their concept of the AHA as the "dominant organization in the cardiovascular field in the country." Aside from exaggerating the number of organizations (there was just the one, the ACC), the letter raises questions about the group's values. It makes no mention of actually improving public health. Among the contributors to this letter were several men who would later serve leadership roles in the newly restricted organization. They spoke openly about eliminating "competition." According to internal documents, "AHA leaders hoped to suppress the new organization" and attempted "to discourage physicians from joining the ACC."[29] Achieving sole authority status seems to have been at least as important as doing the necessary research to provide useful information to the public.

By 1948, the expansionists within the AHA had failed to suppress the other organization, but they had accomplished a coalition within their ranks. After all the saber rattling, "the reformers were galvanized into action."[30] That year, the expansionists put their proposition to start soliciting money from the public and industry to a vote.

Let's consider who might have been in a position to make the largest donations. The obvious answer: giant multinational companies. AHA members who objected to the proposal argued, somewhat prophetically, that the organization might be tempted to make "unjustified claims about the cure of heart disease."[31] After intense debates about the pros and cons of opening themselves up to conflicts of interest that might impede scientific progress, a narrow majority voted in favor of reframing the organization's financial structure from member-based to donation-based in order to "broaden its scope."[32]

A journalist, Nina Teicholz, has painstakingly examined the AHA's meeting minutes from that time period to unravel its early industry entanglements. For a 2014 book, she wrote, "For decades, the American Heart Association was small and underfunded, with virtually no income. Then in 1948, it got lucky."[33] In 1948, the AHA received a cash infusion of $1,740,000 from a fundraising campaign tied to a popular radio contest, called "Walking Man." The company sponsoring the contest was Procter & Gamble—the world's largest manufacturer of cottonseed and other edible oil products. The AHA had just partnered up with vegetable oil.

The impact on the AHA's ideology was immediate. Before 1948, the AHA president and one of the most ambitious reformers, Dr. Paul Dudley White, did not believe saturated fat caused heart disease. According to his colleagues, he was initially critical of Dr. Keys. After 1948, he followed the money, joined with Keys, and changed his tune. He would become the first president of the new AHA. Those against the reform would have been watching their worst fears being realized, and in fact, several of them abandoned the AHA for its competition. Because, as history shows, the new AHA immediately started making "unjustified claims about the cure of heart disease."[34]

And it has continued doing so ever since.

A DEAL WITH THE DEVIL

The AHA had gotten lucky, but it wasn't dumb luck. It was the brilliance of the man at the helm of the PR firm P&G had retained, Edward Bernays.

Bernays is widely recognized as the de facto inventor of the public relations industry, and he's probably the twentieth century's most influential person that most of us learn nothing about. He wielded influence behind the closed doors of the most powerful corporations and political leaders in the world, including at least four presidents, several multinational companies, and the Central Intelligence Agency. He'd begun in advertising, where he revolutionized the industry. Before Bernays, many advertisers tended to tout the practical, rational aspects of their products, things like durability and effectiveness. Bernays taught advertisers to manipulate people's emotions instead. He'd learned about the power of emotions from an uncle he'd grown up admiring, none other than the father of modern psychiatry, Sigmund Freud.

Bernays took Freud's theories about the inner workings of the individual mind and applied them to groups of individuals, so that those in power, his corporate and government clients, could better control the population. Bernays wondered, "If we understand the mechanism and motives of the group mind, is it not possible to control and regiment the masses according to our will without their knowing it?"[35] For Bernays, gifted with mind-control skills befitting an Orwellian villain, the answer was clearly yes.

It may be impossible to overstate the degree to which Ed Bernays influenced the culture of the twentieth century, for better or worse. In the late 1920s, he'd had a hand in ad campaigns for the American Tobacco Company calling cigarettes "Torches of Freedom." This equated smoking to an act of emancipation, thus elevating women who smoked from their status as "trashy" while also giving them a sense of power. The Virginia Slims advertisements of the 1970s built its brand concept on Bernays's initial image of female smokers as modern, liberated women.

If your tap water is fluoridated (as it is for nearly three-quarters of the US population[36]), that's thanks to Bernays. In the 1940s and 1950s, he worked on behalf of the US Public Health Service to convince the American public that water fluoridation was safe and beneficial to human health. The industry needed some good PR to clean up its image because of where fluoride comes from. One of the most common forms of fluoride added to our water here in the United States is fluorosilicic acid, which is derived from the scrubbing systems of the phosphate fertilizer industry. In other words, chimney soot from industrial plants. Of course, strict regulations ensure it gets cleaned up and rendered safe for consumption.

His influence was not limited to the United States. In the early and mid-twentieth century, Bernays's work on behalf of the United Fruit Company impacted a vast swath of the political landscape across Central and South America. Bernays used many tools from his kit of public relations techniques to promote the interests of United Fruit. He worked with the CIA and other agencies to create a propaganda campaign portraying the democratically elected president of Guatemala as a communist—and a threat to US interests—which ultimately led to his removal from power. This had a chilling effect on democracy and social justice movements in those countries, as governments were more likely to be overthrown if they pursued policies that were seen as threatening to US business interests.

Bernays not only knew how to manipulate people, he knew how to get people excited about being manipulated, a process he describes in detail in his 1947 book, *The Engineering of Consent*. The book enumerates a variety of persuasive techniques, including propaganda, advertising, and other forms of mass communication, that he used to create seemingly any desired response from the public. While today we might think differently, he didn't see any problem with using psychology for these purposes and in fact believed his work was essential and beneficial. He felt it was important for educated elites to control the people he considered uneducated. It was good for commerce, capitalism, and the democratic process itself. "The conscious and intelligent manipulation of the organized habits and

opinions of the masses," he had written in an earlier book, "is an important element in democratic society."[37] In other words, he and his clients
know better about what's good for us than we do.

One of Bernays's favorite manipulative techniques involved tapping
into the immense psychological power of medical doctors. Doctors were
a key instrument for Bernays to choreograph behavior "because a doctor
is an authority to most people, regardless of how much he [the doctor]
knows, or doesn't know."[38] Citing his 1993 interview with Bernays (who
was 102 at the time), journalist Christopher Bryson wrote, in a book about
fluoride, "'You can get practically any idea accepted,' Bernays told me,
chuckling. 'If doctors are in favor, the public is willing to accept it.'"[39] One
of Bernays's favorite tactics for promoting new ideas and products to the
public was to stress a claimed public health benefit. He described its effectiveness as "child's play."

By catching Bernays's attention, the AHA hit the jackpot. Thanks to
Bernays, the AHA's many budgetary concerns evaporated overnight. Certainly, companies had paid individual doctors to endorse products before.
But this was a whole other category of relationship. The AHA represented
an entire specialty of medical doctors with ambitions to lead the conversation on heart disease. The money would be used for everything the AHA
had hoped to accomplish. It was enough to fund both cardiovascular
research and nutrition education programs for the public. Dr. Keys and
the AHA had unknowingly become the benefactors of more than money.
They'd been handed the golden ticket: a proven and winning formula with
a track record of phenomenal success.

In one fell swoop, Bernays helped take the AHA "from its unimpor-
tance," as he described it during the 1993 interview, "and made it a large,
effective organization."[40] The $1.74 million that the association received
because Bernays selected its name from the pile of possible contest benefi-
ciaries rocketed the newly reformed AHA off to a stellar start, converting
it from a collection of egotistical cardiologists into a national power-
house. This infusion of money, worth about $30 million in today's dollars,

provided the AHA with the funds it needed to become the dominant force in cardiovascular research, just as the ambitious expansionists had envisioned. More than just a professional society with a research and education arm, the AHA had joined the ranks of true influencers. Or, as Bernays described it, "those who manipulate the unseen mechanism of society [and] constitute an invisible government which is the true ruling power of our country."[41]

The ideas that Ancel Keys and the AHA were promoting about saturated fats were especially valuable to Procter & Gamble because at that time the edible oil industry had a serious marketing problem. Remember, consumers had resisted these oils since their introduction in the early 1900s.[42] That resistance had no doubt frustrated the entire edible oil industry, particularly as oil production ramped up in the early postwar period. Bernays couldn't have done better for P&G than to pick the AHA from among the heap of other nonprofit organizations the company might have donated to. Since the AHA was already saying that saturated fat was unhealthy, it might even agree to say that vegetable oil, which contained virtually no saturated fat, was healthy. Of course, Bernays may not have known about Ancel Keys, but he was probably confident the investment would pay for itself, since, "by the law of averages, you can usually find an individual in any field who will be willing to accept new ideas, and the new ideas then infiltrate the others who haven't accepted it."[43] In other words, knowing how the world works, Bernays gambled that some doctor would figure out how to take advantage of the money in ways that would benefit the company.

And the gamble paid off handsomely. As history shows, the AHA was not only willing, but it opened the floodgates. Remember the Prudent Diet, the AHA's 1956 program promoting vegetable oil? It specifically cited saturated fat as the cause of heart attacks and promoted vegetable oil—virtually free of saturated fat—as the antidote to heart attacks. Coming from the nation's top doctors, the new dietary recommendations made a powerful (if unfounded) argument compelling the growing numbers of housewives, gravely concerned about their husbands' health, to give up their traditional ingredients for good. (It also offered a more actionable step than convincing their spouses to stop smoking.) Suddenly, the old "inexplicable prejudice against the use of vegetable oil" vanished. P&G, one of the leading producers of vegetable oils, reaped the rewards as its products started flying off the shelves. *The Prudent Diet* eventually became a book that sold millions of copies, went into multiple reprints, and is still in use today.

Unlike the other organizations Bernays had helped, the AHA didn't actually hire him, and so the AHA's decision-makers and scientists may never have had any direct conversations with the puppet master who'd pulled their strings. As far as they knew, the money the AHA received from Procter & Gamble was a lucky break, and it was a no-strings-attached scenario.

Except that it wasn't—if they wanted more. And no doubt Ed Bernays, who continued to work for Procter & Gamble for many more years, knew what the future would hold. His client, P&G, would continue to benefit from the relationship, and the AHA would continue to come back to the industry till. There was no reason not to. After all, if Dr. Keys was right and their product was healthy, then why not develop a closer relationship? The AHA made friends of many companies selling vegetable oil, who would later make hefty payments directly to the AHA for the use of its "Heart Healthy" checkmark emblem.[44]

Their course was now fixed. The people at the AHA would continue to work within the oil-is-better-than-traditional-fats paradigm to serve their own ambitions and the needs of their newfound friends in the vegetable oil industry. Some within the AHA must have felt it was a deal with the devil, but it probably seemed like a dream come true to a man like Ancel Keys, on his mission to prove his detractors wrong. Unfortunately for everyone alive today, whenever Dr. Keys failed to substantiate his theory he was unable to admit he was wrong. As we saw in chapter 5, he even chose to suppress his own data rather than publish the results of the failed (to him) Minnesota Coronary Experiment.

Ancel Keys passed away in 2004 at the age of one hundred. The AHA founders have long since retired, having successfully captained the AHA to the position of dominance they'd aspired to. There's no one left to suffer the embarrassments of having been wrong. True leadership might be best defined by willingness to recognize mistakes and change directions when necessary. But the AHA is staying the course. So this flawed theory would seem to be kept alive for financial reasons *only*.

As we will see in the next chapter, the fear of cholesterol is now a key mechanism powering the vast economic engine of the American medical system, a system that grows stronger, larger, and more profitable the more we depend upon it. Whether you're healthy or not, the failed diet-heart hypothesis is costing you money, and, chances are, it has cost people you know their lives.

CHAPTER 7

The Sicker You Get, the Richer They Grow

IN THIS CHAPTER YOU WILL LEARN

- The fear of "high cholesterol" has greatly enriched the health-care industry by creating opportunities to sell drugs for this fabricated problem and for the real problems caused by vegetable oil.
- Because of their great wealth, drug companies now control, to an alarming degree, how doctors get educated.
- Doctors have no idea they prescribe many drugs that are likely to do most of us more harm than good.
- We can escape both sickness and harmful drugs by rejecting the idea that high cholesterol is unhealthy—and by avoiding vegetable oils.

As recently as 2001, health news headlines were generally positive. People were living longer; some speculated that newborn babies might live 120 years or more. This rosy outlook was most often attributed to better preventive medicine, including our healthier, lower-saturated-fat diets.

Meanwhile, my overwhelming daily experience as a primary care doctor with a waiting room full of medication-dependent adults and children told me that the opposite was true. It looked to me like human health was in midst of a precipitous decline. Type 2 diabetes was becoming increasingly common. More women were experiencing pregnancy and delivery complications, driving escalating cesarean rates.[1] Food allergies were becoming more prevalent every year. Learning disorders in children were on the rise, along with behavioral problems, joint problems, chronic allergies, asthma, brain cancers, congenital growth anomalies, and more. The statistics were there, and obvious, but for a long time, nobody was even talking about it.

Then, in 2003, we got a wake-up call. An article in *JAMA* titled "Lifetime Risk for Diabetes Mellitus in the United States" announced that our century of lengthening life spans had come to an end.[2] The authors explained that type 2 diabetes would chop 11.6 years off a man's life, and 14.3 years off a woman's. In a related interview, Dr. William Klish of Texas Children's Hospital warned, "If we don't get this epidemic [childhood obesity] in check, for the first time in a century children will be looking forward to a shorter life expectancy than their parents."[3]

You might expect this to have taken some wind out of the argument that avoiding saturated fat has been helpful. But instead, authorities doubled down, claiming our diets were still too high in saturated fat, and we needed to eat more vegetable oils. Today our polyunsaturated fat consumption exceeds the AHA's recommended 10 percent of our total calories—it's between 12 and 15 percent. In defiance of their own guidelines, our experts still tell us we need more vegetable oil in our diets.[4] While (as we saw in chapter 5) scientists have called the low cholesterol paradigm into question, probably not coincidentally, not one of these reports has been published in any of the fourteen AHA-affiliated journals. Nor have they been picked up by any major media outlets. The paradigm remains unshifted.

In this chapter, we're going to see how the AHA has joined forces with Big Health Care and Big Food to create a trifecta of power so encompassing that it now controls how doctors get educated, how they behave, and what they get paid. Today, chronic illness is big business—and as long as doctors believe high cholesterol is a health problem, there's money to be made in medications to bring cholesterol levels down.

CHOLESTEROL-LOWERING DRUGS: INEFFECTIVE AND DANGEROUS

If the science on low cholesterol and the dubiousness of the diet-heart hypothesis aren't enough, the history of cholesterol-lowering drugs should give us pause about the safety of lowering cholesterol. In 1959, the US Food and Drug Administration approved the world's first cholesterol-lowering medication, triparanol, made by the William S. Merrell Company. By 1962, the FDA discovered that the company had provided falsified laboratory data in order to earn approval, and the agency removed triparanol from the market.[5] The falsified data had omitted reference to cataracts and serious skin problems found in rats and dogs during trials performed to assess the drug's safety. And unfortunately, some patients who had taken the drug for more than a year had also developed cataracts and serious skin problems. While the drug was a complete bust, it taught the industry a key lesson about side effects.

From the point of view of the pharmaceutical industry, it's best to release a drug that causes a whole lot of vague side effects, not just one that's easy to see. That may seem counterintuitive, but think about it this way. It took many years to recognize HIV/AIDS as an infection because the virus causes so many symptoms over such a long span of time that doctors had no idea they were all related. On the other hand, the recent mpox (monkeypox) virus was easy to recognize because it quickly causes a characteristic rash. HIV/AIDS didn't behave like a typical infection. Mpox does.

Triparanol directly blocked cholesterol production—and only cholesterol production—by blocking the last step in the body's process of building a cholesterol molecule. This quickly caused a buildup of the second-to-last molecule, called desmosterol. Desmosterol built up in the skin and eye tissues, where it caused cataracts and rashes. This chemical was a telltale sign that the drug was causing the side effects.

The next cholesterol-lowering drug, clofibrate, would lower cholesterol without leaving a telltale signature. It did that by working in a very roundabout fashion. Clofibrate was released in 1967 by the Imperial Chemical Company.

Clofibrate works in such an indirect way that it's hard to even describe what it does, but it's related to modifying the expression of multiple genes in the liver. Imperial Chemical—not the government—had designed and paid for the prerelease trials that the FDA used to evaluate whether to approve it. It took many years before a respectably sized, non-industry-funded study could be completed. The first such study, published in 1984, revealed that, while clofibrate slightly reduced deaths from heart attacks over a five-year period, it also increased overall mortality during that same time frame by a whopping 47 percent. These deaths were "due to a wide variety of causes other than IHD [ischemic heart disease]."[6] After more years and legal battles—and deaths—clofibrate was finally removed from the market in 2002. However, another cholesterol-lowering drug very similar to clofibrate, called fenofibrate, is still on the market. Like clofibrate, fenofibrate lowers cholesterol by an indirect, super-complex series of drug-gene interactions. Like clofibrate, it seems to reduce heart attack deaths but not a person's overall chance of dying—based on results from a systematic review of fifteen trials.[7] Like clofibrate, fenofibrate *increases* overall mortality. But unlike clofibrate, the FDA has not required its removal. So doctors continue to prescribe it.

In 2011, it was announced that research on a drug called evacetrapib was underway. Evacetrapib was supposed to be a miracle pill. It was the first drug that could actually raise your HDL, the so-called "good" cholesterol, while at the same time lowering your LDL, the "bad" cholesterol. It worked remarkably well to shift the numbers right where cardiologists were saying they should be. But by 2018, after twelve thousand people had taken the drug for more than two years, the study was stopped early "for futility," according to official reports, and the drug was withdrawn from further use. What does that mean, "for futility"? Technically, it means that "the likelihood of finding a treatment effect is low." But that's not quite accurate. They'd found a treatment effect, all right. The people on evacetrapib had had 25 percent *more* heart attacks than those in the control group who were taking a placebo, and 58 percent more of the evacetrapib patients died.[8]

How did the cholesterol theory survive this explicit sign of failure? Well, we've already seen one piece of spin, the claim of futility, suggesting it had no effect. The medical and lay media failed to acknowledge the mortality problem. That made the rest easier. It was shrugged off as a mystery in one article titled "The Mystery of Evacetrapib."[9] Another labeled it a "paradox" that had "dumbfounded many experts."[10] That article actually blamed the manufacturer for chasing "surrogate endpoints" (meaning raising HDL rather than preventing heart attacks) and called for greater oversight. Of course, lowering LDL is a surrogate endpoint, too, yet the authors of this article failed to point that out.

This history of the difficulty of identifying a safe cholesterol-lowering strategy should be an obvious red flag warning that lowering cholesterol might be a really bad idea. Unfortunately, the fear of cholesterol is so ingrained that most doctors can't see it that way. Fear of cholesterol also prevents doctors from recognizing the devastating side effects of the most popular category of cholesterol-lowering drugs, called statins.

A statin called Zocor was the first-ever true blockbuster drug. Today, there are more than a dozen statins on the market, and they are among the top ten most prescribed medications on the planet.

Statins lower cholesterol quite indirectly, by blocking one of the enzymes involved in building cholesterol molecules at a point much earlier in the process than the now defunct triparanol. Statins block the formation of a small molecule called mevalonate. This blockage reduces the body's ability to make cholesterol, which can cut some people's serum cholesterol levels down by half. Statins also block the production of all the larger molecules that the body makes from mevalonate. Cholesterol is just one of them. Others include isoprenoids, farnesyls, geranyls, and coenzyme Q. Some of these molecules help the immune system function. Some of them form the skeleton of the cell, giving it structure and mobility. Some help cells hold on tight to their neighbors, forming barriers to bacterial invasion and blocking entry of unwanted materials. Missing any of these molecules could cause a wide variety of side effects.

Indeed, side effects printed on the package insert taped to bottles of brand-named statins include headaches, sleep problems, vision problems, memory problems, depression, pancreatitis, liver inflammation, skin rashes, a kind of nerve damage that causes tingling or burning pains, dizziness, weakness, fatigue, and digestive problems, including constipation, diarrhea, or bloating. On top of the sheer variety of potential problems, the symptoms may take a while to start. Or they may fluctuate. Moreover, statin drug side effects overlap with symptoms of aging—including fatigue, muscle weakness or stiffness, memory problems, mood changes, and word-finding difficulties. All of this makes it difficult for people to mentally connect starting the drug to the start of their new discomfort.

Many statin side effects bring people to their doctor's office. But doctors have repeatedly been reassured that statins are safe. So, all too often, side effects are misdiagnosed, and medicated accordingly—something that I have seen many times in patients who come to see me after other doctors piled on prescription after prescription. If you have muscle aches, that's probably arthritis, and you'll be advised to take anti-inflammatories. If you get a skin rash, that might look a bit like eczema or psoriasis, so you'll get a steroid cream or other immune-suppressing agent. If you get recurring infections, you'll be treated for those. Diabetes is one of the few accepted complications of statin therapy, but doctors are convinced that the drug is worth it. So instead of being told to drop the drug, you may be given a medication to reduce your blood sugar.

The Statin Slippery Slope

I've met many people on multiple drugs to alleviate unrecognized statin side effects. One such patient is a man I'll call Steve, a construction manager who was sixty-two when I met him. His doctor first prescribed him a statin in his mid-forties. Shortly thereafter, without having made any dietary changes, Steve developed persistent heartburn. But his doctors didn't consider that the statin might be the reason he suddenly developed heartburn, even though it's listed as a possible adverse reaction on the pamphlet accompanying every statin prescription, under the heading "dyspepsia." Instead, his doctor prescribed an acid blocker, which alters the microbiome, reduces bone density, and increases risk of a variety of infections. Fortunately, Steve did not suffer any of those. Several years later, however, he developed depression. So Steve went on an antidepressant. Even though depression is listed on the package insert, the issue was attributed to a difficult divorce. The antidepressant caused sexual side effects, as they commonly do. So Steve went to a urologist. The urologist gave him testosterone shots because his testosterone was low—but remember, cholesterol is a building block for testosterone. Next, he developed high triglycerides, which is a common side effect of testosterone shots. His doctor said he needed to up his dose of statin, which he tried to do, but it caused miserable muscle aches.

That was when he came to see me. We worked together to successfully take him off everything, including his statin. However, now he has another problem: his cholesterol is high and his other doctors are unhappy with him. This is a bigger problem than it sounds like, as having a good therapeutic relationship with your doctor is known to improve health outcomes. If your doctor is unhappy with you, that can disrupt the patient-physician relationship, and it may prevent you from going to the doctor when you need one.

Statin-induced side effects are not recognized enough—even though nearly three-quarters of people who take statins will develop at least one form of side effect.

STATIN-INDUCED MUSCLE PAINS AND HEART FAILURE

According to some reports, 74 percent of people given statins develop aches and pains.[11] In my own experience, about half the people taking a statin experience minor aches and pains but stick with the drug anyway, because they're told they'll die if they don't.

A much smaller proportion develop muscle weakness or myopathy severe enough that they find it hard to "climb stairs, get up from a sofa, get up from the toilet," says Dr. Robert Rosenson, a cardiologist at Mount Sinai, in an interview for *The Atlantic* magazine.[12] He's had patients fall down on the street because they couldn't lift their leg over a curb. The number of people who experience such severe problems in clinical trials is reportedly less than 1 percent. In these trials, only about 3 percent need to stop the medication due to side effects. But outside of clinical trials, when surveying the general population, that figure is around 30 percent.[13]

Dr. Peter H. Langsjoen, a fellow of the prestigious American College of Cardiology, has pointed out that one of the most important muscles in our bodies is the heart, and that it is not immune to statin-induced problems. He's written several papers on the condition called "statin-induced cardiomyopathy" (cardiomyopathy means heart failure). In one, he reported on 192 patients who came to his clinic with heart failure possibly related to their statin.[14] He treated them by stopping their statin and starting a supplement called CoQ10 to replace the missing coenzyme Q (one of those molecules that our bodies can't make efficiently when taking a statin), and it's essential for normal mitochondria function. After an average of 2.8 years off their statin, more than half of the patients experienced dramatic increases in activity and visible (by ultrasound) improvements in the strength of their heartbeat. Without their statin, however, their cholesterol levels increased significantly. How many dropped dead after stopping their statin? At the one-year point: none. 2.8 percent had died by year three. Typical one-year mortality rates in patients with similarly severe heart failure are over 25 percent.[15] In spite of the widespread use of statins, the clear link between statin use and muscle damage, and evidence that at the very least statin users with weak hearts should be given CoQ10, the cardiology community has largely ignored the problem. As currently practiced, cardiology is not a science. It's dogma.

STATINS, BRAIN HEALTH, AND MENTAL HEALTH

Quite a few studies have raised concerns about statins' effects on the brain and nervous system. One actually used a statin to create animal models of dementia.[16] A few human studies show direct evidence that statins worsen brain health. For example, taking statins after age sixty speeds cognitive decline.[17] And lowering cholesterol below 160 impairs speaking ability in people with Parkinson's.[18] Many people report problems with memory, mood, speaking, and coordination that thankfully resolve after stopping statins, although it can take years.[19] (For a personal narrative of what it's like to live with statin-induced brain damage, I recommend a YouTube video called "Statins Made Me Stupid."[20])

Dr. Beatrice Golomb is a professor of medicine at the University of California, San Diego, who has been concerned about statins since the late 1980s, before they were actually released. Her worry began when she was a medical intern, after two early studies testing their safety and effectiveness had shown that statins reduced heart attacks but increased rates of violent deaths. When she brought up her concern to one of the doctors who supervised her, he dismissed the issue, saying, "We know statins can't do that." But in her mind she asked, "How do we know that?" So she dove into the literature and to her great surprise found a "massive amount of evidence that had just never been assembled." Primate studies showed that animals became more aggressive. Human studies showed increased accidents, aggression homicides, and suicides.[21] Over the years, she's assembled quite a series of cases where people developed short tempers, irritability, and violent tendencies. She has met several professionals whose careers were jeopardized by these changes.

The people affected often have no idea. She learned this early on. Once, she asked a gentleman who'd been hospitalized with severe muscle weakness about whether he was more irritable after starting statins. The man said no, and his wife chimed in, "Oh yes you are," to which he replied, with no sense of irony, "You've just become more irritating." The muscle weakness, not to mention the irritability, was later determined to have been brought on by the statin.

For Dr. Golomb's work in this area, she has received a great deal of pushback from colleagues who, as she puts it, "are heavily drug company funded." One individual "goes around telling everybody that I am the devil," she said. Another has tried to get her removed from her position at UCSD.[22]

Despite these troubling associations, statins are some of the most commonly prescribed drugs in the United States. If you aren't taking a statin, chances are someone you care about is.

HOW TO MAKE STATINS LOOK MORE EFFECTIVE: RELATIVE RISK

Statins, despite the evidence cited above, have become de rigueur to the practice of cardiology. Doctors believe they can prevent heart attacks, heart valve disease, and aneurysm ruptures. It's the same in neurology, where they are thought to prevent strokes and dementia related to strokes. Primary care doctors prescribe them, too, to patients with diabetes, kidney failure, high blood pressure, and, of course, high cholesterol.

The latest US guidelines on preventing heart attacks were released in 2018. They increased the portion of the adult population over the age of forty who are supposed to be taking statins from about 15 percent to *over 40 percent*.[23] In England, if doctors follow their latest set of guidelines "almost all males >60 years and all females >75 years, would be eligible for statin therapy."[24] You don't even need to have high cholesterol anymore for your doctor to put you on a statin; you will get one if a risk calculator says you are at high risk for heart attacks.

These risk calculators use factors such as age, sex, race, smoking status, blood pressure, and total and HDL cholesterol levels to calculate your chance of having a heart attack in the next ten years. There are several, all known to overestimate heart attack risk. The most commonly used calculator overestimates the relative risk by "37–154% in men and 8–67% in women," according to research from 2017.[25] It overestimates people with various risk factors differently, having the worst exaggerating effects in people with low to moderate risk. If your true risk of having a heart attack in the next ten years is, say, 7 percent, the calculator will bump it up to 12. That moves you from average risk to high risk, and it's likely that your doctor will heavily pressure you to take a statin.

One of the studies that led to this recent uptick in statin prescriptions claims that taking a statin for high LDL cuts the risk of fatal heart attacks by 27 percent even among people with zero risk factors.[26] But in reality, the study showed that taking a statin actually cut heart attacks by just 0.12 percent in this low-risk group.[27] To translate that into plain English, the article claims the drug is 225 times more effective than the data says it is.

They get away with that by using a concept called "relative risk reduction." Relative risk reduction tells you how much the risk is reduced in a treatment group compared with a control group. In the study mentioned above, the death rate among people with zero risk factors who didn't get statins (people randomized to the placebo control) was 0.45 percent. In the test group (people randomized to take the statin) the death rate was 0.33 percent, or 27 percent less. The 27 percent number obviously looks a lot better, so this is what gets reported. And it sounds quite exciting! So this is what most doctors believe and remember. But the truth is very different.

Let's take a look at an example using money, which is more fun to think about than drug side effects. Let's say your 401K is worth $100,000,

---

HOW TO MAGNIFY A TINY RISK TO IMPRESS DOCTORS

ABSOLUTE RISK	RELATIVE RISK
Statin cuts heart attacks by 0.12% (From 0.45% without the drug to 0.33% with the drug)	**Statin cuts heart attacks by 27%** (0.33 is 27% less than 0.45)

Figure 7–1: Absolute risk gives a better sense of the true impact of a drug, but relative risk is what's reported because bigger numbers sell more drugs. For the source used to create this figure, see the endnotes for this chapter.

and your money manager gave you a 4 percent return in 2020. That earned you $4,000. For the sake of easy math, let's say in 2021 you start with the same $100,000, but this year your money manager gives you a 5 percent return, earning you $5,000, which is 20 percent more than he earned you the year before. That's a relative improvement of 20 percent in his performance. But the absolute increase in dollar value of what the money manager earned for you in 2021 compared to 2020 was $1,000, or just 1 percent.

Now, if your money manager tried to convince you that in 2021 he increased the value of your entire portfolio by 20 percent, you'd fire him. Because 20 percent of your entire portfolio of $100,000 would be $20,000. It's a dishonest representation. But that's what the drug companies do.

Statin studies typically report relative risk instead of absolute risk, which falsely magnifies the benefit of the drugs. By using relative risk reduction they make everyone think their drugs do much more than they actually do.

Still, you might think cutting your risk by 0.12 percent is a good deal if it means staying alive. Chances are, that's not anything close to the truth. Most statin trials report statistically "adjusted" survival data. By 2015, just eleven large, multi-year studies reporting raw, unmanipulated data existed. When a group of physicians analyzed the raw data, they found taking statins does little to nothing to prolong your life, adding just four extra days, at best, and in some analyses *subtracting* days.[28] The pharmaceutical industry wants you and your doctor to be afraid to stop statins, so you'll keep refilling your prescriptions. And so far, it's working marvelously. Unfortunately, the more our health deteriorates, the more powerful our healthcare industry grows.

Health care is now the number one income-generation industry in the United States, representing 18.3 percent of the gross domestic product in 2021, out-earning food and agriculture (5.4 percent), defense (3 percent), and technology (0.3 percent).[29] This does more than enrich and empower the industry. It impoverishes and disempowers American families, who now spend 11.6 percent of their income on health care, a shade higher than the 11.3 percent spent on food.[30]

HIJACKING SCIENCE AND MEDICINE

In a classic episode of *Gilligan's Island*, a wooden chest full of radioactive vegetables floats ashore and everyone who eats them develops magnified nutrition-based abilities. Mary Ann eats carrots and develops long-range vision. Gilligan eats spinach and develops superhuman strength. If there were one more vegetable in that chest and it magnified skepticism, you could say I gorged on it when, in 2008, I read the book *Overdosed America: The Broken Promise of American Medicine*. The author, John Abramson, MD, described in a clear and systematic way how medical knowledge itself has been commercialized. The broken promise originates in the breakdown of the system designed to prevent moneyed interests from hijacking the scientific process. He explained how record-high prescription rates had so enriched the pharmaceutical industry that the normal and necessary checks and balances that had operated in the past had essentially been vaporized. As a result, the industry gained control over aspects of research that it really shouldn't control.

We've all heard of drug company representatives visiting doctors' offices, schmoozing, passing out pens with the drug names, inviting doctors to sponsored dinners. But those strategies are not at all representative of the real problem. The real problem is that drug companies have created an infrastructure that *shapes our knowledge about drugs.*

The drug companies no longer pay just for research and development to create a drug. Government has been playing a smaller role in medical research, so drug companies are now paying for most of the cost of the clinical trials designed to test the effects of their products.[31] In other words, people with a vested interest in making the drug look good are doing the "research" into the drug's benefits. This has been compared to basketball players acting as their own referees.

Drug companies now control the messaging as well. Articles describing the clinical trial results tend to magnify any drug's benefits and downplay its risks. In many cases, the articles are actually written by ghostwriters hired by the drug companies, and the official authors, who generally hold positions at prestigious institutions, just rent out their names.[32] It's like Michael Jordan endorsing Hanes athletic underwear. And medical journals are incentivized to publish these articles because they are kept afloat by pharmaceutical advertising.

It's not just drugs or drug companies. Everything I've said here also applies to makers of surgical and medical devices, such as robotic instruments and heart stents.

From our earliest days, medical students are taught to trust the research published in peer-reviewed journals because they are the best, richest, most timely and reliable source of evidence-based medicine. Publishing in a peer-reviewed journal requires submitting your paper to a committee of medical experts who will rigorously evaluate it to make sure it's worthy of publication. Or at least, they are supposed to. Disturbingly, Dr. Abramson discovered that editors of multiple peer-reviewed journals have, for some time, been skipping the data-review part of the peer review.[33] Why? They are more interested in selling reprints of the articles back to the drug companies to the tune of tens of millions of dollars. The companies, in turn, use the articles in marketing their products to doctors who have no idea how the sausage gets made.

Now that industry has paid for the studies it needed to convince doctors that statins are life-saving drugs, physicians can be financially penalized if they don't write enough prescriptions. Insurance companies can determine the payment they will give to medical organizations in part by how well they meet certain performance standards. These performance standards come from a government agency called the National Committee for Quality Assurance. The collection of standards is called the Healthcare Effectiveness Data Information Set, or the HEDIS measures, and there are many of them. Many are good ideas, that do things like reducing inappropriate use of antibiotics for viruses and ordering screening tests. But some of the standards are based on problematic research funded by drug companies. Every insurance company can decide what standards their doctors should follow, and then they can track doctors' behavior. They then use these measures as standards of performance by which they will rate individual doctors, medical groups, and hospitals. Because the entire group is affected by each individual doctor's behavior, some medical groups will pay doctors meeting these standards quite a bit more money, and they will also financially penalize doctors who don't.

Insurance companies can effectively require doctors to prescribe statins to patients *regardless of their cholesterol levels* if they have diabetes or cardiovascular disease. In fact, that's now a nearly universal standard, and there are others pertaining to cholesterol and statins.

So if you feel like your doctor squeezes you a little too hard to take a statin, that's why. It's more than money on the line for your doctor. Doctors who continually fail to "perform" can get fired.

Statins are just the beginning. The further you dig into how the drug companies push drugs for various diseases, the more you will want to take care of your own health by relying on diet and lifestyle and weaning yourself off of drugs that may do more harm than good.

Do Nutrition Researchers Even Know What They're Researching?

By now you have a pretty impressive understanding of precisely why eating more than just a little bit of PUFA is radically unhealthy. Dietitians are not on board with this idea, largely because they don't learn enough about oxidation. But another reason they're not on board is that thirty clinical trials show that people who eat more PUFA are healthier.[34] Those thirty trials are standing in the way of the ideas in this book being accepted. The most convincing among these trials test people's bodily tissues for PUFA content. These select studies (supposedly) show that people with more PUFA in their body tissues are healthier. So I want to demolish those keystone studies right now by telling you how they are flawed.

First, healthy people tend to avoid deep-fried foods. They get PUFA from whole foods like nuts, fish, and seeds. On the other hand, unhealthy people tend to eat deep-fried foods soaked with oxidized oils.[35] The journey of PUFA from where it exists in the natural world to your body's cells matters. For a delicate PUFA molecule, a deep fat fryer is a cauldron of destruction. Therefore, people who eat deep-fried PUFA are *actually* imbibing large quantities of oxidized PUFA byproducts, not intact PUFA. As a result, their tissues contain less PUFA. Eating those oxidized PUFA byproducts depletes their tissues of protective antioxidants, leaving any intact PUFA in their tissues vulnerable, and thus lowering measured PUFA levels further.

Additionally, these studies are flawed by a failure to account for the fact that saturated fat resists oxidation. Therefore, when PUFA gets oxidized into oblivion, saturated fat remains behind where it can be measured. This explains why people who eat more junk food tend to have relatively more saturated fat in their tissues. It's not that they're eating more butter. It's the fact that saturated fat is more resilient and less oxidizable, which leaves it intact to be detected in these tests and then blamed for your heart disease.

The lipid scientists who could explain all of this to dietitians are not invited to help with these studies. They're simply not welcome at the table. And that's a darn shame because this stuff is really complicated and the details matter. They make the difference between scientific papers that say something meaningful and those that double down on the falsehoods that lead to millions of deaths every year.

HOW TO ESCAPE THE SYSTEM

What we've seen so far is how the 1960s-era public health imperative to eat more seed oils is built on a fiction created by a man who may not have been as interested in improving public health as he was in proving himself correct. The organizations that decided to support this fiction have managed to keep it alive for decades, and in doing so, they've also held back medical science. If the AHA were ever to admit it's been wrong about cholesterol, other organizations would likely take the cue and change their positions, too. Needless to say, I'm not holding my breath for this to happen. For one thing, there's a lot of money being made. But the bigger reason has to do with culpability.

A good legal firm might very well be able to build an international, multitrillion-dollar case against the AHA by arguing that it willfully suppressed the truth and that in doing so it had sickened and killed billions of people around the world. Think about it this way. Without the cholesterol theory, vegetable oils would never have been promoted as "healthy," and chances are good we'd no longer be using them in our food. Actuaries calculate that at least 80 percent of our health is determined by how we live our lives, and I suspect that underestimates it. In a world without vegetable oils, there would be less inflammatory disease, less degenerative disease, and less metabolic disease. There'd be fewer hospitalizations and premature deaths. Less money would be wasted on pointless medical research and more money would be available to help solve myriad other pressing problems.

Fortunately, we don't need to wait for a judicial ruling to kick-start our own personal health revolution. If you want an escape valve to exit this unhealthy cycle, here it is: learn to stop worrying about saturated fat and embrace cholesterol. No amount of money can make us follow a diet we don't want to follow or take a cholesterol-lowering drug that we don't want to take. It's up to us. All we have to do is take control.

Until those eighty-year-old conflicts of interest are more widely recognized, they will continue to blindside millions of doctors, who will continue believing that cholesterol causes heart attacks, and that the answer to our health problems comes from factory oils that didn't exist before the industrial era. Thanks to this twisted paradigm, most of what doctors learn about nutrition is almost exactly backward, and "preventive" medicine now creates illness rather than curtailing it—it's like we're living on the wrong side of Alice's looking glass. In the final chapter of this section, I want to show you what life on the right side of the mirror looks like. We're going to see just what a wonderful world we could be living in after we and our healthcare providers free ourselves of the oppressive fear of cholesterol that's been holding us back from the kind of diet and the kind of health we deserve.

CHAPTER 8

Reason for Hope

How Cutting Vegetable Oils Leads to Healing

IN THIS CHAPTER YOU WILL LEARN

- Thanks to the growing popularity of the keto diet, researchers are finally getting the funds to study the health benefits of eating nutrient-dense, cholesterol-raising foods.
- Scientists who revived the one-hundred-year-old idea that cancer starts in our mitochondria, not in our DNA, are using keto to battle cancer—but are unaware how vegetable oils damage mitochondria.
- The new field of metabolic psychiatry optimizes mitochondrial function using a keto diet, and practitioners are just starting to add vegetable-oil avoidance to their recommendations.
- Beyond keto, other whole-food-based diets have been clinically shown to help reverse diabetes, but no diet works unless it also cuts down on vegetable oils.
- The keto diet has drawbacks that we can avoid by tweaking it just a little, creating a diet that works better for everyone.

Something amazing happens when doctors lose their fear of cholesterol. They begin to embrace ways of eating that actually improve human health, which has the potential to start correcting the dangerous and dysfunctional aspects of both medicine and food production. Over the years I've been in practice, I've seen that when my patients are given permission to eat the cholesterol-raising foods they've craved, foods packed with nutrients that recharge our energy, they can recover from conditions that few people would ever think might be influenced by diet. Once this happens on a grand scale, it will wake doctors up to the idea that nutrition is far more powerful than what we learned in school. One example of how this is already starting to happen, albeit on a small scale, comes to us by way of a popular diet known as the keto diet.

If you're not familiar with it, the keto diet is very low in carbohydrate. It takes away sources of empty-calorie carbs such as soda, juice, candy, and bakery treats as well as plates of pasta, bowls of rice, and big piles of mashed potatoes. It promotes protein-rich, high-fat meats of all kinds, cheese, butter, eggs, and seafood while steering us toward vitamin- and mineral-rich low-carb vegetables. Studies of keto show amazing promise. But keto also elevates cholesterol, so only the very boldest, most dedicated scientists and practitioners have been willing to even consider rigorously studying it or recommending it to their patients. But this tiny sliver of the medical research world is packed with disruptive evidence that nourishing foods can reverse diabetes, alleviate a variety of mental health issues, and even stave off cancer.

I've been making the case that our chronic disease epidemics are not highly complex, unsolvable problems. The story is simple: we've eaten our way into them, and we can eat our way out. So far, I haven't highlighted my own experience as a physician using diet to transform people's health. In this chapter I will start to introduce you to some of the remarkable stories I have witnessed or learned about from other practitioners that show how people can ditch the vegetable oils and reconnect to their real-food roots.

Clearing Arterial Fat

Dr. Sean O'Mara has worked in the White House serving President Bill Clinton, Vice President Dick Cheney, three secretaries of state, and other senior government officials and high-level foreign dignitaries. After retiring from military service, he opened a weight-loss practice. Many of his patients were not severely overweight but were severely "skinny fat." Being an advocate for the idea that seeing is believing, he started using an MRI machine to show his relatively normal-weight patients how their inflammatory, visceral fat was choking out their internal organs. He also used it to demonstrate how dietary changes could melt the fat away from their hearts, livers, kidneys, and so on, allowing organs and muscle to emerge in clear definition. Seed-oil avoidance is central to his dietary strategies.

Because his patients also reported thinking more clearly and noticing improved memory, he and his team realized there might be brain changes happening, too. So they started doing brain scans at every visit. They found example after example of arteries opening up and blood flow improving as the visceral fat cleared away. One of the most striking improvements was a gentleman who had a 100 percent blockage of one of the large blood vessels in his brain, the left middle cerebral artery. (The brain tissue itself was surviving thanks to healthy flow from the right side making its way across.) Needless to say, this motivated his patient quite a bit. In ten months, after losing thirty pounds and all of his excess visceral fat, his brain scan showed that he'd completely restored flow through this previously blocked artery.

RETHINKING CANCER

Cancer is quite possibly the most feared disease in the nation today. It's almost always looming in people's minds when they come to see me worried about a new, unexplained pain or concerning lump. Cancer is particularly scary because of a common conception that all it takes is a genetic mutation in a single cell to seal your fate. But what if cancer is not, in fact, a genetic disease? One cancer researcher has turned this widespread doctrine on its head. His approach to cancer offers great hope to survivors around the world currently living under the specter of recurrence, as well as to anyone newly diagnosed. Let me introduce you to Dr. Thomas Seyfried.

Dr. Seyfried should be a household name. To the elite group of medical doctors who know his work, he is a rock star. To the many hundreds of patients who still walk this Earth today thanks to Dr. Seyfried's work, he is a miracle worker.

Dr. Seyfried is a professor of biology at Boston College, but when you listen to him talk, you might be reminded more of a street-smart, seasoned cop than an academic. He's been studying metabolism, genetics, and cancer for more than forty years, and he has hundreds of publications to his name, plus a few books. He came to cancer research by a rather indirect route, having started out studying the genetics of epilepsy.

Throughout the 1980s and 1990s, Dr. Seyfried had meticulously mapped the genes involved in seizure disorders. He'd been passing his information up the research chain to scientists who would translate his basic research into therapeutic drugs. As is typical with this sort of research, very few of the drugs ever worked, and even the best didn't work all that well. Still, he kept at it. Then one day in the early 1990s, he was involved in a kind of epilepsy think-tank convened by, of all people, a Hollywood movie producer with a son affected by epilepsy. Dr. Seyfried learned, to his amazement, that in 1924, a Mayo Clinic doctor had devised a diet to treat epilepsy that actually worked. This diet drastically reduces carbohydrates, making up for the missing calories with fat instead. When we drastically cut back our sugar and carb consumption, our insulin levels drop, enabling our livers to produce a very special sort of fuel called ketones (introduced in chapter 4). Since this sort of very low-carb, high-fat diet supports the body's production, or genesis, of ketones, the doctor who invented it called it a *ketogenic* diet.

Dr. Seyfried already had epileptic mice, so all he had to do was rustle up a keto diet for them and test it out. It didn't take long to see that the keto diet blocked seizures amazingly well, better than any drug he knew of, and, he speculated, possibly better than any drug ever could. Of course, that meant the end of his days studying epilepsy genes in order to develop drugs, but he was perfectly okay with a career pivot for the cause. In interviews discussing the success of keto for seizure prevention, he puts his decades of hard work sorting out the genetics of epilepsy for the drug companies into the proper perspective: "Sure, we mapped all those genes. But the thing of it is, the diet blocked the seizures." Instead of fighting a new paradigm for treating epilepsy, he rolled with the punches—and thought about what else he might apply it to. It wasn't long before he came up with an idea that, as luck would have it, turned out to be the beginning of an even bigger story: the cause of cancer.

Dr. Seyfried knew that keto diets worked for epilepsy because they provided the brain with energy—and seizures are often brought about by inadequate cellular energy supply. The moment he saw how ketones helped his epileptic rats, a genius idea had popped into his head. *Why not try a keto diet for cancer?*

Jumping from epilepsy to cancer may seem like a random move, but it isn't if you know the history of cancer research in the early twentieth century. Dr. Seyfried knew that in the 1920s a cancer researcher named Otto Warburg—a German doctor of medicine who also had a PhD in chemistry—had made a fascinating observation about cancer. While studying a variety of cancer cell types, he found a common link between all of them: every last cancer type, every individual cell, had abnormal mitochondria. *Severely* abnormal mitochondria. This meant that cancer cells couldn't generate energy like normal cells. They could only do it by fermenting sugar. Sugar fermentation is an ancient method of energy production, a metabolic holdover from before mitochondria existed.

Fermenting sugar allows cancer cells to survive without fully functional mitochondria. (Cancer cells can also use other small molecules including an amino acid called glutamine, but sugar is the important one for our purposes.) If you take sugar and some of these small molecules away from cancer cells, they will starve and start to die.

Dr. Warburg made these stunning observations about cancer back in the 1920s. But he had no way to prove the idea, so it remained a hypothesis. Today its referred to as the Warburg Hypothesis.

Dr. Warburg would go on to win a Nobel Prize in 1931 for his related work, discovering how mammalian cells use oxygen to generate energy. Basically, he discovered why we breathe. Tragically, after World War II, this brilliant man's research was almost completely ignored for a purely political reason: he was German. The world no longer wanted to hear from German scientists. Meanwhile, Allied scientists had made great advances in our understanding of DNA, unlocking the structure of our genetic code. As a result of our fascination with DNA, and an intense distaste for anything that put Germany in a favorable light, the Warburg hypothesis was replaced by the idea that has become so commonplace today: that cancer is a genetic disease. Under this paradigm, fighting cancer requires disrupting DNA replication, thus killing all rapidly dividing cells in the body, not just cancer.

Even though few cancer specialists ever hear about it, support for the Warburg hypothesis kept rolling in as the decades passed. For example, cancer-causing genes, including the BRCA1 breast cancer gene, typically cause cancer by disrupting mitochondrial metabolism.[1] Likewise, carcinogens typically damage mitochondria (and mitochondrial DNA) long before they damage our human DNA.[2] Radiation, too, causes toxicity largely by damaging mitochondria.[3] We also now know that cancer cells are not, in fact, clones of each other.[4] Nor is there just one random mutation: cancerous cells in a single melanoma, for example, may contain thousands of different mutations.[5] And as we saw in chapter 3, dysfunctional mitochondria release high-energy free radicals that can mutate DNA.

A defining characteristic of cancer cells is their immortality; they have an ability to reproduce seemingly without end. This, too, comes down to mitochondria, which must be functioning normally for the cell to undergo what's called "programmed cell death." When mitochondria inside a cell are not working right, cells can start dividing faster and faster until they form a giant, unruly mass—a cancerous tumor visible to the naked eye. During the last one hundred years of research, whenever scientists have evaluated the mitochondria within cancerous cells, they have found evidence of dysfunction. On the other hand, some malignant tumors show no sign of gene mutation—which makes no sense at all if cancer is a genetic disease.[6]

While the Warburg hypothesis handily explains the observed DNA mutations, the gene theory of cancer has no simple explanation for the observed mitochondrial abnormalities. Nor can the gene theory explain why cancer cells require so much sugar. Cancer cells have such a voracious appetite for sugar that radiologists pinpoint the location of cancerous tumors using a form of radioactive sugar, which shows up as black nodules on PET scans. Only the Warburg hypothesis can make sense of all these observations.

For these reasons and more, it made a great deal of sense to Dr. Seyfried to revive Dr. Warburg's ideas. He recognized that a cancer cell's lack of functional mitochondria would make it overly dependent on sugar fermentation, and that a diet nearly devoid of sugar might slow or stop cancer growth. He had just finished his research using keto to treat seizures, so the next logical move was to find out what kind of effect the keto diet had on animals with cancer.

It just so happened that Dr. Seyfried already had the perfect group of mice to test out this idea, because he'd also been doing research into brain cancer. He describes the results of feeding his cancerous mice a keto diet as so "unbelievable" that he wondered how "a simple diet change could be so effective."[7] While the cancers in the animals fed a regular diet could grow into giant tumors, some squishing the rest of the brain into half its normal volume within the confines of the skull, switching to a keto diet at any point in the experiment halted cancer growth in its tracks. After making further refinements to the protocol, he was able to shrink advanced deadly brain tumors down to nearly invisible dots.[8]

Shrinking tumors with a keto diet is already an incredible feat. But Seyfried went several steps further. He designed an elegant sequence of experiments that could disprove the gene theory of cancer once and for all. He performed microsurgery on cancerous cells, showing that mitochondria from cancer cells transmitted cancer, while mutated DNA from cancer cells did not. He also designed experiments to test where the DNA mutations came from. Those experiments showed that mitochondrial dysfunction was causing DNA mutations rather than the other way around. This is irrefutable evidence that cancer comes down to mitochondrial dysfunction, not DNA mutation, exactly as Warburg predicted. And it demands we use a radically different strategy for beating cancer than what we've been pursuing for the past three-quarters of a century. We've been killing rapidly dividing cells when what we should be doing is healing our broken metabolism.

Dr. Seyfried explains his revolutionary rediscovery of this important one-hundred-year-old cancer hypothesis extremely modestly: "Otto Warburg had said many years ago that tumors can't burn ketones for energy because the mitochondria are defective. They need glucose. On a keto diet, the glucose is low, the ketones are elevated so, wow, it makes perfect sense."[9] The keto diet effectively starves just the cancer cells. It's a beautiful, completely nontoxic way to treat cancer.

Dr. Seyfried made this initial discovery twenty years ago. In the intervening years, he and his team have tested the keto diet in mice with multiple types of cancer. He published a book called *Cancer as a Metabolic Disease* in 2012, and today he regularly hears from readers who "should be dead" but who read his work, adopted the keto diet, and outlived their prognosis by years—some were still alive decades after diagnosis. Dr. Seyfried has shown that you can treat cancer by starving it. And you starve it by reducing blood sugar while ensuring that your brain has access to an alternative energy source, namely ketones. When our blood sugar drops, we need ketones as brain fuel because, as we've seen, our brains cannot easily burn large fatty acids.

The cancer starvation strategy has worked for every type of solid tumor cancer he's studied so far, including the most common (and most commonly fatal) ones: colon, breast, bladder, and kidney cancers, as well as brain cancer in adults, and increasingly in children—childhood brain cancer is on the rise. Blood cancers such as leukemia and lymphoma also involve damaged mitochondria, but their growth is less often driven by sugar and more often by one of the other fermentable metabolites, the amino acid glutamate. In animal studies, his team has even developed other metabolic therapeutics that further block the cancer cell's access to energy by depriving it of glutamate as well. This strategy magnifies the effectiveness of the keto diets and produces superior results to keto alone. However, these metabolic blockers are only available for veterinary use, and his requests to study them in human cancer have repeatedly been denied.

Starving cancer with a ketogenic diet and minimally toxic metabolic therapies sounds almost too good to be true, doesn't it? You might be tempted to presume that, if it were truly this easy for people with the deadliest forms of cancer to radically lengthen their lives, we'd have heard about it. Could it really be so simple?

What gets Dr. Seyfried going more than anything else is exactly that—the fact that it could all be so simple. "We want to show the world how we exploit that and manage this disease without toxicity, but that's a hard sell, because everybody wants this thing to be so complicated and so involved." Thanks to that inertia, "the field of oncology has not yet accepted the mitochondrial metabolic theory as the origin of cancer."[10]

One criticism of the Warburg theory is literally that "it's too simple," and that because Dr. Warburg didn't know about the structure of DNA at the time, he couldn't study it the way we can today. While it's true that we have learned a lot more about genetics since Dr. Warburg passed away in 1970, I'm not sure why not knowing everything we know today about genetics would invalidate the discoveries he made.

Another criticism Dr. Seyfried hears is that metabolic therapy doesn't always work. But these failures are coming from laboratory experiments, not from tests on people. The animal experiments where keto fails use animals that are genetically engineered to develop cancer. No human has been engineered to develop cancer, nor have the animals Dr. Seyfried uses. His team uses animals with cancer that has developed spontaneously, the way it does in humans. So to this criticism, he simply says, "I don't know why a mouse that's been genetically engineered to get cancer doesn't respond to metabolic therapy, but I think I'll leave it for the next ten thousand years [of research] to figure that out." Dr. Seyfried explains this dysfunctional state of medical research as only a New Yorker can. "No matter what level of scientific evidence you could present, it would be discounted because of the ideology that they [other academics] are afflicted with." The ideological affliction he is referring to is the idea that cancer is a genetic disease.[11]

Because oncologists believe cancer is a genetic disease, they keep using the standard chemotherapies that indiscriminately kill all the rapidly dividing cells in the body, an approach that tragically sometimes also kills the patient. Dr. Seyfried wants to target just the cancer cells. The amazing thing is that we already have metabolic therapies capable of doing just that, and they cost much less than standard chemotherapy. Dr. Seyfried is using them successfully in his animal models, and for now, he conducts this work in a small university lab. If the American Cancer Society were to back him—and others who share his ideology—the war on cancer might finally become winnable.

Fortunately, we don't need to wait for the field of oncology to accept the theory. If you want to protect yourself from cancer starting today, there is a clear path forward: keep your mitochondria as healthy as possible.

Sick-Care Out. Health Care In.

Meet Dr. Shawn Baker, founder of a virtual health company, Revero, that treats autoimmune and inflammatory diseases, including lupus, rheumatoid arthritis, inflammatory bowel diseases, and more. All these diseases are now recognized to originate in mitochondrial dysfunction and oxidative stress, as we discussed in chapters 2 and 3. In spite of breakthroughs in our understanding of the root causes, most clinics still rely on long-term use of immune-suppressing drugs like steroids, and—lately—biological infusions. Biological infusions can cost thousands of dollars for a one-week supply, and they can cause cancer and death from infections. Steroids are much less expensive, but they can cause cataracts, severe bone loss, and more.

As an orthopedic surgeon, Dr. Baker was disturbed by the number of young people needing multiple joint replacements due to the combination of medication failure and steroid-induced bone damage, and this was part of what inspired him to start his new company. The other part was that he was inundated with testimonials from people following the type of diet he recommended. These individuals had gotten off medications for these serious and life-limiting conditions while feeling better than ever. Revero uses strict seed-oil avoidance and an easy-to-understand elimination diet called the carnivore diet—which eliminates most foods other than animal fats, organs, and meats. Revero faces a lot of challenges given the current healthcare model, in which the costly infusions have become huge profit centers for hospital systems and private rheumatologists. Revero is currently in start-up mode, but it is one man's creative answer to the shortcomings of the medical system that we discussed in chapter 7.

BECOMING CANCER-PROOF: MENDING YOUR MITOCHONDRIA

Right now, most people believe there's not much they can do on a practical level to avoid cancer other than avoiding cigarettes and perhaps a few other habits. This fatalistic attitude is a natural outgrowth of the idea that cancer starts in our genes due to random mutations, exposure to nearly unavoidable environmental contaminants, or a bad family history. But if cancer is a mitochondrial disease, as it seems to be, then it means that if your mitochondria are healthy, you can't get cancer. We have more than one hundred years of cancer research showing this statement to be true.

The flip side of that reality is that when we damage our mitochondria, we open ourselves up to cancer. The worst thing we can do to our mitochondria is subject them to oxidative stress. And now you see where I am going with this (and maybe you got it from my first mention of mitochondria in this chapter): on a high-vegetable-oil diet, there's no such thing as healthy mitochondria. What's more, the insulin resistance that a high-PUFA diet creates also elevates your blood sugar, ensuring that any hungry cancer cells will get their favorite food.

At this point, you may be wondering if you need to follow a keto diet in order to *prevent* cancer. To answer that, we need to turn our focus back to the root cause. The Warburg hypothesis tells us that mitochondrial dysfunction is the root cause of cancer. That means keeping our mitochondria healthy should prevent cancer from ever forming. Ketones support mitochondrial health, but there is no evidence that they are *required* for mitochondrial health. So my answer is no, we don't need to focus on ketones for cancer prevention. We need to focus on reversing the nearly universal metabolic disease, insulin resistance, which raises our blood sugar in an attempt to adapt to damaged mitochondria. And avoiding vegetable oil is a key piece of the insulin-resistance reversal plan.

Cancer certainly existed before the modern era, so it's not all down to vegetable oil, but cancer does appear to come down to oxidative stress. It's impossible to fully prevent oxidative stress—it's simply a part of normal life. But our modern diet invites oxidative stress far in excess of what our biology was designed to withstand. Not just from the vegetable oil, although I believe that is the single most important factor, but from the fact that the standard American diet is almost devoid of nutrients, and nutrient deficiency also promotes the oxidative stress that harms our mitochondria. In essence, our diet is *forcing* cells to become cancer cells *if they want to survive.* The more we damage our mitochondria, the more likely some cell somewhere in our body will revert to this ancient fueling strategy. It just so happens that in order to make this shift, the cell must also reject its membership in the body. It reverts to a primitive, bacteria-like lifestyle: Divide. Divide. Divide.

What that means is that you have incredible power to prevent cancer from developing, no matter your genetics. It means that our war on cancer has already been mostly won—all you have to do is change how you've thought about fighting it.

New Possibilities for Cancer Treatment

Once cancer develops, we're out of prevention mode and into different territory where flooding the body with ketones may become essential to continued survival. Anyone diagnosed with stage 4 esophageal cancer has just a 20 percent chance of being alive one year later. These were the odds facing eighty-year-old Guy F. when he first came to see me. He'd already completed chemo and radiation, and the question at this point was whether he should undergo surgery to remove most of his esophagus and stomach. The procedure would remove his cancer but leave him weakened and reliant on tube feedings for the remainder of his days. He was also taking insulin for type 2 diabetes, but was otherwise in good shape for his age.

I told Guy I'd met others with dire diagnoses who'd survived for years and attributed it to keto, but that I'd not personally used it to treat cancer. After watching some of Dr. Seyfried's videos, a few days later he decided to forgo surgery and try his luck with keto.

He was so motivated to follow the program to a T that, despite having diabetes for decades, he got off his insulin and his other diabetes drugs *over a weekend*. He cut vegetable oils and carbs, radically changed his diet, and shrank his cancerous tumor to the point that it was invisible on a PET scan just ten weeks later. He enjoyed two more years of incredible health, able to carry his grandson around on his shoulders after T-ball games, mow his five-acre property, and go for regular walks. Unfortunately, after a traumatic car accident where he hemorrhaged half his blood internally, his cancer did regrow rapidly, and he quickly deteriorated. He soon passed peacefully in his home surrounded by his family and love. His son told me they were grateful to have had the extra time, as was he.

Guy was a good man. If organizations like the American Cancer Association had focused on researching Dr. Seyfried's metabolic therapies—instead of questionable chemotherapies—he might still be alive today.

NEW DISCOVERIES IN PSYCHIATRY

Unlike cancer, where the role of mitochondria and metabolism have been actively ignored, in the field of mental health it's starting to be actively explored. Leading scientists have recently formed a hypothesis that mental illness is rooted in mitochondrial dysfunction and should be considered a metabolic disease, not just genetic or random. And this hypothesis suggests that improving our mitochondrial health may help with mental illness in ways that drugs do not.

Psychiatrists have long recognized the link between metabolic and mental illnesses. In 1879, a prominent English psychiatrist name Sir Henry Maudsley wrote in his textbook *Pathology of Mind* that "diabetes is a disease that often shows itself in families in which insanity prevails." (Today, we no longer use the term *insanity*, and now recognize the behaviors Maudsley was referring to as the severest manifestations of two distinct but in many ways similar disorders, bipolar disorder and schizophrenia.) In the 1950s, psychiatrists observed that people with bipolar disorder and schizophrenia had abnormal levels of lactate, a hallmark of abnormal energy metabolism. In the 1990s, MRI-based technology called functional neuroimaging revealed that people with a variety of psychiatric conditions suffer from altered energy availability in multiple brain regions.[12] Recently, scientists have homed in on mitochondrial structure and function. Using genetic markers, they've learned that the more disabling a person's psychiatric symptoms, the more distorted their mitochondria become, and the fewer they have per cell.[13] (Remember, mitochondria produce energy for our cells.)

Christopher Palmer, MD, who holds an assistant professorship in the Department of Psychiatry at Harvard Medical School, has been researching the root cause of psychiatric illness for much of his twenty-seven-year career. He has come to the conclusion that most, or maybe all, mental disorders are actually mitochondrial metabolic disorders that disrupt the brain's access to energy. He believes that restoring mitochondrial health is the key to restoring mental health, and, like Dr. Seyfried, that the keto diet can help. He is part of a new movement—metabolic psychiatry—that addresses the root cause rather than medicating chemical imbalances (that remain unproven).[14] Thanks to this growing movement, the keto diet has gained some recognition.

For example, a small study conducted by a Canadian psychiatrist, Dr. Albert Danan, showed that keto manifested as "unprecedented improvements in mental and physical health" in patients hospitalized for major depression, bipolar disorder, and schizophrenia.[15] Nearly two-thirds of the patients ultimately went home from the hospital on *fewer* medications than they needed before they went in, which is unusual. Dr. Georgia Ede, a Harvard-trained psychiatrist who coauthored the study, has been using a keto diet for over a decade in her practice, and now trains other doctors in its use. In her experience, 50 percent of patients will benefit so much from keto that they can slowly reduce and sometimes even stop their medications.[16] She's getting these outstanding results without any focus on seed-oil avoidance, and I suspect adding that component would improve the results significantly.

To understand why the keto diet works so well for mental health, let's take a step back in time to revisit how the keto diet came to be used for epilepsy.

Doctors have treated people suffering with epileptic seizures using fasting regimens since as early as 500 BC, but they had no idea why fasting worked. In the early 1920s, Drs. Stanley Cobb and W. G. Lennox at Harvard Medical School noticed that people's seizures typically improved about two to three days into a fast, precisely when they observed that people started producing urinary ketones. At about the same time, Dr. Russell Wilder at the Mayo Clinic suspected that dietary manipulation might produce ketones without the need for fasting. He soon worked out a formula for what became the keto diet: fewer than ten grams of carbs, the minimum amount of protein to prevent muscle wasting, and the rest of the calories coming from fat. Throughout the 1920s and 1930s, the keto diet was used to help thousands of epileptics. But scientists never made much progress on sorting out how it worked because, in 1938, a team of neurologists named Houston Merritt and Tracy Putnam had discovered a drug called diphenylhydantoin, still in use today and known as phenytoin. With that, physicians and researchers shifted focus from understanding and implementing the keto diet to understanding and prescribing antiepileptic drugs. A new era had begun, and the keto diet fell by the wayside.[17] Even today, with the resurgence in scientific interest in the keto diet, we lack a clear understanding of exactly how the diet works.

Most of the focus has been on the ketones themselves, which certainly makes sense. But there's another variable that I think might be just as important, if not more so, which relates to the metabolic damage induced by vegetable oils. That has to do with blood sugar dips. As we've seen, vegetable oils bring about insulin resistance, and when we're insulin resistant, our brains are frequently subjected to blood sugar swings.

Blood sugar fluctuations reliably bring on seizures—even in people without epilepsy.[18] Blood sugar dips disrupt brain energy, and scientists highlight this "disruption of energy availability" as a key problem. Blood-sugar spikes cause problems, too, for entirely different reasons that have to do with how high blood sugar disrupts the ability of nerve cells to sustain an electric charge. Being virtually free of carbs, the keto diet effectively blocks spike-related energy disruptions while at the same time providing a steady supply of cellular fuel in the form of ketones, thus preventing energy dips. So the benefits of a ketogenic diet may have less to do with ketones being particularly beneficial than with the fact that they give cells an alternative to burning the high-PUFA body fat that causes insulin resistance and blood sugar problems.

When doctors first noticed the link between insulin resistance and bipolar disorder, they assumed it came from the medications used to treat bipolar, which can promote significant weight gain. When a research group in India tested people newly diagnosed with bipolar, they found evidence that insulin resistance actually comes first. Folks with bipolar disorder had average HOMA-IR scores of 3.5, while an age- and weight-matched control group averaged a much healthier 1.19.[19] (Recall, from chapter 4, that I proposed 1.0 or less as normal.) Since it takes years to progress from insulin sensitive to insulin resistant, the metabolic problem must have preceded the psychiatric one. This suggests that reversing insulin resistance may delay or even prevent the development of bipolar disorder.

Seizure statistics further link insulin resistance to detrimental brain consequences. The number of US children diagnosed with epilepsy increased 4.44 percent between 2007 and 2015, even while the total number of US children dropped slightly during that time, by 1.4 percent.[20] I should point out that the problem of insulin resistance in children approaches that of adults, with nearly zero children aged eight and up scoring a HOMA-IR of 1 or lower.[21]

So doctors are increasingly recognizing that metabolism plays a role in brain-related disorders of all kinds. But unfortunately, they are not often recognizing that when people go keto, they're doing more than just cutting carbs. They're often cutting seed oils. This means that they're not just producing ketones, they're also cutting the main source of oxidative stress in our diets, and oxidative stress disrupts brain function in several ways: First, by depleting our brains of the antioxidants required to keep mitochondria running smoothly. Second, by promoting insulin resistance, which causes blood-sugar spikes and energy dips that disrupt brain function. And third, toxins from vegetable oils actually enter our brains, where they promote oxidative stress and brain-cell inflammation and destruction.[22]

While the very low carb diets that support ketone production may be important for treating epilepsy and starving cancer, cutting carbs may not be the factor behind keto's success that many people currently assume. This point becomes crystal clear when we look at studies comparing different diets for type 2 diabetes.

TYPE 2 DIABETES: THE SO-CALLED INCURABLE DISEASE THAT PEOPLE ARE CURING

As we saw in chapter 3, nearly everyone in the United States—and increasingly the entire world—is insulin resistant. This means nearly everyone is on the way to developing type 2 diabetes or already has it. Fortunately, the same diet that reverses one will reverse the other and could help billions of people alive today.

But first, let's talk about the kind of diet that the American Diabetes Association (ADA) trains dietitians to recommend, called MyPlate. MyPlate is very similar to the Prudent Diet that the American Heart Association has been promoting since the 1950s, encouraging low-fat meats and dairy, and emphasizing fruits and starchy foods such as breads and pasta as long as they are "whole grain." But wait... Isn't diabetes a disease of high blood sugar? And don't starchy carbs and sugary fruits raise blood sugar? Of course, the answer to both questions is yes. It seems counterproductive to the point of irresponsibility to recommend these sorts of foods to people with diabetes, since they can dramatically increase the need for blood-sugar-lowering medications. It's not particularly surprising that the ADA does so. After all, the organization relies on drug companies to fund its research, publications, and educational outreach.

As a result of these business relationships, anyone who visits the ADA website today will find themselves being subtly discouraged from trying to heal their metabolic disease with anything but drugs. The ADA website warns that "there is no magic diet that can cure diabetes."[23] The use of the term "magic" undermines the very idea that diet matters. Elsewhere, the website states that "there's no one size fits all diet" for treating diabetes. Indeed, dietitians are encouraged to use this phrase when counseling clients.[24] This makes it sound like you're in for a lengthy trial-and-error process, which is both dispiriting and not strictly true. Just about any diet will work *as long as it reduces oxidative stress.* And this means that just about any diet that gets people off high-PUFA vegetable oils will help make a dent in diabetes severity.

For example, studies using whole-food vegan diets have helped some people to get off their diabetes meds.[25] What often goes underreported is that vegetable oil is not considered a whole food, and these diets are vegetable-oil free. Cutting PUFA appears to be the secret to making other popular diets work, too. Another study that put some people's diabetes into remission got similar results using either a Mediterranean diet, that used olive oil instead of vegetable oil, or a diet that was similar to MyPlate but much lower in fat—with just 10 percent of calories coming from fat, versus the usual 30. So for different reasons, both of these diets reduced people's PUFA to less than 6 percent of total calories, which is much less than our baseline average of 15 percent. Both types of diets also worked better than the standard ADA advice.[26]

What about diets that cut carbs? Those should be a slam dunk, right? Well, not always. Unfortunately, doctors and dietitians are not paying attention to the vegetable oil variable, so that when they look at the most logical candidate for diabetes control—namely, diets that cut out blood-sugar-raising carbs—the results are mixed.

CUTTING PUFA: THE OVERLOOKED FACTOR NECESSARY FOR LOW-CARB SUCCESS

Doctors who specialize in using low-carb diets like keto have had incredible successes reversing diabetes. We currently have six well-designed clinical trials run by some of the country's top "low-carb" doctors. These studies show that diets low in carbs consistently outperform the standard ADA diet.[27] However, we also have six equally well-designed studies showing that low-carb diets do not work any better than the standard ADA diet.[28] What's going on here? How could cutting carbs ever fail?

Given what we discussed about scientists for hire in chapter 7, you might suspect some sort of foul play, and that we need to follow the money to get to the truth. But a close look at the differences in the low-carb diets provides the scientific explanation. It comes down to oxidative stress—which, once again, comes down to vegetable oils. In the six studies showing that low-carb diets worked better than MyPlate, people ate much less PUFA. In the six studies where they failed to work any better than the generally poor-performing MyPlate, people got most of their fat in the form of PUFA, and very little of it from the foods we typically associate with a keto diet. In these studies, the cholesterol-raising butter, cheese, and fatty meats were forbidden, and vegetable-oil-rich foods were encouraged instead.

If you've been on a keto diet yourself, you might be surprised to learn that some keto diets restrict animal fats. This is partly a result of ideological disagreements between most dietitians and the select few doctors in the country who have overcome cholesterol-phobia. As a result, there are actually two different "brands" of keto, corresponding to two different outcomes in the research. When a study's keto diet is designed by practitioners who no longer believe cholesterol-raising foods cause heart attacks, the guidelines allow study participants to enjoy the usual list of cholesterol-raising foods—butter, meat, cheese, and so on. This type of keto diet was popularized in the 1970s by Dr. Robert Atkins and used to be called the Atkins diet. The other brand of keto looks more like a low-carb version of the AHA's Prudent Diet and is used when a study's keto diet is designed by practitioners who are more concerned about choles-terol. In this case people are told to choose skim milk, low-fat yogurt, and lean meats and to avoid coconut oil, butter, and full-fat cheese and dairy. Because AHA-compliant keto keeps saturated fats below 10 percent of total calories, while Atkins puts no limits on saturated fat, the two diets can differ greatly in their PUFA content.

But even Atkins doesn't specifically steer people clear of vegetable oil. Remember, for many decades "keto" has simply meant "very low carb," and seemingly anything goes when it comes to dietary fats. Atkins simply didn't know about vegetable oils and never specified what "oil" to use in the sauces, dips, and mayonnaise his cookbooks encourage folks to eat. Therefore, fol-lowing an Atkins-style diet is not a guarantee that your diet is vegetable-oil-free. The first keto book to highlight the vegetable oil problem was called *The Keto Reset*, published in 2017. (The authors interviewed me extensively on the subject.) Unfortunately, it seems not everyone paid attention, and many "keto" resources still include vegetable oils among their recommended cooking fats. (For instance, on its "How to Build a Keto-Friendly Grocery List" webpage, the popular grocery chain Whole Foods Market prompts readers to "keep a stock of cooking fats like ghee or olive, sunflower, grape-seed, and rapeseed oils" among their keto "pantry essentials.")

Reducing people's blood sugar levels requires addressing both of the factors that increase it: blood-sugar spikes and the elevated baseline need. Most of the focus is on the spikes, which improve by cutting carbs. But medical science ignores the elevated baseline need, which is driven by oxidative stress and is best resolved by cutting PUFA (as discussed in chapter 3). So when keto fails to outperform high carb, it may be exchang-ing fewer blood-sugar spikes for a higher baseline blood sugar. When keto works, it's combating both the short-term blood-sugar spikes and the oxidation that drives our fasting blood sugars higher over the long run. The differentiator is oxidative stress—something that most doctors are not yet fully aware of. So they've attributed the diets' successes to ketones. Or, alternatively, to insulin itself, which some believe promotes oxidative stress. In reality, it's oxidative stress that promotes insulin resistance (as seen in Chapter 3).

As you can imagine, missing such a big piece of the insulin-resistance puzzle has caused a great deal of frustration within the ranks of doctors promoting keto. It's led to this situation we have now, where keto only works when pro-keto doctors write the reports. It's caused fights between advocates for low-carb and neutral researchers, with both sides accusing the other of questionable conduct.[29] The discord trickles down through the media to the healthcare consumer and leads to unnecessary confusion among people just trying to improve their health.

Unhealthy Ways to Produce Ketones

Ketones in our blood do not necessarily indicate we're in good health. *For one thing, ketones in our blood may indicate we're breaking down muscle!*[30] Furthermore, one of the most reliable ways to start generating ketones is to fall ill with a fever.[31] Another way is to eat a lot of vegetable oil. It turns out that when our diets contain large amounts of PUFA, we actually produce far more ketones than when our diets are low in PUFA. In one study, people on a high-PUFA version of keto developed ketone levels nearly three times higher than people on a lower-PUFA version.[32] But, as we just saw, high-PUFA keto performs worse than low-PUFA keto in reversing diabetes. Remember all the bad things that happened to the soy-oil-fed mice in Dr. Sladek's experiments we discussed in chapter 3? Those mice actually achieved higher ketone levels than the relatively healthier mice

---

fed coconut oil.[33] In another mouse study using corn-oil-based keto, mice produced plenty of ketones but developed insulin intolerance— in just three days.[34] If ketones were the thing that reversed insulin resistance, that wouldn't be possible.

The ultimate ketogenic diet—in terms of ketone production only—may be alcohol based. Most people on keto diets only produce ketone levels of between 0.2 and 5 millimoles per liter (mmol/L).[35] In a one-week study where participants replaced all dietary carbs with alcohol, ketone production increased to a level of 10 mmol/L.[36]

While ketones are a better cellular fuel than sugar, they are not superior to healthy body fat.[37] My point is, there may not be anything magic about ketones beyond the fact that they get into our brains (and perhaps other cells) when fat can't. I think the magic comes from having a healthy, flexible metabolism.

Having Ketones In Your Blood Doesn't Mean You're Getting Healthier

We've just discussed several unhealthy ways to produce ketones. The healthy way to produce ketones is for your liver to make them from mobilized body fat between meals. But for this to happen, you need metabolic *flexibility.*

Metabolic flexibility is the holy grail of metabolic health, and the opposite of insulin resistance.[38] When you are metabolically flexible, your body can easily switch from burning the calories coming into your bloodstream from your last meal to burning your body fat. If you are exercising or go long enough between meals when your blood sugar drops, your liver can convert your body fat into ketones. You won't get hypoglycemia symptoms even if your blood sugar drops below normal. This happens even when you are not following a keto diet.

How do you know if you're metabolically flexible? You'll be able to go for long periods without eating and engage in heavy activity without experiencing any of the eleven symptoms of pathologic hunger. That's why I ask you to start tracking the eleven symptoms of pathologic hunger that we learned about in Chapter 3. Those eleven symptoms mean your body is not producing energy efficiently, your mitochondria are being damaged, and your cells are experiencing inflammation. And their absence means that you've prevented mitochondrial damage and inflammation.

Remember, metabolism is all about energy. So focusing on energy levels is the most accurate way to gauge your metabolic recovery.

SO SHOULD WE ALL GO KETO?

Given the promising literature on keto we've just discussed, you may be wondering how important it is to follow a keto diet. If you've investigated keto in any depth for yourself, you may have even run into passionate keto devotees who've made it sound like we *need* to follow a keto diet because ketones are essential for basic cellular function. But there is no evidence for this. Ketones themselves do not appear to play an especially important role in improving metabolic flexibility or reversing insulin resistance. More to the point, however, we do not need to produce ketones to be healthy, nor does producing ketones indicate good health. (See box "Unhealthy Ways to Produce Ketones.")

In fact, for those who are insulin resistant, there may be drawbacks to cutting carbs down to keto diet levels. Therefore, although I do recommend the keto diet to some people, there are three reasons why I don't recommend it for everyone. First, variety. It must be said that the keto diet is very restrictive of carbs, and having worked with thousands of patients, I've seen that many people struggle to replace the familiar, carb-laden dishes they rely on in their weekly meal rotations; on a keto diet, they end up limiting themselves, getting bored, feeling deprived—and giving up. Allowing strategic use of a few carbohydrate-containing foods can really make their new lifestyle more enjoyable. (It helps to use a continuous glucometer device so you can see for yourself how various foods affect you since everyone is different. This is especially helpful for diabetes reversal.) Second, I think keeping our bodies' cells abundantly energized is a more important first goal than keeping our dietary macros in the keto range. Abundant cellular energy makes us feel really good—even before we lose any excess weight we may have. It also helps to prevent the hypoglycemia symptoms that drive bad moods, pathologic hunger, and insulin resistance. Third, there is reason to believe that restricting carbs to keto levels when someone is insulin resistant might even be harmful.

Although it is true that a *healthy* human body has no biological need for dietary carbohydrate, when we are insulin resistant, we are no longer healthy. That completely changes the usual carbohydrate equation. When we are insulin resistant, yanking almost all the carbohydrates away from our sugar-dependent cells may force the liver to accelerate the process of gluconeogenesis and muscle breakdown, and of course we wouldn't necessarily feel this as it's happening. However, I think some people do feel it, but they don't realize what it means. Let me explain.

When starting a low-carb or keto diet, many people feel bad, experiencing sugar cravings (hunger), fatigue, headache, foggy brain, fatigue, irritability, leg cramps, and nausea; it's sometimes called the "keto flu." These symptoms are assumed to come from fluid shifts as the body adapts to a new diet. To beat them, keto experts recommend staying well hydrated, getting extra salt, and taking a few mineral supplements. Since these symptoms often go away in a few days, there's been little serious discussion as to the cause. If they don't go away, people usually give up, blaming themselves. However, you may recognize these symptoms. Many are symptoms of hypoglycemia—and they represent unhealthy hunger reflecting our metabolic sugar dependence. Is the keto flu the body sending a distress signal, warning that in our insulin-resistant state, our cells still *need* sugar?

I think it might be. And that means when the keto flu doesn't go away, it's not our fault; it's our metabolism. Indeed, the fact that the keto flu does go away might be lulling us into a false sense of security, because there's evidence to suggest that its symptoms resolve only if a person's body can adapt to the lack of sugar by burning more protein instead. And this may mean that going keto while we're still insulin resistant forces our bodies to break down relatively more muscle than we otherwise would.

Doctors who use keto have assumed that people on a ketogenic diet are burning more body fat than they would following a higher-carb diet, thanks to the insulin-lowering effects and the appearance of ketones in the urine. In recent years, one of the most respected metabolic researchers in the United States, Kevin Hall, PhD, performed a series of studies to put this idea to the test. What he found was disturbing. When the people in his studies started a keto diet, their insulin did go down while their ketones went up, but this shift did not translate to burning more body fat. In fact, the study participants actually burned *less* body fat on keto than they did on low-fat diets.[39] How is that possible? Following a keto diet does enable you to burn *dietary* fat, but it doesn't necessarily mean you're burning your body fat. It may even make you burn protein.

Remember, as we saw in chapter 4, our cells will burn sugar as an alternative to burning PUFA. This is likely true whether the PUFA comes from diet or body fat. Cutting carbs while one still has high-PUFA body fat forces the cells to seek out an alternative to the alternative, and that leaves protein. The carb-starved, PUFA-overloaded body will have no choice but to convert muscle protein into energy. In fact, studies in diabetes suggest that, when someone is severely insulin resistant, any ketones produced are as likely to be coming from muscle as from body fat.[40] This is not what we want. All of this supports the idea that, in order to avoid burning PUFA, cells undergo a profound metabolic shift—one that may make following a ketogenic diet counterproductive. (Importantly, the keto diets in Dr. Hall's studies contained more PUFA than is ideal. This may have made keto look worse than it would have were the diet lower in PUFA, and highlights the paramount importance of avoiding vegetable oil.)

The nearly carbohydrate-free keto diet was initially created in the 1920s, when there was very little vegetable oil in the food supply. Most likely, nobody in the world at that time was metabolically dependent on sugar the way most of us are today (as we discussed in chapter 3), and so anyone could cut carbs without metabolic repercussions. That is not true today. So, in my view, the keto diet needs modification to work with our radically different metabolism.

For these reasons, I recommend a lower-carb diet that is not low enough to qualify as keto and includes specific kinds of carbohydrates— slow-digesting carbs—at least once a day. (We'll learn about those carbohydrates in chapter 10.) These carbohydrates may be the only way that some people can escape the metabolic vicious cycle. They may also help accelerate our metabolic recovery and prevent some of the problems folks can have when cutting carbs too far and too fast while they are still insulin resistant (see Figure 8–1).

A widely publicized human clinical trial reported in the *American Journal of Clinical Nutrition* in 2022 supports the idea that it might not be great to jump from a typical diet of vegetable oils and processed foods to keto without some sort of preparatory phase first.[41] This study fed people either a whole-food-based keto diet or a whole-food-based Mediterranean diet (Med diet) for twelve weeks, then switched them to the other diet for another twelve weeks, for a total of twenty-four weeks of diet intervention.[42]

Both study diets were far healthier than the average American baseline diet; they were free of junk food and empty calorie sugars and flours. When eating the Med diet, folks were allowed fruits, legumes, and whole (intact) grains. Thus, the group that did the Med diet before keto had a chance to improve their nutrition before starting a diet that would force their sugar-addicted cells to cope with much less incoming sugar. The keto

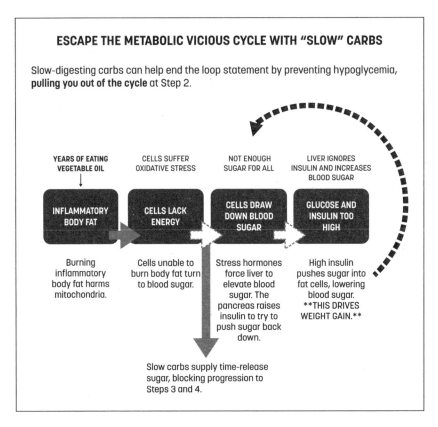

Figure 8–1: Insulin resistance hijacks our willpower and drives us to want foods that we know not to be healthy, trapping us in a vicious cycle of worsening health. **Cutting carbs reduces insulin levels *after* a meal**, which helps us to burn our body fat between meals. However, it may not reduce **fasting** insulin levels enough to allow the liver to generate ketones from body fat, thus leaving the brain without ketones or sugar. This would **cause some people to experience pathologic hunger, which is often called "the keto flu."**

Worse, stress hormones enable our bodies to make both sugar and ketones from our muscle tissue. This means **some people on a keto diet may be getting energy from sugar and/or ketones that originated in dietary protein or muscle tissue.** This is not desirable, either.

Fortunately, slow-digesting carbs can give us the energy without the after-meal insulin spikes.

first group had no such opportunity, and the final HOMA-IR scores suggest that jumping right into keto may actually have *harmed* their health!

In the beginning, both groups were markedly insulin resistant, with HOMA-IR scores of 5.3 (keto first) and 5.6 (Med first). By the end, the group that jumped into keto first was more insulin resistant than when they started, with HOMA-IR scores averaging 5.9. Meanwhile, the group that was allowed to recover from the standard American diet for twelve weeks before cutting carbs to keto levels had dramatically improved their scores to 3.4.

The kind of carbs and fats that people were permitted during the Mediterranean diet phase is revealing. During this phase, people avoided added sugars and refined grains. Olive oil was their primary fat source, so most of the PUFA they got was coming from whole foods that would also contain important antioxidant vitamins, including C and E. (It would have been helpful if the participants had also been asked about hypoglycemia symptoms.) The point I'm making is that if you want to try keto to see what all the buzz is about, it would be wise to take a few weeks or months to first fortify your mitochondria against the oxidative stress produced by burning high-PUFA body fat. The kind of diet we will learn about in the next section is the best way to do that—and you can continue it indefinitely, because, as we've seen, the magic comes not from ketones, but from having healthy body fat and a healthy, flexible metabolism that can produce energy efficiently. I'm going to give you the tools for creating three meals a day that sustain your energy (so you won't need to snack) and enable your mitochondria to more easily use body fat for fuel, as nature intends. This diet is lower in carbs than the Mediterranean diet because I think the moderate carb restriction can more efficiently control your hunger, improve your energy, and rehabilitate your metabolism.

In this chapter I have only scratched the surface of what's to be gained by losing our fear of cholesterol. In the next section, in addition to discussing exactly what to eat, we'll also hear from more people who have improved their health in myriad ways. It's more than freedom from illness. It's also relative freedom from a medical system that is more than happy to continue business as usual, selling everyone drugs and procedures with questionable value. If you're ready to join the growing ranks of people escaping this predatory system, let's find out exactly what to eat and how to get started.

PART THREE

TAKING BACK OUR HEALTH

Good food is very often, even most often, simple food.

—ANTHONY BOURDAIN

CHAPTER 9

How to Ditch Vegetable Oils for Good

IN THIS CHAPTER YOU WILL LEARN

- How to distinguish good fats from bad.
- How to identify two other categories of problematic ultra-processed food ingredients: protein powders and refined carbohydrates.
- How to spot the Hateful Eight before you buy, and how much is too much.
- How to avoid vegetable oils while dining out.

By now, you may have already rounded up all the vegetable oils in your kitchen and tossed them—good riddance! In this chapter, we're going to cover everything you need to clear the oils out of your house, because they may be hiding where you least suspect. We'll also see that when we're avoiding vegetable oils, we're automatically cutting down on two other important categories of ultra-processed ingredients that also harm our health. Then we'll cover the essentials for avoiding these oils everywhere else, with essential tips for dining out in a variety of venues.

The following chapters in this part of the book will walk you through a better way of eating to support your body in healing, along with a Two-Week Challenge to get you started.

Before we jump in, a note: I know that getting rid of a bunch of food can be an emotional (and expensive) endeavor. You may wish to take smaller steps. Instead of throwing away a lot of food from your cupboard and fridge in one fell swoop, you might commit to not buying any more, and replacing any vegetable oils and vegetable-oil-containing foods with healthier options as you finish them. If you'd like to do the Challenge in this book, you won't have to buy a lot. It's up to you—whatever feels right for your budget, your comfort with risk, and your family's health.

While (as mentioned in chapter 3) it might take years for PUFA to fully clear from your body, the good news is that usually people feel better within a couple of weeks of cutting out vegetable oils. Are you ready to take these next exciting steps for your health? Let's begin.

> "I used to feel hopeless about ever being able to lose weight or getting rid of my migraine headaches that pained me almost on a weekly basis. I felt like I was taking too much medication and still they were very debilitating. After seven months of avoiding the Hateful Eight seed oils, I've been migraine-free with only two very minor headache episodes and I'm also down forty pounds."
>
> —Jennifer S.

THE DELIGHTFUL DOZEN COOKING FATS

Happily, avoiding seed oils opens you up to a variety of healthier (and tastier!) options. Consider the "Delightful Dozen" your antidote to the Hateful Eight.

Except as noted, all the fats in the Delightful Dozen can be used for cooking. Unlike vegetable oils, which are almost tasteless, you do need to choose the oil that matches the cuisine, and I've made some notes on that below. For that slight extra thought process, you'll be rewarded with a much tastier dish. Some people worry about smoke point. I discuss this in-depth later in this chapter, since their high smoke point is a tactic used to sell vegetable oils (see "Understanding Smoke Point" on page 225).

All of these options may seem overwhelming, but you don't need all of them. To get through your Two-Week Challenge, you'll probably only need three or four. In the United States, most people use butter, olive oil, and peanut oil most of the time, as these are readily available and relatively inexpensive. They are also amazingly versatile and tend to go with a variety of cuisines. If you like to make East Asian–style dishes, you might want to add coconut oil and/or toasted sesame. As your repertoire expands, you'll probably want to have more than just three on hand.

Butter

Butter is hands down my favorite cooking fat. I use it with simply flavored foods such as eggs, steak (together with olive oil), and chicken livers. When it browns slightly it creates a delicious nutty, slightly butterscotchy taste. Butter burns easily, so if you want a nice brown sear on your meats and veggies, you will need to lower the temperature if you see the butter starting to smoke before the food has had a chance to cook. Real butter has only one ingredient: cream. (Unless it's salted, in which case it has two.) Grass-fed butter is best, as it contains more omega-3 fatty acid, vitamin A, and, in the spring and early summer, vitamin K2. It also has a more complex—and I think better—flavor than regular butter from grain-fed cows.

Extra Virgin Olive Oil or Unfiltered, Unrefined Olive Oil

I use olive oil for robust-flavored dishes, including homemade pasta sauces and anything Italian, Mediterranean, or Mexican. I also use this versatile oil for roasting vegetables and making dressings, marinades, and mayonnaise. You can get unrefined olive oil, also known as extra virgin olive oil (EVOO), or, even better, look for unfiltered, unrefined olive oil, which is higher quality than ordinary extra virgin. These types of oils are cold pressed to remove the oil and there is no additional refining that would reduce their nutritional value.

Unrefined Peanut Oil

I use peanut oil instead of olive oil when I'm cooking with soy sauce or miso. Unrefined peanut oil is best; it should be very flavorful. Some people recommend against using peanut oil because it does have a higher PUFA content than most others on this list, but I keep it on the list because peanuts have been bred for thousands of years to be high in oil, which makes the final product more nutritious. If you or someone in your family has a peanut allergy, allergists will tell you that refined peanut oil is actually safe because all traces of protein are removed. Unrefined oil is not safe for those with allergies.

Unrefined Coconut Oil

Boldly flavored, coconut oil goes amazingly well with East Asian and Indian flavor profiles. Coconut is extremely heat stable, and a little goes a long way. It's also great for your skin—you can use it like moisturizer, and a little goes a long way here, too!

Unrefined Avocado Oil

Avocado oil is a new kid on the block. It's not a traditional culinary oil; however, its fatty acid profile makes it good for culinary uses. Unrefined avocado oil is expensive and will have a strong flavor. Avoid the "private label" companies (i.e., the store brands) as there is currently no regulation in this facet of the industry, and about 70 percent of these are adulterated or oxidized.[1] Examples of good quality, non-private labels would be Chosen Foods and La Tourangelle.

Ghee

Ghee is simply butter that has been clarified, a process that involves heating the butter to coagulate the milk solids and then skimming them off. This is a traditional practice throughout India; it helps to preserve the butter in the hot climate. It is actually less healthy than regular butter because the additional heating destroys some of the more fragile nutrients, particularly omega-3 fatty acids. But it's still a healthy and flavorful culinary ingredient, and it's gaining in popularity across the world.

Sesame Oil

This is a high-PUFA oil. What is it doing here? Similar to peanut oil, it's a traditional oil that has been cultivated for thousands of years. This has imparted special properties that make it more suitable for use as a culinary oil, and sesame is now an essential component of many cuisines. If your dish calls for more than than five or ten minutes of cooking, it's best to combine sesame oil with more stable oils, like coconut or peanut. Because it's high in PUFA, it's not a good oil to cook with day in and day out, even if it is better than other vegetable oils.

Tip: Try an Asian oil medley made by combining sesame with peanut and/or coconut oil in roughly equal parts.

Unrefined Palm Oil

This is a traditional, low-PUFA oil, but it's not often used in many areas of the world, perhaps because of its flavor, which is sometimes described as earthy and carrot-like. It's a great choice for making soups and sauces and sautéing, especially if you like the spices and flavor profiles of the African continent. Red palm oil has a much stronger, more bitter taste than other types, so make sure you know which one you're getting. (Most palm oil in processed foods is refined and falls into the third "okay but not great" category discussed next.)

Bacon Fat

Use bacon fat to cook eggs, steak, burgers, and anything else you want to give a bacon flavor. I like to warm it up, drizzle it over spinach, and add a splash of apple cider vinegar or lemon for a quick salad dressing. Unlike other recommendations on this list, bacon fat isn't something you need to buy at the grocery store. After frying bacon, pour off the fat into a clean heatproof jar or grease can, cool it, and store it in the fridge. (It should be used just once, so if you have any bacon fat leftover in the pan after cooking with it, discard it.)

Tallow

Tallow is simply beef fat. It's extremely heat stable and has a high smoke point, making it the best cooking fat for extensive high-heat frying, particularly shallow pan or deep frying. Even so, after two or three uses in a deep fryer, it should be discarded.

Lard

Lard is pig fat that's been rendered by a process similar to making ghee that helps to preserve it. It has a high smoke point but is less heat stable than tallow, coconut oil, and butter. It's great for baking and making pie crusts.

Chicken Fat

Rendered chicken fat is a huge part of Jewish cuisine, where it's called *Schmalz*. If it's made from the fat of pasture-raised chickens, it will have a better omega-3 to omega-6 balance than when it's from confinement animals.

Unrefined Tree Nut Oils

Any nut can yield oil, but the most popular tree nut oils are almond, hazelnut, and pecan. (Do not use walnut oil for cooking, as it is too high in easily oxidized omega-3.) I've experimented with these oils for pan frying fish, poultry, and other meats, and it seems like they taste good with just about anything. Unrefined nut oils are generally very expensive specialty items, so I don't include them in the Delightful Dozen. Although they are probably not going to become your go-to cooking fats, they are a fine and nutritious choice. That said, if you or someone in your family has a tree nut allergy, you should skip these.

OKAY (BUT NOT GREAT) REFINED FATS AND OILS

This category includes oils that are chemically more stable than the Hateful Eight, but that have been subjected to extensive refining. Refined oils are far cheaper than unrefined because the raw materials can be significantly lower in quality, since the refining will strip out unwanted components. They are also less flavorful, less nutritious, and more prone to oxidizing, because many vitamins and antioxidants are also stripped out. They do typically have higher smoke points as a result, although this is not a nutritional benefit (as discussed below). Refined and hydrogenated oils are the empty calories of the fat world.

These oils are not nourishing, but they're not as bad as the Hateful Eight, so they fall into a middle category, "okay but not great." You don't need to avoid them, but if you can, find an alternative that would be more nutritious.

Refined Avocado Oil

This product can be useful for making mayonnaise, since it lacks the strong flavor of olive and unrefined avocado oil that some mayonnaise aficionados object to. "Private label" brands are often adulterated.

Refined Peanut Oil

Refined peanut oil has a more neutral flavor than unrefined, making it more suitable for making mayonnaise if olive and avocado are too strong for your tastes. Some restaurants have started using refined peanut oil as their cooking fat, which is much better than a Hateful Eight oil but still not ideal. Refined peanut oil is generally devoid of peanut allergens, but this is one of the least healthy of the oils in this "okay but not great" category.

Refined Olive Oil

Refined olive oil contains more PUFA and fewer vitamins and minerals than EVOO and unrefined oil. This, too, is on the unhealthy end of the "okay but not great" collection of oils.

Refined Coconut Oil

Coconut oil that has been refined is often slightly coconut flavored, but less so than unrefined coconut oil. It is also less beneficial, although it is very heat stable and oxidation proof. Like unrefined coconut oil, it works well as a skin cream.

Refined Palm Oil

This type of palm oil is used in many baked goods and nut butters. The refining processes now used reduce the formation of carcinogenic byproducts that were a problem until around 2015. If you see an item in your cabinet that contains "non-hydrogenated palm oil," it probably falls into this category—it is likely refined palm oil, and thus okay but not great to include in your diet.

Hydrogenated Fats and Oils

You may see hydrogenated coconut oil, palm oil, or lard listed as ingredients, especially in peanut butter and baked goods such as pastries, cookies, cakes, and donuts. The two most commonly used hydrogenated fats are palm oil and lard. Hydrogenated fats and oils contain mostly saturated fat and are therefore safer than the partially hydrogenated fats and oils, which contain mostly trans fat. Hydrogenation takes away the double bonds, turning unsaturated fat into saturated fat. Partial hydrogenation takes away *some* double bonds, and those it leaves behind have been distorted into an unnatural configuration that chemists call *trans fats*. Both processes improve the fats' resistance to oxidation, thus lengthening shelf life, which makes foods that are made with them cheaper. If the label says "hydrogenated," that means it's fully hydrogenated.

"I had been suffering from an increasingly common condition where I had terrible difficulty swallowing. Not in my throat, but in my lower esophagus. Food would get lodged, sometimes for an hour or two. Choking—or should I say, drowning—would ensue if I tried to wash the food down with a liquid. This condition is called eosinophilic esophagitis, or

EE. Various physicians told me it was likely caused either by excess stomach acid (take omeprazole, they told me) or a food allergy/intolerance. After about eighteen months of trying omeprazole and numerous food elimination diets, I stumbled onto the real culprit: industrialized seed oils. I have avoided these oils as much as possible and completely eliminated the swallowing issues! I've told my primary physician and asked him to share [your teachings] with his other patients also suffering from EE. Thank you!"

—Dennis V.

BAD FATS AND OILS

Ditch products with the following bad fats whenever possible, unless the amount is minimal (see "Understanding the Ingredients List" on page 235). If a product does not list any of the fats and oils on this list, it's free of toxic seed oils. However, it's not entirely free of oxidized, toxic PUFAs. Let me explain.

In addition to the Hateful Eight, there are now many different products made from seed oils that you'll see on labels, including lecithin and interesterified products, which I'll discuss below. Unlike the oils listed as "bad fats" themselves, the seed-oil derivatives are not absolute deal breakers, as they are generally present in smaller amounts.

The Hateful Eight

I've discussed these at length in chapter 1. So that you can easily spot these on ingredient labels, look for any of the following:

- Corn oil
- Rapeseed oil

- Cottonseed oil
- Soy oil
- Sunflower oil
- Safflower oil
- Grapeseed oil
- Rice bran oil

Also avoid:

Vegetable oil (a general term for any of the Hateful Eight)

Partially Hydrogenated Oils

Partially hydrogenated fats are rarely used since the trans-fat ban. Only the Hateful Eight will be partially hydrogenated. Believe it or not, partially hydrogenated oils are actually worse than fully hydrogenated ones (see "Hydrogenated Fats and Oils" on page 222). These are less oxidation-prone than PUFA, but trans fats have a kind of double bond that nature rarely makes, and eating a lot of trans fats can have toxic effects.

Vegetable Lecithin

Lecithin is an emulsifier that helps blend fats and water together. It is getting harder (but not impossible) to find chocolate made without soy, sunflower, or other vegetable oil lecithin. Vegetable lecithins are not at all healthy. However, if there is no alternative product, it's still okay to buy it, because for the most part only very small amounts are used. Mayonnaise and salad dressings are notable exceptions. It's better to get mayonnaise made the old-fashioned way, with egg yolk—or make it on your own at home with an oil you like.

Other Artificial Fats

A growing collection of engineered vegetable-based fats are being used in our foods. These go by a variety of names that you might read about in health-oriented publications, including structured lipids, tailor-made fats, designer lipids, modified fats, restructured fats, and novel triacylglycerols (TAGs). More seem to be popping up every few years. Unfortunately, right now we can't usually tell when they're in our foods. The only ones currently listed on labels are the *interesterified fats*, made by rearranging the *ester* bonds of the fat molecules. All are best avoided because they are essentially experimental chemicals that food manufacturers have invented to comply with various government recommendations about avoiding cholesterol, saturated fats, and more recently trans fats. (You can thank the American Heart Association for these experimental foods.) The good news is that they're expensive, and so they're not (yet) being added in particularly large amounts.

"My hip pain was so debilitating I couldn't walk without a cane and I would sit and cry. I believe it was mostly due to inflammation. I have changed my diet and my energy level is way up. I'm also losing weight. I have told friends and family about how and why vegetable oils are so bad. Thank you."

—Sue D.

UNDERSTANDING SMOKE POINT

If you've heard the term "smoke point," you should know it's a marketing angle for the oil industry. It does not tell us anything our own common sense wouldn't tell us.

The term *smoke point* refers to the temperature at which a fat starts to smoke. At the smoke point, you might see a thin wisp of light blue smoke, and heating the fat past that point will fill the air with bitter smoke and ruin the food. Smoke point says nothing about the chemical stability of the fatty acids to oxidation. While cooking with a high-smoke-point oil allows for higher heat and makes things go faster in a busy restaurant kitchen, using high heat makes foods cooked in these oils potentially more toxic than they would be otherwise. To understand why this is so, it helps to understand where the smoke comes from.

The smoke is coming from the combustion of proteins and free fatty acids. The Hateful Eight oils have zero protein and very few free fatty acids compared to unrefined oils, and so they tend to have higher smoke points for that reason. But their higher smoke points allow them to be heated to the point they oxidize and become more toxic.

The lower smoke point of healthy fats and oils will prevent you from eating them after they've been oxidized (so you aren't eating toxic food). Most foods should not be cooked at super-high temperatures anyway, because heat also destroys the nutrition in the food: the higher you heat something, the less nutritious it becomes.

A low smoke point also helps make food taste better. If you want a nice browning on your steak or your scallops, for instance, you'll get that faster using butter. Part of honoring the ingredient is learning how to cook it just right, and that applies to the fat you're using as well.

Contrary to popular belief, you can actually deep fry in oils with a low smoke point right at home in a deep cooking pan because it doesn't take extreme heat to crisp batter and cook the interior. (Italian chefs often deep fry eggplant, for example, in a suitably deep pan filled halfway with olive or peanut oil.)[2] However, you do have to watch much more closely, since, if it does start to smoke, the hot oil can boil over the pot and make a dangerous mess.

VEGETABLE OIL'S LITTLE SIBLINGS

Vegetable oils are the worst ingredients in our food supply, but they're not the only ingredients worth avoiding. Two other components of processed food also make it very unhealthy: protein powders and refined flours and sugars. I group these last two together because they are chemically nearly identical, being composed of sugar molecules. Together with vegetable oils, these three ingredients represent more than three-quarters of the average American's diet.

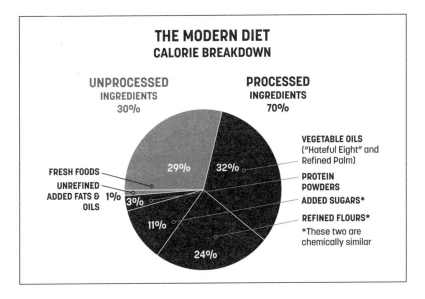

Figure 9-1: This is the modern diet. **We don't need MyPlate, or the Food Pyramid, or Tufts University's new "Food Compass" to guide us to healthy food.** We just need to learn about the big three processed ingredients: vegetable oils, protein powders, and refined sugars and flours.

Note: These data sources appear to lump fruit juice, nut milks, hot dogs, and frozen prepared dinners together with fresh food, so Americans are eating less truly fresh food than this. Unrefined fats include butter, tallow, lard, olive oil, and avocado oil. Palm oil use has increased more than ten times over since 2000 due to the trans-fat ban.

For sources used to create this figure, see the endnotes for this chapter.

There is a lot of talk about what constitutes processed food that makes the issue much more complex than this, but this is really the crux of the problem. Having been convinced that cholesterol, saturated fat, and salt are harmful, we're now living on three industrial products. Enough is enough. It's time to identify them clearly and learn a little bit about what they are doing to us.

REFINED CARBS: EMPTY CALORIES THAT AGE OUR TISSUES

Carb is short for carbohydrate. Carbohydrates include fiber, starches, and sugars. Many foods are naturally high in carbs, particularly potatoes, rice, and fruits, but those are not what I'm talking about here. Here I'm talking about the factory-refined sugars and flours. Unlike vegetable oils, these ingredients have their uses, so we don't need to categorically avoid them. It comes down to the dose.

These kinds of carbs are empty calories, meaning they are devoid of nutrition. They lack other complex nutrients that take a while for our digestive systems to process, so they can get absorbed very quickly. When we eat foods made mostly from refined carbs, they spike our blood sugar—and our insulin. High blood sugar isn't good for our tissues and can accelerate a process called *glycation*. Glycation accelerates the aging process in many tissues, especially our joints and skin.

Foods made with sugars and refined carbs are also problematic for the simple reason that they are also easy to overeat. Remember that sweet foods and foods full of starchy carbs can be addicting, so it's very easy for our plans to eat just a little bit to turn into regrets that we ate too much. Still, even these bad carbs are not as bad as vegetable oil. If you do not have diabetes (or prediabetes), enjoying them in small quantities from time to time is not especially harmful. The key is to feel you're in control.

A lot of people think of sugary foods and beverages as a source of instant energy, but it's a very short-lived energy burst. Blood-sugar spikes cause insulin spikes, which help us clear that extra sticky sugar out of the bloodstream. Since insulin works quickly to get the extra sugar into your fat cells, rather than thinking of sugar as instant energy, it's more accurate to think of sugar as instant body fat. After a blood-sugar spike, the big spike of insulin often pushes the blood sugar back down a little too far, making us hungry or tired. If you get hungry or tired a few hours after eating something full of carbs, think of that as the feeling of your fat cells filling up with more fat.

Spotting Refined Flours

The most ubiquitous refined flour is wheat flour. You will see this on the label as wheat flour, whole wheat flour, or simply "flour." Both wheat flour and "flour" are actually just white flour, and the vitamins listed on the nutrition label are artificially added, not naturally present. You might expect whole wheat flour to be better, but the reality is that flour labeled "whole wheat" has actually been extensively milled and processed. Let me explain what I mean so you can understand why the kinds of breads I recommend provide significantly superior nutrition.

Most flour in the United States is processed into three parts: the endosperm (starchy and nutritionally bereft) and the germ and bran (both nutritious). This is done for supply chain reasons, since most products are made with white flour, and millers usually need to sell the germ and bran separately. In the minority of foods that also contain the two nutritious components, manufacturers will simply recombine the three back together, and the reconstituted product label can say "whole wheat flour." The problem with processing wheat like this comes down to oxidation. As long as the seed remains intact, the vitamins and fats are protected from oxygen. Disassembling and reassembling the wheat kernels exposes them to oxygen. After just a few weeks or months (depending on storage conditions), most of the nutrients are oxidized. As we've seen, oxidation both reduces nutritional value and creates toxins. The oxidized compounds impart a bitter flavor that is often assumed to be an indication that bread is "healthy."

For whole-wheat flour to be truly healthy, it needs to be eaten shortly after being milled, and this can only be guaranteed by bakeries that do their own milling onsite. I recommend choosing either bread sold right where the flour is milled, or bread made with intact grains that have never been processed or oxidized, called "sprouted-grain" breads (more on this in the next chapter).

Due to the fact that whole wheat flour is oxidized and white flour has very little nutrition, I recommend limiting foods made with mostly flour, such as baked goods and pastas. I personally avoid them, because I don't have space in my calorie budget for the empty calories. White flour is fine if it is a minor ingredient, but I do avoid most pasta, cookies, cakes, crackers, pretzels, chips, muffins, cereals, pie crust, donuts, and pastries—as well as breads in general (see chapter 10 for recommended breads).

The vast majority of these foods also contain the Hateful Eight vegetable oils. However, if you are looking for an occasional treat, in the Resources section at the back of the book I've included a link to my Shopping List, where you can find better brands that at least are not made with vegetable oil.

USING FLOURS AT HOME

I want to point out that even white flours have their uses. For example, if there are super-healthy foods that you do not normally like, a recipe using a little flour might turn them into a favorite. A couple tablespoons of flour can make a roux for thickening bone broth into gravy. Coating chicken livers in a bit of flour before frying them up in butter gives them a delicious nutty flavor. Of course, making your own sourdough bread is another great use of flour, and here freshly milled whole wheat is a better choice (ancient grains such as barley, spelt, and teff are even better).

Spotting Sugars

Cane sugar, beet sugar, honey, maple syrup, and fruit juices are all examples of ingredients that are essentially pure sugar. There are dozens of other names for sugar that you'll find on labels, and I don't expect anyone to memorize them all. The most important terms to look for, besides plain "sugar," "syrup," or "juice," is anything with those words in them, such as "date sugar," "barley malt syrup," or "cane juice." Another trick to finding secret sugar is to look for words ending with the suffix *ose*, as in "sucrose," "fructose," "xylose," or "dextrose."

"I struggled with my weight ever since I was a kid. I used to crave junk food and had to finagle money out of people at school for the vending machines. In college I was always riding on the razor's edge of discipline. The minute I lost focus on my calorie-restriction and six-mile daily running, I regained. In medical school I couldn't do that, and I got up to 280 pounds. The minute I cut out seed oils and processed carbohydrates, I lost 60 pounds like it was nothing. It was like a silver bullet for me."

—Paul Grewal, MD, author of *Genius Foods*[3]

Protein Powders: The Protein Equivalent of Sugar

Modern food-processing practices extract protein from its original source and concentrate it into a powder. This reduces the nutritional value of the protein. All processed proteins are best avoided, for several reasons.

First, they have been separated from the whole food. In addition to being stripped of fats and carbohydrates, many of them have been stripped of the vitamins, minerals, and other nutrients that were present in the original food. Thus, they are relatively empty-calorie proteins. Second, extracting the protein from the whole food often destroys and distorts a portion of the amino acids, which is very similar in concept to how vegetable oil extraction and refining distorts PUFAs.[4] Third, when added to foods, they react with other components in ways that are more likely to generate oxidative-stress-inducing toxins.[5] This is an especially serious problem for babies. Protein powders have been shown to damage intestinal cells but they are nevertheless ubiquitous in infant formulas.[6] (Shame on the American Academy of Pediatricians for accepting money from formula companies, failing to inform parents of the problematic ingredients they contain, and failing to deveop an alternative for the millions of women who are unable or choose not to breastfeed.)[7] Fourth, they can be adulterated and contaminated, and consumers have no way to know.[8] Fifth, the protein content can be overstated.[9] Currently, manufacturers are not required to assess or disclose the degree of amino acid destruction or toxin formation that occurs during the production of processed proteins.[10]

Finally, these processed proteins tend to get absorbed into our bloodstreams very quickly, spiking the amino acid content of our blood in ways that our biology is unprepared for. Just as sugar spikes can glycate and age our tissues, amino-acid spikes can, too. Given their chemical properties, I worry they may damage our kidneys if we eat very much, and may contribute to declining kidney function, high blood pressure, kidney stones, or gout.

SPOTTING PROTEIN POWDERS

The most obvious sources of protein powders are literally called "protein powders." These include the athletic supplements sold under the guise of muscle building, diet drinks sold as "protein shakes," products sold as "protein smoothies," and nutrition boosters for the elderly, toddlers, and people on the go. Even though it's a small portion of our average calorie intake, protein shakes and supplements were worth about $7 billion in total revenues in 2022, reflecting an extraordinarily high profit margin.[11] (Compare this to the $13 billion in revenues for the twenty-six billion pounds of soy oil produced in the United States the same year.[12])

Protein powders are essential to the protein bar industry, including vegan, low-carb, and keto products. Vegan meats are particularly likely to contain a form of processed soy protein called textured vegetable protein. Frozen food manufacturers often save money on ingredients by filling their products with processed proteins that cost far less than actual meats. And lately, manufacturers catering to protein-seeking and low-carb consumers will use protein powders in their pastas, breads, wraps, and other baked goods. All of these protein-powder-containing foods overstate their nutritional value for the reasons described above. Worse, they are likely to contain compounds with at least mild toxicity to our gut flora.[13] Due to these low-level toxins, I worry that regular consumption of highly processed proteins may cause later development of food allergies and autoimmune diseases.

Fortunately, they are easy to spot because they are listed on the label with the term "protein" (the exception is casein, a kind of milk protein, which will be listed simply as casein). Common processed proteins listed on labels include milk protein, whey protein, soy protein, egg white protein, pea protein, brown rice protein, and textured vegetable protein. The least processed form of processed proteins is called protein concentrates, as in milk protein concentrate or soy protein concentrate. The most processed form is called protein isolate, as in whey protein isolate and soy protein isolate.

FOOD VALUE of the BIG THREE PROCESSED INGREDIENTS

INGREDIENT	NUTRITION PER CALORIE	POTENTIAL TOXICITY
VEGETABLE OILS	MINIMAL	VERY HIGH
PROTEIN POWDERS	ACCEPTABLE	LOW
FLOURS & SUGARS	MINIMAL & ABSENT	HIGH

Figure 9-2: **This is why the modern diet is making us chronically ill.** These three ultra-processed ingredients lack the nutrients of the whole foods they came from, and they have a variety of toxic effects in our bodies that increase our exposure to oxidative stress. Our failing health is not that mysterious. **We don't need more research; we need better food.**

Even if you don't try to reduce your intake of refined carbs or protein powders, and only focus on avoiding vegetable oils, you will be eating less processed food. And so you will be cutting back on these other two ingredients almost automatically. Now that you know about the two other bad players in our food supply that you'll largely be avoiding as a byproduct of cutting out seed oils, you're ready to learn how to expunge these oils from your life completely.

HOW TO SPOT THE HATEFUL EIGHT

When you're shopping, or if you're undertaking a kitchen detox and weeding out the seed oils in your pantry, fridge, and freezer, look at the ingredients list of every product that has a nutrition label. Every. Single. One. In fact, if you want a suggestion for a first, easy step to getting healthy, I would like to recommend that you make a habit of turning around every package and reading the label every time you go shopping.

Reading labels is necessary because you simply can't predict what will have vegetable oil. You might think that dried fruits, for example, wouldn't have vegetable oil, but they do. Or peanut butter. Or the "butter" on your microwave popcorn, or nuts, rotisserie chicken, mayonnaise and dressings that say "made with olive oil," granola (even "healthy" high-protein brands), canned tuna, olives, sun-dried tomatoes and other vegetable preserves, even random things like vitamins and spice blends. The only exceptions are things like bottled water and beverages such as juice, soda, and tea—although these may contain unhealthy amounts of sugar, so I'm not recommending you drink them.

The ingredients list is not in the box labeled "Nutrition Facts," and it's generally not going to be located on the front of the package. To find the ingredients list, you need to look *under* the black-and-white "nutrition facts." Some awkwardly shaped packages will place them next to this label, or on the side. The writing is tiny, unfortunately. So if you're over age forty, you might need your reading glasses or a magnifying glass.

Price Check

One way to save time on your search for products made with healthier oils is to start by looking at the price tag before drilling down into the ingredients. If a product costs twice as much or more than its neighbors on the shelf, that's (unfortunately) a good indication that it

---

might be made with a healthier oil, or without added vegetable oils. This is often the case with salad dressings, mayonnaise, nut butters, canned seafoods, and pasta sauces. But always read the ingredients to be sure!

UNDERSTANDING THE INGREDIENTS LIST

Once you've spotted a member of the Hateful Eight, the next step is to figure out if the food contains a deal-breaking amount or a minimal amount. To do that, you need to understand a few basic principles of the ingredients list.

List Order

The *first* ingredient on the list is the one present in the largest amount by weight. The *second* ingredient on the list is the one present in the next largest amount by weight. And so on. The order rule applies to the ingredients listed within parentheses, too. This helps us to guess how much vegetable oil is in a product.

Fat Calories

When vegetable oils are the only source of fat calories, you can directly calculate the percentage of calories coming from vegetable oil (see Figures 9–3 and 9–4). When there are multiple fat sources, it's more difficult, but knowing the list-order rule can help you take a guess.

"Less Than ___ Percent"

The number in the blank is either going to be 1, 1.5, or 2 percent. Any oil listed after this is, by definition, present in less than that percentage by weight. You'll see a lot of chemical names listed here. Most of them will be your classic, hard-to-pronounce chemicals, including flavoring agents, antioxidants, stabilizers, preservatives, and texturizers. Oils listed here are generally not present in high enough concentrations to worry about.

UNDERSTANDING THE INGREDIENTS LIST
LIST ORDER, EXAMPLE 1

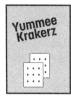

- The FIRST ingredient on the list is present in the largest amount by weight. The SECOND ingredient on the list is present in the next largest amount by weight. The rule applies within parentheses, too.

- Although vegetable oils may look like a minor ingredient based on their position about halfway down the list, once you notice the parentheses you can see they are actually the second ingredient.

- As you can see by reading the first three ingredients, these crackers are mostly flour, seed oil, and sugar. Sugar appears again in the form of corn syrup and malted barley flour.

- Conclusion: AVOID.

(This list comes from a popular brand sold in the US.)

Ingredients:

UNBLEACHED ENRICHED FLOUR (WHEAT FLOUR, NIACIN, REDUCED IRON, THIAMINE MONONITRATE (VITAMIN B1), RIBOFLAVIN (VITAMIN B2), FOLIC ACID), **VEGETABLE OIL** (SOYBEAN AND/OR RAPESEED AND/OR PALM AND/OR PARTIALLY HYDROGENATED COTTONSEED OIL), **SUGAR**, SALT, LEAVENING (BAKING SODA AND/OR CALCIUM PHOSPHATE), HIGH FRUCTOSE CORN SYRUP, SOY LECITHIN, MALTED BARLEY FLOUR, NATURAL FLAVOR.

UNDERSTANDING THE NUTRITION FACTS
PERCENT OF FAT CALORIES IN YUMMEE KRAKERZ

Nutrition Facts	
Per 6 crackers (20 g)	
Calories 100	% Daily Value*
Fat 5 g	7 %
Saturated 1.0 g	5 %
Trans 0 g	
Carbohydrate 12 g	
Fiber 0 g	0 %
Sugars 4 g	2 %
Protein 1 g	
Cholesterol 0 mg	0 %
Sodium 160 mg	7 %
Potassium 20 mg	0 %
Calcium 30 mg	2 %
Iron 0.75 mg	4 %
*5% or less is **a little**, 15% or more is a lot	

- In this example, vegetable oils are the only source of fat calories.

- When this is the case, you can easily calculate the percent of calories coming from vegetable oil.

- Total fat is 5 grams. Fat has 9 calories per gram. So six crackers (1 serving) contain 45 fat calories.

- 45 out of 100 is 45 percent. So nearly half of the calories in this box of popular snack crackers are coming from vegetable oil.

Figure 9–3

UNDERSTANDING THE INGREDIENTS LIST
LIST ORDER, EXAMPLE 2

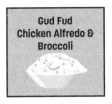

Gud Fud
Chicken Alfredo &
Broccoli

◎ Soy oil is listed before any other fat and again in the ingredients for the cream sauce.

◎ Other fat sources: cream, cheeses.

◎ Okay to ignore everything after the "2% or less."

◎ Guesstimating: Half the fat calories come from vegetable oil.

◎ Conclusion: AVOID.

(This list comes from a popular brand sold in the US.)

Ingredients:

Cooked Enriched Pasta (Water, Enriched Wheat **Flour** [Durum Wheat Semolina, Niacin, Ferrous Sulfate (Iron), Thiamine Mononitrate, Riboflavin, Folic Acid], **Soybean Oil**, Dried Egg Whites), Sauce (Water, Cream, **Soybean Oil,** Parmesan Cheese [Part-Skim Milk, Cheese Culture, Salt, Enzymes], Romano Cheese from Cow's Milk [Cultured Part-Skim Milk, Salt, Enzymes], Sherry Wine, Nonfat Dry Milk…[remainder of sauce ingredients all "less than 2%"]), Boneless Chicken Breast Strips (Boneless Chicken Breast with Rib Meat, Water…[remainder of chicken strips ingredients less than 2%]), Parmesan Cheese (Pasteurized Milk, Cheese Culture, Salt, Powdered Cellulose, Potato Starch, Enzymes), Dried Parsley

UNDERSTANDING THE NUTRITION FACTS
PERCENT OF FAT CALORIES IN GUD FUD DINNER

Nutrition Facts		
1.0 servings per container		
Serving size		**1 meal (369g)**
Amounte per serving		
Calories		**440**
		% Daily Value*
Total Fat 18g		23 %
Saturated Fat 6g		30 %
Trans Fat 0g		0 %
Cholesterol 60mg		20 %
Sodium 1040mg		45 %
Total Carbohydrate 43g		16 %
Dietary Fiber 4g		14 %
Sugar 6g		
Includes less than		
1g added sugars		1 %
Protein 27g		47 %
Calcium 200mg		15 %
Iron 2.8mg		15 %
Potassium 710mg		15 %
Vitamin D 0mcg		0 %

◎ In this example, vegetable oils are just one source of fat calories. Cream and two types of cheeses are the other three sources.

◎ Given that dairy fat is mostly saturated and soy is mostly PUFA, we can guesstimate that (very roughly) a third of the fat calories come from dairy fat.

◎ 2/3 of 18gm is 12gm.

◎ 12gm fat has 108 calories.

◎ So about 1/4 of all calories come from PUFA.

Figure 9–4

Spice Mixes and Seasoning Blends in Other Foods

Many spice mixes and seasoning blends used in packaged foods are blended with oil to prevent caking, so that the final mixture is usually around 1 percent oil by weight. Sometimes the oil's purpose is explicitly stated, as in "added to prevent caking." Sometimes the label also explicitly states "seasoning blend" or "spice blend" or a similar term, and then lists all the various spices, including the oil within parentheses. (If no oil is listed, it is safe to assume the spice mix doesn't contain any.) But sometimes you'll have to figure it out yourself, by noticing that the term "vegetable oil" is surrounded by spices, salt, pepper, and other ingredients that are usually part of a spice mix. In all of these cases, the oils are not present in high enough concentrations to worry about.

Oils Added to Dried Fruit

Many dried fruits are given a light coating of oil to prevent clumping. In some cases, the amount is significant. One way to tell is by looking at the total fat content on the nutrition label. If the number is zero, it's probably insignificant. But even 1 gram can be significant. For example, a brand of dried blueberries called Foods to Live contains 1 gram of sunflower oil per serving, which equates to 9 calories of fat, meaning that 10 percent of the total 90 calories per serving will be derived from the oil.

KITCHEN DETOX ASSIST

Now it's time to get into your kitchen, roll up your sleeves, and start clearing out the toxic food. Many people have found it helpful to have a list like what I'm showing you here. It provides a plan of attack to jump-start the project. Other people don't feel that they need a list to follow. In fact, you don't even need to throw out all your old food for the Two-Week Challenge (in chapter 11) if you don't want to. Either way, reading through this list will help you to better understand the scope of the problem, and reveal how seed oils find so many ways to seep into our lives.

How to Use This Worksheet

- Pull items from your cupboards, fridge, pantry, and anywhere else you store food and ingredients by group (each heading is a group).
- Review ingredients for seed oils and make notes as follows:

    ◦ Mark ✓ to indicate that you've checked the product(s) and found no seed oil.
    ◦ Mark R to indicate products in this category that need to be replaced.

- Use the Shopping List link in the Resources section to help find replacements.
- Consider discarding or donating products with seed oils (most folks just toss them).

"Life changing....I got rid of the Hateful Eight vegetable oils....I've been decreasing the grains and the sugars—which I didn't think I could ever do—and now I have trained my body to [burn fat] instead of me running to the pantry for the sugary stuff....I'm no longer bloated at night! What woman isn't bloated at night? We're all bloated at night. I've had fifty-one years, bloated at night. My god. It's working!...It's game changing. You're not hungry."

—Megyn Kelly[14]

KITCHEN DETOX WORKSHEET
Condiments, Spreads, and Toppings

___ ☐ Peanut butter
___ ☐ Pasta sauces (e.g., marinara, Alfredo)
___ ☐ Salad dressings
___ ☐ Mayonnaise
___ ☐ Hummus
___ ☐ Dips
___ ☐ Store-bought guacamole
___ ☐ Barbecue sauce
___ ☐ Hot sauce
___ ☐ Chocolate spreads (e.g., Nutella)
___ ☐ Chocolate sauce
___ ☐ Whipped cream and whipped topping (e.g., Cool Whip)
___ ☐ Coffee creamers
___ ☐ Frostings
___ ☐ Mustard spread (regular mustard does not need added oil)

Snacks and Desserts

___ ☐ Trail mix
___ ☐ Candy
___ ☐ Cookies
___ ☐ Donuts and pastries
___ ☐ Brownies
___ ☐ Muffins
___ ☐ Crackers
___ ☐ Chips (including veggie chips)
___ ☐ Pretzels
___ ☐ Microwave popcorn

Fats and Oils

____ ☐ Cooking oils and sprays
____ ☐ Shortening (e.g., Crisco)
____ ☐ Butters, spreads, and margarine
      (e.g., Smart Balance)

Frozen and Refrigerated Meals and Sides

____ ☐ Waffles
____ ☐ Entrees (e.g., Lean Cuisine,
      Marie Callender's)
____ ☐ Breaded meats (e.g., chicken nuggets,
      fish sticks)
____ ☐ Burritos, burgers, and sandwiches
____ ☐ Stuffed pastas, pierogies, and pot stickers
____ ☐ Soups
____ ☐ Vegetable sides (e.g., french fries, tater tots, sauced
      vegetables)
____ ☐ Frozen pizzas
____ ☐ Desserts (e.g., cakes, pies)
____ ☐ Ice cream (especially ice cream with any mixed-in
      components, such as cookie dough)

Cereal and Food Bars

____ ☐ Boxed cereals
____ ☐ Granola
____ ☐ Breakfast bars
____ ☐ Protein bars
____ ☐ Energy bars
____ ☐ Toaster pastries (e.g., Pop Tarts)

Canned and Preserved Foods

____ ☐ Canned tuna and seafood
____ ☐ Canned soups and stews
____ ☐ Canned vegetables and beans
____ ☐ Dried fruits (e.g., cranberries, raisins)
____ ☐ Beef jerky and other kinds of jerky
____ ☐ Marinated vegetables (e.g., artichoke hearts, roasted red peppers)
____ ☐ Sun-dried tomatoes

Miscellaneous

____ ☐ Mac and cheese
____ ☐ Nuts (e.g., almonds, peanuts)
____ ☐ Seeds (e.g., sunflower, pumpkin)
____ ☐ Chocolate chips
____ ☐ Drink mixes (e.g., hot cocoa)
____ ☐ Meal replacement drinks and protein shakes
____ ☐ Toddler formulas*

*Note: Infant formula is another source of vegetable oil; however, as of this writing, there is no good, easy alternative for those who are not breastfeeding. I do, however, provide a recipe on my website. See the Resources section.

You may find vegetable oils in many of the foods you've come to depend on, particularly breakfast foods such as muffins and protein bars, snacks (pretzels and microwave popcorn, for example), and convenience foods (pasta sauces, frozen dinners, and take-out). Don't panic. In the Resources section, you'll find a link to my Shopping List, which gives you brand-name recommendations for alternatives to just about everything you could possibly need.

Be patient. It will take time to go through every product in your kitchen. And it may take you a few grocery trips before you find your new go-to foods, so that you can just grab a familiar item without reading the label. (Though, be careful here, too—sometimes brands will change their ingredients without warning, so it's good to check even if you think you've picked up an old standby.) With time, you'll become adept at spotting these ingredients on labels and will be able to quickly move on to a better choice.

Protect Your Mitochondria

Since seed oils are the worst mitochondrial toxin in the food supply, avoiding them is the single most powerful thing you can do to protect your mitochondria.

If you want to keep your mitochondria healthy, you simply must avoid vegetable oils. Here are a few more essential dietary strategies for keeping your mitochondria healthy by controlling oxidative stress:

- Pursue protein: Assess and boost your whole-food-based protein intake. You can assess your portion intake with the protein intake calculator in Appendix A, which also provides guidance about how much you need. (Chapter 10 will go into depth on sources of protein.)
- Mind your minerals: Your body's antioxidant enzymes require a variety of minerals, including iron, magnesium, selenium,

---

manganese, and copper. If your dietary intake of these is inadequate, you should supplement. To assess your mineral intake, see the Resources section.

- Avoid omega-overload: I don't recommend supplementing with fish oil unless you've been tested and are critically deficient in omega-3. (For tips on avoiding fish oils that are oxidized, see the Resources section.)
- Eschew environmental toxins: There are literally thousands of environmental toxins affecting our mitochondria, so I'm only going to list the most potent ones here: smoking legal or recreational drugs; air pollution; phthalates (from eating or drinking out of plastic containers); heavy metals (such as lead, mercury, and arsenic); and PABA (in sunscreen).
- Sleep and exercise are also key to keeping your mitochondria healthy and functional.

AVOIDING THE HATEFUL EIGHT WHEN DINING OUT

Very often when I warn patients about the toxicity of vegetable oil, they reassure me that they're not eating any, saying, "I don't cook with any of those oils. I only cook with olive oil." Even if you consider yourself a health nut, chances are you're loading up on enough of these unstable oils to harm your body in a big way—because other people are preparing food for you in restaurants, at the grab-and-go section of the grocery store, and at shopping malls, airports, hotels, dining halls, and so on.

Restaurants also take advantage of the fact that vegetable oils cost less than traditional fats and oils like olive oil and butter. Since many customers choose and rate restaurants based on price, and vegetable oils help keep that dollar figure down, they're now in foods at every type of restaurant, from fine dining to fast food. You can spend $600 a plate in the Napa Valley's famous French Laundry restaurant and still be fed seed oils, or $16 at a local ethnic restaurant that uses only traditional fats. So it's not always about how much money you are spending; it's about finding restaurants that cook with traditional fats and knowing what to order. Your server may not even know which foods are made or cooked with vegetable oil.

Restaurants use vegetable oil in all deep-fried, pan-fried, and batter-fried foods (including crispy noodles, onion rings, fried shrimp, chicken nuggets, chicken fingers and fillets, and Japanese tempura). Restaurants love serving deep-fried food because the process is so simple that you can hire folks without any culinary skills whatsoever. Dump, dip, cool, and serve. Since it's so easy, deep frying is often applied to as many menu offerings as possible, even those you might think are pan fried or sautéed, such as chicken parmigiana, battered chicken, and breaded prawns. Deep-fried food is the worst of the worst, because the vegetable oils in deep fryers are continuously heated and reused over and over for days. US law requires changing fryer oils after a week, but since the law is not easy to enforce, it's usually that long, if not longer, before the oils in fryers are replaced. A friend of mine who spent years working over a Fryolator at a fancy French bistro (while putting herself through business school) told me she can't remember seeing the oil ever getting changed.

Restaurants also use vegetable oils in sauces traditionally made with butter or olive oil, including hollandaise sauce and aioli. Most salad dressings contain vegetable oil in place of olive oil or cream, and lecithin derived from vegetable oil in place of egg yolk. (Any dish that contains mayonnaise will also contain vegetable oil, since mayo is rarely made from olive oil.)

Restaurants often par-cook vegetables early in the day and finish the cooking later. Most of these par-cooked foods are already sautéed in vegetable oil, so asking for alternative cooking fats would require major disruptions in the kitchen. Vegetable oils are also already baked into donuts, Danishes and muffins, and numerous other kinds of desserts and confections.

My patients often tell me that they feel physically unwell after big vacations, and they've assumed it was because of their various vacation overindulgences, or perhaps lack of sleep. If you feel bad after traveling, or after you've eaten out more than usual, there's another factor to consider: how much vegetable oil you consumed.

That said, we can't always cook at home, and sometimes we want to socialize. The next section summarizes the most important foods to avoid when dining out to reduce your exposure to toxic fats. It also gives you a few tricks of the trade for maxing out on healthy, energy-sustaining fats while you're on the go.

Avoid Anything Deep Fried

Avoiding deep-fried food is the number one rule for restaurants and grabbing food out. *As mentioned earlier, anything battered or breaded and fried is typically deep fried*, and in fast-food restaurants and many other establishments, it's often fried twice, once at the factory and a second time just before you are served. More than half the calories in some deep-fried foods are in the form of the most oxidized and disease-inducing heat-deformed seed oils you can possibly find. If in doubt, ask, but here are some of the most popular deep-fried foods that you should avoid:

- Battered or breaded shrimp, calamari, clams, and fish
- Breaded chicken, including nuggets, fingers, and cutlets
- Chips, including corn chips, potato chips, and veggie chips
- Chicken-fried steak
- Crunchy taco shells
- Donuts
- Deep-fried cookies and pastries (e.g., churros, rice fritters, and funnel cake)
- French fries
- Fried chicken
- Hash browns
- Onion rings
- Tater tots
- Tempura sushi or vegetables (tempura means "batter fried")

Choose Baked or Steamed

Choosing entrees and sides that are baked or steamed are preferable to entrees and sides that are fried.

Pick Smarter Toppings and Sides—and Watch the Sauce

Avoid mayonnaise and anything made with it (cole slaw, potato salad, macaroni salad, egg salad, and tuna salad), tartar sauce, oil-based sauces, dips, dressings (creamy dressings like ranch are especially problematic), sauces, and finishing oils (such as Subway's oil and vinegar), as these are most often made with seed oils. Most establishments carry a few options that will help boost the flavor of your selections, so be sure to review the menu or ask what sides and toppings are available. (McDonald's now offers real butter to go with its pancakes, but you can ask for butter at any time of the day and it dresses up any of their entrees.)

To boost flavor, ask if the following are available when dining out (asterisks [**] indicate good sources of healthy fats):

- Avocado**
- Bacon
- Butter**
- Coconut**
- Cheese (sliced, cubed, or shredded)**
- Cream**
- Cream cheese**
- Guacamole**
- Hot sauce
- Lettuce
- Mustard (brown, Dijon, etc.)
- Nuts (raw or dry roasted)

- Olives**
- Onions
- Pepperoncini
- Peppers
- Pickles
- Relish
- Salsa (green or red)
- Seeds (raw or dry roasted)
- Soy sauce
- Sour cream**
- Sriracha sauce
- Tamari sauce
- Tomatoes

Order High-Protein Foods

Choose burgers, grilled (non-breaded) chicken, fish fillets (not fried or shredded, like tuna salad), or slices of roasted meats and cold cuts. Solid chunks of meat (such as steak) are better than shredded meats (such as carnitas).

Choose Salads with Lots of Flavorful Ingredients

Pick a Cobb or chef's salad, but skip the dressings. (See above for topping suggestions.)

Try the Soup

Soups usually contain very little oil. Cream-based soups, miso, pho, and bone broth are best. (Upscale hotels often make chicken soup with real bone broth!)

Skip the Popcorn at the Movies

The "butter" is simply butter-flavored seed oil. It is also often cooked/popped in a mixture of rapeseed and coconut oil.

Avoid Premade Baked Goods

Cookies, muffins, and non-dairy-based cakes and desserts are often made with seed oils.

Safer Fast-Food Choices

Seek out the following whenever possible:

- Poké bowl franchises
- Korean BBQ
- Sushi
- Arby's (their meats are higher quality than most)
- Grocery stores selling rotisserie chicken or meaty soups

Restaurant websites are a great resource and offer an opportunity to get information without the added pressure of an "audience" in the form of your server and dining companions.

Read the Menu Before You Go

Many restaurants post their entire menu online. After reviewing the menu, I suggest calling ahead to ask about specific dishes. You can use the information in the rest of this chapter to guide the conversation.

Call Ahead, If Possible

This is a good solution for anyone who really dislikes asking questions during the ordering process. Calling ahead allows you to become comfortable with the whole process of Q and A—basically, you can practice your routine this way but without the extra pressure of having your friends as an audience. The best time to call is generally between 2:00 and 4:00 p.m., to avoid the lunch and dinner rush hours.

Whether you're calling ahead or in the restaurant, there are four things you need to communicate:

- You need to avoid seed oils.
- The oils you need to avoid (corn, rapeseed, cottonseed, soy, sunflower, safflower, grapeseed, rice bran).
- You are fine with butter, cream, and olive oil.
- You don't expect your server (or whoever answers the phone) to know, but you do expect that he or she will ask the kitchen.

Reasons to give for avoiding seed oils can include intolerance, allergy, and dietary restrictions. Here's a script you can use:

"Can you tell me if there are any menu items that I can order that can be prepared using only 100 percent olive oil, not a blend, or real butter, not butter oil or margarine, and that will be completely free of any vegetable oils or blended oils? If you have to ask the kitchen I can wait." Depending on the response, you may need to add, "I am intolerant to soy oil, rapeseed oil, rice bran oil, and the other factory-refined vegetable oils."

Here's a shorter version that I recommend when you're already at the restaurant: "Do you have anything that you can cook in butter?" You may need to specify real dairy butter and not butter oil.

Be sure to show your appreciation, whatever the answer is (but be prepared to be disappointed). A hearty "Thank you so much for looking into it for me, it really helps," or anything similarly positive, often makes a big difference to the staff; it relieves any built-up tension around the table, too, if you're asking in person. In addition, if the restaurant actually does have at least one seed-oil-free option, please take a moment to express what a rare gift their chef is offering to the world and that you truly appreciate the extra effort required to use healthy fats and oils.

Think of your whole Q and A conversation as an opportunity to help expand the no-seed-oil movement. Let's earn a reputation for kindness, patience, and truth-seeking!

Eating to Heal

Welcome to the next phase of your culinary life, where you develop a new relationship with food. *Real* food. The kinds of foods our human bodies all need.

Right now, most people live in a nutrition paradigm that lacks a center. It's more defined by what *not* to eat than what we need to eat. In our current, rootless nutrition paradigm, just about every sort of food has been dressed down as the latest dietary boogeyman for one reason or another. Medical doctors tell you to avoid salt, fat, and cholesterol, while other practitioners tell you to avoid eggs, yeast, meat, nightshades, legumes, dairy, grains and wheat, sugar—and the list goes on. If we listened to all the warnings, we'd be left with a very short list of acceptable options to choose from, making it almost impossible to get the nutrition we need. The folks telling us to avoid these foods are trying to help, but they don't understand what you've just learned about vegetable oils in the last nine chapters. If they did, they'd realize that many real foods have been wrongly blamed for problems caused by vegetable oils, and that, unless we have rare digestive issues or clearly diagnosed allergies, we have nothing to fear by including these foods in our diets. Indeed, I've worked with patients who were told they needed to cut numerous foods from their diet but were unable to do so, and were left feeling hopeless about their health. Worse, some people developed illnesses or life-changing injuries stemming from protein or mineral deficiencies caused by avoiding nourishing foods.

In this chapter I want to celebrate the nourishing and delicious foods that you *can* feel good about enjoying. These are foods that will help to support your mitochondria, optimize hormone function, and quiet inflammation, enabling your body to restore its balance.

I will also address some of the most prominent fears around salt, fat, cholesterol, dairy, and meats, to help you understand why you can actually enjoy these foods in spite of the fact that many well-meaning practitioners say they're unhealthy. By the time you've finished, you'll be able to tell the difference between the factory foods that assault our biology and the real foods our bodies need.

THE ANCESTRAL APPROACH

Avoiding vegetable oil and its two little siblings, refined carbohydrates and protein powders, keeps the worst ingredients out of your diet and opens up a whole lot of caloric "space" for healthy food. So what can you fill it with? Some would say "everything in moderation." But our healthiest ancestors did better than that, and so can we.

The kind of diet I recommend is nothing like what you'll find in a typical diet book. It's not based on my own ideas. It's based on our healthiest ancestors' knowledge. It's not "the latest thing" or a fad. It's the oldest, most proven approach for optimal health.

The ancestral approach is born of respect for the wisdom of the past—specifically, the culinary principles and practices that enabled humanity to thrive across the globe. The philosophy holds that if we want to be healthy, then we need to understand how our ancestors ate. The idea is that humans have evolved to eat a certain way, and that we would be healthier if we ate similarly. This intuitive idea is also supported by science (a branch of genetics called epigenetics). Whether they followed a settled-farming, nomadic-herding, or hunter-gatherer lifestyle, it's thanks to our ancestors that we exist today. What's more, although the average human life span was shorter in times past, this was likely not due to diet but rather to life being significantly more physically demanding, often violent, and lacking in the basic medical resources that we have today, such as antibiotics to fight infections and anesthesia for surgeries. By all accounts, our ancestors enjoyed a far greater *health span* than we do today, living independent, active lives well into their eighth decade.[1] In contrast to *life span*, which means the length of time a person (or animal) lives, *health span* refers to the span of a person's life in which they are generally in good health. In the United States, our average health span is just sixty-six years, two decades shorter than our life spans, and it's getting shorter still with each passing generation.

Two popular diets exemplify the ancestral philosophy, the paleo and carnivore diets. Both aim to mimic the diets of our ancient ancestors, specifically those who lived as hunter-gathers during, for example, the Paleolithic era—which ended around ten thousand years ago. That said, these diets are based on relatively limited evidence. Although anthropologists have uncovered thousands of artifacts widely scattered across every continent except Antarctica, it's still very difficult to guess what these ancient people actually ate. More to the point, the paleo diet philosophy also assumes that human health has been in decline since the end of the Paleolithic period, which may not be true.

There's another, more practical ancestral approach that has advantages over paleo, and which I prefer. It's a more modern-day ancestral approach. The approach doesn't assume we need to go back so far in time to rid ourselves of chronic disease. We can instead emulate our more recent, pre-industrial ancestors who lived before our disease epidemics began. Over the course of my career I have evaluated eighty such pre-industrial cuisines around the world and identified the strategies common to all of them, which I call the Four Pillars of a Human Diet:

1. Eat fresh, uncooked food.
2. Eat meat. Include recipes that slow-cook skin, tendons, and bones to extract the special nutrients in these collagenous tissues (for example bone broth).
3. Eat fermented and sprouted foods, including yogurt, kefir, kombucha, kimchi, and sprouted nuts, seeds, and beans.
4. Eat nose to tail, making use of all the animals' organs.

Keep in mind, our ancestors ate animals that enjoyed a species-appropriate diet and time in the sunshine outdoors. And they survived by extracting as much nutrition as they could from the landscapes wherever they lived—and in every form possible, be it animal, vegetable, or mineral. This is what we've done for hundreds of thousands of years, and it is what we still need to do to build healthy human bodies and keep them running right.

"Your [advice] really changed me. Lost weight. Feel better. Enjoy procuring fine products. It's a lifestyle. Just eating a lot of eggs and fruits and veggies and fresh whole wheat sourdough toast for breakfast...then healthy lunches of soup and maybe some salad or protein—then dinner of ribeyes and lamb chops and pork chops and chicken and halibut and branzino…with potatoes and broccoli sides— pasta sometimes—and have been having small amounts of high-quality chocolate for dessert. I put chicken fat on liver and then lightly rolled on flour before searing. It was actually really good. And fun and easy to make. Not a single minute of exercise besides an occasional walk—and I lost 5–10 lbs. I don't get it. Is diet *The* most important element?"

—Jesse Watters, American conservative political

commentator on Fox News (Via text message.

My answer to his question was *Yes. 100%.*)

MACRONUTRIENT RANGES

I often get asked what portion of daily calories the macronutrients (i.e., the fat, carbs, and protein) should represent, and here, too, we can look to ancestral wisdom for guidance. The answer for you, personally, varies depending on your metabolic health. When we are metabolically healthy, we can tolerate a wider range of macros. If not, we need to be stricter with our carbohydrate intake. Here are my recommendations for each situation:

- **Fat Calories:** 50 to 80 percent of your daily total.
- **Carb Calories:**
  o *With moderate insulin resistance (HOMA-IR score 2.5 or over):* 15 to 20 percent of your daily total (roughly 50 to 100 grams). It's important to divide these between at least two meals instead of eating them all in one meal.

- ○ *With mild or no insulin resistance (HOMA-IR score 2.4 or less):* 0 to 40 percent of your daily total (roughly 0 to 150 grams).
- **Protein Calories:** 15 to 25 percent of your daily total (roughly 60 to 150 grams).

Note: See the Resources section for information on HOMA-IR testing.

This breakdown is based on our ancestral eating patterns. Our ancestral diets range most widely in terms of carbs, and not surprisingly there are more disagreements about high versus low carb than almost anything else in the nutrition world. Remember, people used to eat what was available to them where they lived. Since protein- and fat-rich animals were generally abundant year round, but plants were not, the macro that comes from plants—carbohydrate—varied the most. There is a lot of anxiety about this macronutrient, but the truth is that what matters to our metabolic recovery is building meals that prevent pathologic hunger, and a wide range of total carbs can do that. The *kind* of carbs, however, matter a good deal, and we'll discuss those later in this chapter. First up, though, are those healthy fats we've been discussing.

FAT: OUR CONNECTION TO HEALTH AND CULINARY RICHES

The only kind of fat that I recommend *against* is vegetable oil. Otherwise, fat is part of a healthy diet. (For a detailed list of good and bad fats, including questions on cooking and more, see chapter 9.)

Most people who lived through the 1980s and 1990s have such an ingrained fear that fat will make them fat, or coat their arteries, or clog their hearts, and have spent so many years avoiding it, that it just seems bizarre to start seeking it out. Fat does indeed have more calories than sugar, so pound for pound it will be more fattening. But fat is more satiating than sugar, so you're more likely to eat less of it. And, as we saw in chapter 5, fat will neither clog nor coat your arteries.

The modern nutrition paradigm has convinced us that these life-giving sources of nutrients are going to riddle us with disease, thus separating us from our collective cultural wisdom. This is tragic. Historical culinary practices represent a great body of nutritional wisdom that enabled us to survive in every corner of the globe. Animal fats were central to culinary practices the world over. By dutifully avoiding these fats, we've deprived ourselves of many foods our ancestors enjoyed, and that enabled them to have healthy children and build healthy, resilient, beautiful human bodies.

Fat Won't Coat Your Arteries

Why would Mother Nature tempt us to eat fatty foods that would build up in our arteries? Answer: she doesn't. But that's exactly what Ancel Keys actually tried to suggest when he said, famously, that "fat builds up in your arteries like hot grease in a cold pipe." That is simply not how the body works.

In chapter 5, I briefly mentioned that your body has fat-delivery vehicles called *lipoproteins* that deliver cholesterol throughout your tissues so it can do its job. These vehicles can be destroyed by oxidation, however. As we've discussed, both smoking and seed oils will oxidize our lipoproteins, and build plaques in our arteries. If you avoid both, your arteries can start to heal.

You might think we should avoid eating fat so we have less fat in our arteries. While that's true with vegetable oils, *avoiding* the healthy fat tends to *increase* the amount of triglyceride (fat) in the blood. Both vegetable oils and carbohydrates (particularly fructose sugar) reliably elevate our blood levels of triglyceride fat. High triglycerides are associated with arterial fat and heart attacks, so this is not a good thing.

Benefits of Healthy Fats

ENERGY

Saturated and monounsaturated-rich foods are ideal mitochondrial fuels. They help to prevent the hypoglycemia symptoms that disrupt brain function and drive so many people to snack. Including healthy fats in our meals helps our mitochondria heal.

METABOLIC HEALING

By providing fuels that heal our mitochondria, we start to restore a normal blood sugar set point. This is the key to metabolic health, and in combination with proper carbohydrate consumption (discussed below) it will reverse diabetes and insulin resistance.

FLAVOR

Every real chef will tell you fat is flavor. And the truly enlightened chefs will tell you that vegetable oil is the exception to that rule. Vegetable oil kills flavor. Sure, when you deep fry starchy foods such as french fries or batter-coated shrimp in vegetable oil, that hot crispness can make for a satisfying crunch. But if you take the same ingredients and deep fry them in a cuisine-appropriate fat, such as tallow, or even pan fry them in butter, I can guarantee the taste will be superior.

Tips for Including Healthy Fats in Your Meals

- Cook with healthy fats—the Delightful Dozen I listed in chapter 9.
- Use butter, cream, cheese, and dairy fat, including whole milk and whole-milk yogurt. You can cook foods in butter, add cream cheese instead of jelly to a peanut butter sandwich, and add extra cream to your coffee instead of fake creamer or milk. Cheese, cottage cheese, and yogurt make for excellent additions to lean meats such as fish and chicken. They are also good as standalone meals or even desserts.

- Use avocados, coconuts, and nuts, especially almonds, pecans, hazelnuts, and peanuts.
- Learn which animals have the highest-quality fats. Some animal fats are relatively high in PUFA, and their higher-PUFA content can contribute to a state of PUFA overload, which is not ideal. Ideally, the animals you buy would also be fed such that their PUFA content is relatively low. Sadly, most of our feedlot pigs, poultry, and farmed fish eat high-PUFA corn- and soy-based pellets. Unless stated otherwise, the list starts with animals with the highest PUFA content first, and PUFA descends as you go down the list, assuming a typical feedlot scenario. (For more about these, see "Good Protein: Whole-Food Animal and Plant Sources of Protein," on page 267.)
  - **Farmed fatty fish:** The fatty acids in farmed salmon or other fatty fish will vary wildly since the feed varies wildly. It's best avoided. (Low-fat fish won't have enough fat to worry about this particular issue.)
  - **Chicken:** Chicken has more PUFA than red meats. Pasture-raised chicken is a better choice, if available to you.
  - **Pork:** There's a big difference between confinement-fed pork and pork fed a species-appropriate diet. A pig in the wild will eat grubs, mushrooms, nuts—especially acorns—in addition to fresh greens. The flavor will reflect its diet, too. Even though pork can be delicious when raised in confinement and fed pelleted corn and soy, it's nothing like what pork tastes like when properly raised. If you have money burning a hole in your pocket, you should try forest-raised pork or Iberico pork (from a traditional breed native to the Iberian Peninsula). Both will also be much lower in PUFA. This doesn't matter much for lean cuts, such as tenderloin, but it matters a great deal for bacon, pork belly, and other delights.

- o **Beef:** Cows can consume a relatively high-PUFA diet but still produce low-PUFA body fat. Cows that get grass and other natural cow-forage are healthier themselves and more nutritious for us.
- o **Lamb:** Lamb cannot be raised on grain, or even indoors. So all lamb is technically grass-fed and pasture-raised. Because of this, lamb is relatively low in PUFA—and relatively high in micronutrients, too.

BENEFITS OF CHOLESTEROL-RICH FOODS: REJUVENATION, UNCHAINED!

Years of cholesterol-lowering seed-oil consumption has suppressed some people's total body cholesterol to the point that it has suppressed their sex hormones, cortisol, and even DHEA (dehydroepiandrosterone, a precursor to hormones such as estrogen and testosterone that is commonly sold as an anti-aging supplement). Our bodies can make cholesterol, but if our cholesterol production has been suppressed for years, it can take some time before our ability to make cholesterol ramps up again. Seeking out cholesterol-rich foods can rejuvenate our hormone levels and help to jump-start our metabolic recovery. I've seen men in their fifties and sixties triple their testosterone levels, and women of various ages normalize their menstrual cycles or dramatically reduce perimenopausal and menopausal symptoms, including mood swings and hot flashes.

Cholesterol is not a fat. Our bodies cannot use it for energy. Still, it suppresses pathologic hunger by two important mechanisms.

How Cholesterol-Rich Foods Prevent Hunger
SATIETY

Cholesterol is such an important nutrient that nature has seen fit to make it one of the most satiating chemicals in the edible world—you could say it's satiety on steroids. This is why eating just three or four eggs feels like plenty, while most of us need many more calories of sugary, high-carb foods such as oatmeal, muffins, donuts, or fruit to feel equally full. Three eggs have just 180 calories but 561 mg cholesterol—and can sustain most people all morning. A Dunkin' Apple 'n Spice donut has 230 calories and zero cholesterol, and often it sustains you for just an hour or so. Incidentally, at least a dozen large epidemiological studies and clinical interventions involving tens of thousands of people have shown that people who eat six or more eggs per week live longer and have fewer heart attacks than people who avoid eggs.[2]

KETONES

Cholesterol-rich foods help support your body's ability to make ketones. The liver is a main source of both cholesterol and ketones, but it cannot make both at the same time.[3] Remember, ketones are made specifically for the brain, which can't use body fat. And studies show that ketones are superior to fueling with sugar.[4] Ketones powerfully suppress hunger, especially pathologic hunger, and will keep us from getting distracted by thoughts of snacks lurking elsewhere nearby. So on a low-cholesterol diet, the liver is busy making cholesterol, which deprives us of ketones—and all the good they do.

Tips for Including Cholesterol-Rich Foods in Your Diet
- **Eggs:** You can eat as many as you like. The healthiest way to cook an egg is to poach it or soft-boil it. If you fry it, leave the yellow part runny. Use butter for best flavor.
- **Liver (chicken, beef, etc.):** I recommend getting four to eight ounces of liver per week. More important than the type of animal is how healthy it was, which you can estimate by looking at the liver's color. Dark maroons are better than pale or dull browns.

- **Crustaceans (lobster, shrimp, crab):** The healthiest way to cook these is to steam them or gently (quickly) fry them in healthy fat.
- **Dairy fat and animal fat:** These are great sources of cholesterol as well as the healthy fats mentioned in chapter 9.

"As I type I'm crying tears of joy and appreciation for all you've done for me and my health! I won't go into my life story but in a nutshell—I am no longer a compulsive over-eating addict suffering under the crushing 'thumb' of all food and alcohol. Neither can control me, I've got health and energy, and I understand why!! Your plan works and I am a testament to it!"

—Polly W.

KNOW YOUR PROTEINS

We need protein for more than just muscle building; we need it for every cell in every organ in our bodies. Our mitochondria need protein to make the antioxidant enzymes that control oxidative stress. Protein plays an essential role in health—and your metabolic recovery.

Yet here in the United States, a third of adults over the age of fifty do not get enough protein, and roughly half of all people with diabetes are significantly protein deficient, according to data from the 2005–2016 National Health and Nutrition Examination Survey.[5] Protein deficiency is far more common than most people realize, because doctors are not well-trained to diagnose it. For example, hair loss, nail breakage, and low white-blood-cell counts are all known to be signs of malnutrition, and I've seen many cases where these issues resolve with adding protein. Short stature, low peak bone density (leading to osteopenia and osteoporosis), and low muscle mass are lifelong consequences of inadequate protein in childhood. Lower protein intake correlates with shorter male height in 105 countries studied.[6] Low protein intake contributes to both the development of type 2 diabetes and to mortality in people who already have diabetes, especially for those over the age of sixty.[7]

The most worrisome aspect of the protein discussion is that the US Department of Agriculture's Dietary Reference Intake (DRI) is likely a whopping 40 to 50 percent too low.[8] The government's Recommended Daily Allowance (RDA) guidelines were set back in the 1940s, before we understood protein metabolism as well as we do now. According to new science, those older techniques "significantly underestimated" how much protein we need. Flawed nitrogen balance equations led to this egregious underestimation, and governmental agencies have not reset their recommendations based on the newer, better calculations.

Most people need a minimum of 60 to 100 grams per day. To more accurately estimate your protein needs and intake, see the calculator in Appendix A. If these numbers seem low to you, keep in mind that websites listing higher protein intakes are often designed for body builders who are trying to hack their biology to make it look a certain way, which is not the same as seeking health.

Protein and Politics

Before we jump into the next section on healthy, high-protein foods, I want to address the arguments that often come up in discussions about our protein needs, particularly the idea that eating animals is bad for the environment and that meat causes cancer.

Let's look at the environmental concern first. These days, there is a common feeling that we should all be eating "lower on the food chain," and especially avoiding beef, because cows promote global warming. These arguments put the cart before the horse. We need to first get clear on our nutritional needs. If we need more protein than the government is currently recommending, and if red meat is one of the most healthful foods in the food system, then cutting these foods will have health consequences that need to be considered and discussed as part of the conversation.

Right now, that is not happening. The assumption is that we eat too much protein and we can safely cut down. But a good portion of the population appears to not get enough protein, especially thin people (including thin children and pregnant women), health-conscious people, people trying to lose weight, and people over fifty, and their health is suffering as a result.

Our health authorities are misleading us into believing that we can all do fine living on a completely novel diet of highly processed ingredients derived from just a few monoculture crops—mostly wheat, corn, soy, rice, and potatoes—as long as we throw in a few fresh fruits and vegetables. This is the trajectory we have been on for decades, and our health is collapsing. If we want to address either the climate concerns or the animal welfare concerns, we need to have an honest discussion about the big picture. The fact is, if we continue on our current trajectories with our food systems and our health, both will collapse.

Ecologists warn that *all* industrial-scale agriculture, whether it produces cows or wheat, disrupts the soil, and our continued reliance on it is unraveling the vital threads connecting the systems that support life. Our health has always depended ultimately on the health of the soil, and ecologists are trained to understand all the various interconnected Earth systems that contribute to healthy soil. Today, many ecologists are saying that animals are part of the solution to our climate crisis. Experts have identified farming and ranching practices that can actually put carbon in the soil seemingly more efficiently than any other method so far identified. These methods also boost the productivity of the soil and the diversity of the ecosystem, while simultaneously improving animal health and welfare.[9] Thus, their solutions can also benefit human health. Simply cutting out animal products and turning to all plant-based foods doesn't solve the problems that giant factory farms introduce.

Animal-based protein has somewhat followed in the footsteps of cholesterol, in that our health authorities make concerning claims that discourage us from eating it. But how valid are those claims?

Let's look at the concern that meat causes cancer. In the early 2010s, the World Health Organization (WHO) convened a working group of twenty-two experts from ten countries to study the available evidence on a possible connection between cancer and meat (both mammalian muscle meat, including beef, veal, pork, lamb, mutton, horse, and goat, and *processed meat*, meaning meat from any animal, not just red meats but also poultry, fish, shellfish, and so on, "that has been transformed through salting, curing, fermentation, smoking, or other processes to enhance flavor or improve preservation").

By 2015, the working group came to the conclusion that red meat will give you cancer. Sort of. Well, maybe. Red meat was added to their short list of Group 2A carcinogens, defined as "probably carcinogenic to humans."[10] To be clear, WHO is not saying we *know* red meat causes cancer in humans—there's no evidence for that. The working group found a faint statistical link between meat eating and cancer, and so it looked at animal studies to see if there was a plausible mechanism by which red meat might generate cancer. The team claimed that there was. But let's take a look at a few key details upon which this determination hinged.

The pertinent part of the report refers to several dozen animal studies. Some of these studies used mice genetically prone to developing a kind of *non*cancerous tumor, called an adenoma. In these studies, beef increased the number of adenomas.[11] But adenomas are not cancers, and these beef-eating, adenoma-forming mice did not get cancer. (It's not clear how a study of mice bred to form adenomas would translate to humans even if they did.) The report also cites numerous rat studies that used tumor-prone rats, and in these studies red meat failed to cause cancer unless other foods were blended into their meat.[12] Those foods were *margarine and corn oil!* I think they should have mentioned that you can only make red meat cause cancer by blending it with some kind of seed-oil-based food.

WHO has also said that *charred* red meat, cooked on an open flame, may be the real problem, not red meat cooked without charring. Charred meat has been partially burnt, creating flecks of black, burned meat (like grill marks). The concern is that this burned material may contain carcinogenic compounds from a family of chemicals called heterocyclic amines and polycyclic aromatic hydrocarbons. However, the doses used in these studies were "equivalent to thousands of times the doses that a person would consume in a normal diet," according to the National Cancer Institute and others.[13] In other words, it appears that the only way these "carcinogenic" chemicals can actually give animals cancer is when they get them in concentrations thousands of times greater than anyone could possibly eat even if they lived off nothing but charred red meat.

One last point. What causes charring? Oxidation. So if we are willing to consider the health effects of oxidation in animal foods like red meat, then we should be willing to consider the health effects of oxidation in the plant-derived seed oils.

Next, let's discuss what the WHO report says about the link between *processed meat* and cancer. The working group determined that processed meat is a Group 1 carcinogen, meaning "it is known that this substance causes cancer in humans." So let's look at what the data showed.

First, the statistical link between processed meat and cancer is barely even there. Processed meat has only been statistically linked to only one type of cancer: colorectal. Not esophageal. Not stomach. Not oral, etc. I get very suspicious when a supposed cancer-causing agent is only linked to a very specific subtype of cancer. That's because if a compound is truly carcinogenic, it causes cancer in most tissues, not just a select few.

Second, it turns out that the colon cancer risk level rises only a small amount *even if you eat processed meat like hot dogs every day of the year* (most of us do not).[14] For a man at an average 5 percent risk, a daily hot dog increases that risk to 5.8 percent. Finally, according to a study that dove into some important details, processed meat does not give women cancer, no matter how much they eat. That same study also found that the men who got cancer were more likely *to smoke cigarettes* than the men who did not get cancer—which again implicates oxidation as the true issue.[15] Another study found a strong link between processed meat consumption, ultra-processed food consumption, and, once more, cigarette smoking.[16]

In summary, the link between these meats and cancer is not there, and the links between oxidation, seed oils, and cancer seem to have been suppressed.

I'd like to wrap up this discussion by pointing out that WHO also states that red meat is good for children and pregnant women, citing it as a good source of protein, iron, and zinc. Children and pregnant moms who avoid red meat are more likely to be deficient in one or more of these key nutrients.[17] As a result, WHO recommends introducing red meat into a child's diet starting at the age of six months.[18]

In other words, WHO recommends red meat for infants and pregnant women, while at the same time warning everyone else not to eat it because it may cause cancer. Is it that red meat is good for us at certain phases of life and bad at others? Of course not. Insects may need different nutrients throughout their life span, starting out as grubs or larvae before metamorphosing into creatures with legs and wings. But we don't do that. As humans, we have the exact same organs throughout our lives and the same or very similar nutritional needs, too.

So now that we've addressed those common concerns, let's look at how to ensure we're getting enough protein.

Good Protein: Whole-Food Animal and Plant Sources of Protein

The best sources of protein are whole foods. The best whole-food sources are going to come from animal proteins, which include not only the muscle meats of land and water animals but also many organ meats. Animal proteins are superior to plant proteins due to the simple fact that our bodies are made from identical building blocks to those of mammals and fish. Plants are built of different building blocks, and thus it requires more careful planning and much more dietary restriction to get enough protein from them. Moreover, since many high-protein plant foods are actually high-PUFA seeds—as explained later in this chapter—it's more difficult to avoid PUFA on a plant-based diet.

ANIMAL-BASED PROTEIN

Beef

All cuts of beef are great, including ground beef, steaks, stew meat, ribs, tails, and the organs, such as liver, tongue, tripe, and heart. Bone marrow is often very fatty, making it lower protein. The best beef is going to come from grass-finished cattle. Note that 100 percent grass-fed meat does taste different from grain-fed and requires adjusting your cooking technique to bring out its best flavors. You can find plenty of good guidance online. See the Resources section for a few webpages that I like.

Chicken

All kinds of chicken parts are great: breast, thighs, legs, wings, back, and of course whole roasted or rotisserie chicken. The best chicken is going to come from chickens given access to pasture, bugs, and sunlight. Skin-on, bone-in has more flavor and more nutrition.

Crustaceans

All crustaceans sold as food are great: crab, crayfish, lobster, prawns, shrimp, mollusks, clams, oysters, and scallops. Many crustaceans are excellent sources of cholesterol, which makes them very satiating. The healthiest way to cook them is to steam them or gently (quickly) fry them in healthy fat.

Dairy

High-protein dairy products include milk, yogurt, cottage cheese, and cheese (see the box that follows).

Duck

Everything I just said about chicken applies to duck.

Eggs

Hailed as the perfect food, eggs are great sources of protein and cholesterol and are very satiating. The best eggs come from the best chickens, ducks, and so on—meaning they had access to fresh air and a species-appropriate diet.

Fish

All fish are great, and every part of the fish you can make use of is also great. Popular fish include salmon, catfish, cod, flounder, halibut, tuna, mackerel, bass, trout, walleye, and mahi-mahi. The best fish are going to be wild caught. Even tilapia can be healthy when it's not farmed. Farmed fish, unfortunately, can be quite full of industrial contaminants.

Lamb

As with beef, all cuts of lamb are great.

Pork

As with beef and lamb, all cuts are great.

Turkey

Everything I said about chicken and duck applies to turkey.

Other

Less popular but very healthy high-protein animal foods include venison, goose, eel, buffalo, ostrich, rabbit, guinea pig, and quail.

Dairy: The Original Superfood

Milk is the only food that nature intended for the sole purpose of nourishing our bodies. Dairy is a superfood that supports bone and dental health and helps us build muscle. It's a natural source of vitamin B12

---

and healthy omega-3 fatty acids. It is also a complex food, with many components that people can develop allergies or intolerances to, a fact that often convinces people we shouldn't be eating it at all. But that is no more an indication that everyone should avoid milk than the fact that many people are allergic to fish, eggs, wheat, and soy means everyone should avoid these foods. It's worth noting that, as more processed foods enter our food supply, more of us are developing allergies to components of those processed foods, including milk.

Another problem people have with milk that is not allergy-related is lactose intolerance. Lactose is the main sugar in milk. When you are lactose intolerant, the lactose does not get absorbed into your bloodstream but stays in your intestine, where it can cause bloating, cramping, and even diarrhea. When we are born, we have a special enzyme to break down lactose and bring it into our bodies, called *lactase*. This enzyme goes away after we stop drinking mother's milk, historically by age five. After age five, it's *normal* to be lactose intolerant; most of the world's population is. And yet people on every continent enjoy a variety of dairy products—because they enjoy mostly fermented dairy. Fermented dairy includes things like yogurt, cheese, and sour cream and traditional foods such as labneh (a kind of strained yogurt) and kefir. During fermentation, microbial cultures consume the lactose sugar, fermenting some or all of it away. The longer the ferment, the less lactose remains. Cheeses like cheddar, Parmesan, and Swiss, which are very low in lactose, are the best choices for people with troublesome lactose-intolerance issues. Fermented dairy is a great way to ensure a proper protein intake.

PLANT-BASED PROTEIN

The best plant sources of protein come from the seeds. (For more on these, see "Know Your Carbs," on page 272.) What botanists would refer to as "seeds" fall into a variety of categories of foods, including nuts, beans, grains, and what we call seeds in everyday parlance.

Plant-based foods with the highest protein levels are as follows (listed as percentage of total calories):

- **Seitan:** 80 percent protein
- **Tempeh:** 45 percent protein
- **Extra-firm tofu:** 40 percent protein
- **Lupini beans, dry:** 39 percent protein
- **Edamame, cooked:** 36 percent protein
- **Japanese black soybeans, dry:** 33 percent protein
- **Split peas, dry:** 29 percent protein
- **Oat bran, dry:** 27 percent protein
- **Lima beans, dry:** 25 percent protein
- **Black lentils, dry:** 25 percent protein
- **Pumpkin seeds, dry:** 22 percent protein
- **Hemp hearts, raw:** 22 percent protein
- **Japanese soba (buckwheat) noodles, dry:** 21 percent protein
- **Spelt (whole grain), raw:** 17 percent protein
- **Wheat berries, raw:** 17 percent protein
- **Wild rice, dry:** 17 percent protein
- **Amaranth, dry:** 17 percent protein
- **Peanuts, dry roasted:** 16 percent protein
- **Buckwheat groats, raw:** 16 percent protein
- **Pistachios, dry roasted:** 15 percent protein
- **Quinoa, raw:** 15 percent protein
- **Almonds, raw:** 15 percent protein
- **Sunflower seeds, raw:** 15 percent protein
- **Bulgur wheat, whole grain, raw:** 14 percent protein
- **Teff, raw:** 14 percent protein
- **Cashews, raw:** 13 percent protein
- **Hazelnuts, raw:** 10 percent protein

- **Brazil nuts, raw:** 9 percent protein

- **Walnuts, raw:** 9 percent protein

Notice that the highest-protein plant-based items in the list are all traditional foods: seitan, tempeh, tofu. Ancestral food-processing practices typically *concentrate* an ingredient's nutrients—unlike modern food processing. It's especially notable that this was accomplished thousands of years before anyone knew the term "protein"!

KNOW YOUR CARBS

Carbs will play an important role in your metabolic recovery because when we are insulin resistant, our bodies need more sugar than is normal to avoid burning muscle protein for energy—but we are also more susceptible to sugar spikes and harmful aging of our tissues as a result. So it is really a delicate balancing act. By eating the right types of carbs at the right time, we can keep our blood sugar steady, keep our brains functioning better, and reduce the wastage of muscle and dietary protein. (If you are trying to lose weight, you may be tempted to go "all in" on cutting carbs, but try to shift that all-or-none mindset from carbs generally to the refined carbs and carb-bombs discussed below.)

Slow-Digesting Carbs: Get the Energy Without the Insulin

Slow-digesting carbs are more nutritious and take a longer time to digest than refined carbohydrates. (Dietitians often call these *low glycemic carbs*, but I prefer the term *slow-digesting* because it more accurately describes why they do what they do.) As they trickle out of the digestive system into the bloodstream over the course of several hours, slow-digesting carbs provide a steady supply of sugar to sugar-dependent cells, preventing the blood-sugar spike as well as the insulin spike. They also prevent the insulin-spike-induced blood sugar dip that makes people feel hungry and tired a few hours later.

SLOW-DIGESTING CARBS

Slow-digesting carbs fall into five categories.

- Whole grains
- Beans
- **Nuts and seeds**
- **Semi-starchy vegetables**
- Select fruits

The slowest of the slow are highlighted in bold.

We've already discussed that refined flours and sugars have an insulin-spiking, energy-crashing effect, but any highly processed grain—including quick cooking oatmeal—can do the same thing. As can rice, potatoes, and most fruits. These foods are basically carb bombs, bred for thousands of years to be a source of calories. As a result, they now offer very little nutrition relative to other whole foods, so it's best to limit them while we're trying to recover from insulin resistance. While they are not off the menu entirely, you'll see that they don't appear very often in the Two-Week Challenge. You'll also notice that where they do appear, they are paired with foods that contain fat, protein, and fiber.

Just as the fiber, fat, and protein in something like a peanut slows down the absorption of the carbohydrate component within a given food, the same applies within a given meal. For example, by itself an apple might spike your blood sugar by, say, 30 points or so (likely higher if you have diabetes). Spreading peanut butter on the two halves of an apple can cut such spikes in half. We can slow the absorption of rice used in a stir-fry by adding plenty of bok choy, celery, snap peas, eggs, shrimp, and peanuts. A slice of dry toast might spike blood sugar by 35 points, but scooping some scrambled eggs onto the toast could cut that in half. These food-combining tricks even work for junk like soda and candy—but not very well. They work much better and in some cases prevent spikes entirely when used with whole grains, beans, and the specific breads and fruits I recommend below.

Everyone's response to carbs and combinations of carbs with other foods is a little different. Remember, the goal is to suppress your pathologic hunger and prevent hypoglycemia symptoms between meals, not to predict exactly what's happening with your blood sugar. If you have either prediabetes or type 2 diabetes, it can be helpful to test blood sugar after eating carbohydrate-containing foods to make sure you're not spiking your sugar; and if you do see a blood-sugar spike, you will know to make different choices or reduce the amounts in the future (see Appendix B, "Simply Counting Carbohydrates," on page 325). The new continuous glucometer (CGM) technology makes understanding how different foods affect blood sugar easy and fun. You usually need a doctor's prescription to buy one; however, a few tech companies have found a workaround for this. (See the Resources section for examples.)

SOAKING AND GERMINATING
Soaking and germinating enhances the nutritional value of all seeds, including grains. You can buy nuts and seeds that have been "activated" in this way already. They cost more than raw or roasted, but they taste better and are better for you. Buying dry beans and soaking them at least overnight is healthier than buying canned. Draining after the soaking process and allowing them to germinate for an additional twenty-four or so hours further enhances their nutritional value.

Good Sources of Slow-Digesting Carbs
SPROUTED-GRAIN BREADS
Sprouting awakens enzymes in the seeds that convert storage glucose to vitamins, fiber, and amino acids. These are the healthiest breads you can buy. They're sold in the freezer section because they contain no

preservatives and mold quickly—so keep them in your fridge. They are flavorful and coarse, and they take some getting used to if you've always eaten fluffy bread. Toasting helps.

YELLOW CORN TORTILLAS

These types of tortillas are made with corn masa, which is slightly less processed than flour, and therefore slightly healthier and cause less of a spike in blood sugar. They're also generally smaller than flour tortillas, so the "dose" of carb is lower. When I say yellow corn tortillas, however, I do not mean the hard taco shells that are sold in a box, which are usually made with vegetable oil.

BEANS

All beans are healthy. The most popular varieties are lima, kidney, black, pinto, split pea, cannellini, and garbanzo. I don't recommend the newfangled bean-based pastas, however, since they're generally highly processed and suspiciously flavorless.

WHOLE GRAINS

These include wheat, oats, rye, barley, buckwheat, quinoa, and wild rice.

NUTS

Popular nuts include peanuts and tree nuts such as almonds, pecans, cashews, walnuts, macadamia nuts, Brazil nuts, pistachios, and hazelnuts.

NUT BUTTERS

All nut butters are great, including peanut butter, almond butter, or any nut butter. The best kind of peanut butter is the kind you can grind yourself right in the store. The next best is all natural with no added oils or sugars, but the natural oil does separate and get annoying. Skippy and Jif both offer peanut butter options without added sugar that use palm oil to prevent separation.

SEEDS

These can be high in omega-3, but also high in total PUFA. The best seeds are pumpkin seeds. Other seeds, such as sunflower and chia, may best be consumed after you've been off seed oils for long enough that your biomarkers have improved.

"This is the first time ever I changed my diet and felt better. I have more energy. I feel stronger. I lost 15 pounds without trying, I am very fit and cut/trim now. This does not feel like a diet. I'm a former Israeli soldier and suffered with PTSD for decades—but that is now almost gone! The biggest surprise and maybe the best part is everything tastes better than it used to. The diet is working, I'm beyond excited, I love the way I feel."

—Ethan G.

SEMI-STARCHY VEGETABLES

Most vegetables are very low carb and don't sustain our energy on their own. Potatoes and corn are very high carb, and I don't recommend eating them on a regular basis. Peas, pumpkin, cooked carrots, and winter squashes such as butternut and acorn squash represent a middle category that can sustain our energy all by themselves without producing a big blood-sugar spike. Even so, it's still better to combine these with healthy fats.

Anything Fruit Can Do, Vegetables Can Do Better

The many varieties of vegetables besides the semi-starchy ones we've just covered are naturally low in carbs and packed with nutrition. In general, you can feel good about choosing vegetables. (Potatoes are the only vegetable I recommend particular caution with—see the aforementioned semi-starchy vegetables section.) That said, there are a few things to keep in mind with these plant foods.

WATCH THE SUGAR CONTENT OF FRUITS

Most fruit today is so full of sugar that getting the vitamins and minerals you need from fruit will come along with hundreds more sugary calories than the same amount of vitamins and minerals from vegetables. The best fruits for metabolic rehab are not the sweetest ones. In fact, the less sweet, the better. Avocados, cranberries, currants, and coconuts are the best. Berries and melons are also low in sugar. Blueberries, raspberries, strawberries, cantaloupe, honeydew, and watermelon are great choices. It's best to use fruit to flavor other, more nutritious foods than to eat it all by itself. My advice to patients has long been to limit their intake of fruit based on how much sugar it contains. A good upper limit is twenty grams of sugar, and I wouldn't push it to the max every day. That would be one banana, orange, grapefruit, apple, peach, or pear; about half a mango or papaya; about three-quarters of a cup of grapes; about two cups of watermelon or cantaloupe; or only about an ounce of dried fruit such as raisins, banana chips, or dried cherries.

I like to think of fruit as a spice. You can add it to a dish to make it flavorful and give something savory that element of sweetness. Or, use it as a dessert. Having fruit as your meal without any accompaniment is very likely to make you feel hungry again a short while later.

PAIR LOW-CARB VEGETABLES WITH FAT AND/OR PROTEIN

Most low-carb vegetables are extremely nutritious. But bear in mind that most of them are also too low in calories to sustain our energy. Be sure to consume them as a side dish or otherwise accompanied by some healthy fats and/or protein. Examples of low-carb vegetables include all lettuces and salad greens, celery, spinach, radishes, kale, peppers, tomatoes, broccoli, cauliflower, green beans, asparagus, and fresh herbs.

When shopping for vegetables, it's important to consider that many of them do not last more than a week in the fridge. If you don't like shopping at least once a week, you can get frozen vegetables, and the vegetables that tend to keep a little longer, including carrots, onions, and celery. Leafy greens like lettuce, arugula, baby greens, and kale tend to go bad quickly, so plan accordingly. For vitamin C, bell peppers beat orange juice every day of the week.

ORGANIC IS IMPORTANT...SORT OF

Testing shows that certified organic fruits and vegetables are generally lower in toxic pesticide and herbicide residues as well as other environmental contaminants, as you would hope. But this may be less important than whether the produce is fresh and tastes like it should.

HOW MUCH CARB IS TOO MUCH?

I don't recommend piles of starchy carbs as the centerpiece of a meal. Instead of a plate of pasta, make it a side. Instead of a heaping pile of mashed potatoes, take a smaller portion. Rice, corn, and potatoes are full of relatively empty calories, and when combined with butter and salt can be so delicious that it's too easy to overeat them. Brown rice is not significantly more nutritious than white rice. Sweet potatoes have an undeserved reputation for being healthier than white potatoes—they are not.

If weight is not a concern for you, and you have not been diagnosed with prediabetes or diabetes, then you can enjoy more of these foods. Just be sure you're not eating so much that they've displaced the nutritious foods your body actually needs.

If you have moderate insulin resistance or diabetes, it's best to limit your *added* sugars as much as possible. I recommend one teaspoon or less per day.

Flour is best used as a thickener for healthy bone-stock gravies and to coat very healthy foods, like liver, before pan frying. Sugars are best thought of as a spice, to be used to flavor otherwise nutritious dishes.

TIMING YOUR SWEETS AND CARBS

The worst time of day to have anything sweet is in the morning. Sweetness is more addicting at that time and more damaging to the metabolism.

The reasons have to do with hormonal circadian rhythms. The same goes for starchy foods that are not sweet, such as breads, bagels, quick-cooking oats, and the like. Although these are common breakfast items, they are also a common cause of mid-morning hunger and hypoglycemia. Keep in mind that if you feel you cannot stay in control, they are best avoided.

BEYOND MACROS: SALT, HERBS, AND SPICES ARE POWERFUL HEALTH ALLIES

Aside from nourishing healthy fats, protein, and carbs, I'd like to discuss a few other foods here because, while they are not the main components of our meals, they can impart healthful properties and make our meals more enjoyable. I'm referring to salt, herbs, and spices.

Salt Is an Antioxidant

We like salty flavors because they indicate the presence of minerals and antioxidants. One of the little-known facts about sodium chloride (table salt) is that it is a potent antioxidant, effectively preventing oxidation not only in our foods but also in our bloodstream. Our blood is very salty, and nature puts salt there to help fight the oxidation that would otherwise damage our arteries.

Salt gets a bad rap and (as with red meat) we often hear we are eating too much of it. But our bodies regulate the salt content of our blood. If we eat too much of it, we get thirsty, which helps our kidneys eliminate the extra amount. (It's actually quite hard to eat too much salt, because when we over-salt our food it's generally so unpalatable that we simply won't eat it.) On the other hand, chronic salt *deprivation* while consuming caffeinated beverages or taking certain medications can lower our sodium levels to the point that we feel absolutely miserable. Unnecessarily avoiding salt causes a staggering amount of unnecessary suffering. Between three million and six million people visit their doctors and roughly one million are hospitalized annually because of low blood sodium levels.[19] Virtually nobody is admitted to the hospital because of high blood sodium, unless they have another serious issue that is causing it, such as severe dehydration or kidney failure.

Salt and Blood Pressure

Dietary surveys have linked salt consumption to high blood pressure. But in doing these analyses, the researchers generally just tally up the salt and pay no attention to what else came along with it.[20] Since processed foods are both heavily salted and laden with seed oils, when you get your salt from processed foods, you're also getting plenty of toxic oils and refined carbs. Furthermore, since health-conscious people avoid salt (unnecessarily), people who eat the most salt are generally eating poorly overall. These methodological flaws completely confound the results. It makes it look like salt is the problem, when the real problem is processed foods.

If you pay close attention, you will notice experts don't usually say salt actually *causes* hypertension, because there is no evidence of this. The American Heart Association's website says salt *"may worsen hypertension"* (emphasis mine); it does not say that it *does*. Just to be clear, if you don't have hypertension, no one can even make the claim that you will benefit by avoiding salt.

However, even the claim that salt "may worsen hypertension" is questionable. Clinical trials have tested the idea that lowering salt intake improves blood pressure, and while some have shown it works, many have not. The more likely reason that a "low-salt" diet shows any benefit has to do with the fact that participants in these studies aren't just eating less salt, but are also given a salt substitute made with minerals that many folks don't get enough of, including magnesium sulfate or potassium chloride. They also benefit by meeting weekly with dietitians who tell them to eat less junk. So while all the focus in these studies is on salt, the real health benefits are probably coming from the other variables that get less attention.[21]

Note: If you have severe heart or kidney failure, then you do need to restrict salt intake. These organs regulate the body's balance of salt, water, and many minerals. When they are failing, everything needs to be calculated and monitored, including not just salt but also water, potassium, and phosphate.

Chefs often say that their number one "secret" ingredient is liberal use of salt. Junk-food manufacturers notoriously use fat, salt, and umami flavors to make foods incredibly delicious. (Umami is the savory flavor we get from, for example, soy sauce, fish sauce, miso, cooked mushrooms, browned butter, and Worcestershire sauce.) Obesity experts warn that salt, umami, and fake flavors make processed foods hyperpalatable, meaning they taste so good that we can't stop eating them. But the reason we can't stop eating them is that the artificial fats and fake proteins don't provide real satiety.

So, why not use these "hyperpalatability" techniques on healthy foods? By combining healthy fats, salt, and real proteins (or real umami flavors), we can make our own healthy meals every bit as crave-worthy as the processed food industry makes their junk. Not only will they taste great, they'll give us real satiety—especially if they contain a bit of cholesterol—so we will be less prone to overeating them. So, go ahead and use salt. Salting healthy food helps you look forward to the main dish, not just the dessert. And those healthy foods will be even more enjoyable with added flavor from herbs and spices.

Herbs and Spices

Herbs are vegetable superfoods, packed with even more nutrition per ounce than most other vegetables. But they go bad really fast, so buying fresh herbs puts the pressure on to use them before they turn into compost. One solution to this problem is buying herbs in a pot and growing them yourself. Herbs that grow easily indoors include mint, rosemary, thyme, basil, oregano, chives, and sage. Success with herbs can be the gateway to a bigger and better relationship with gardening, so give it a go!

If you're not up for that, then dried herbs are amazing, too. A simple Italian herb blend goes a long way to freeing you from dependence on store-bought prepared sauces. Dried herbs retain their minerals, but their vitamins will deteriorate over time.

Like herbs, spices are superfoods: most of them are absolutely loaded with minerals. They are also essential to creating a sense of variety when you only buy a few meats or veggies. By shifting from Mexican to Asian spices, for example, you can make chicken, onions, carrots, mushrooms, and celery taste Tex-Mex or Sichuan. If spices are intimidating, start with a simple blend of something you would eat dining out, such as a curry, a Lebanese 7-spice mix, a dry rib rub, or a Cajun fish blend. Spice blends sold in individual packages are sometimes bulked up with non-nutritive ingredients such as silicon dioxide and maltodextrin, which are not ideal, but not a deal breaker, either. Most spice blends sold in jars in the spice section of grocery stores are absolutely great—sprinkle the world of flavor into your food with a tap of your fingertips.

Now that you're more familiar with the good foods and not-so-good foods, let's take a look at how to incorporate the good foods into some fast, easy meals that will get you started on the road to metabolic heath.

CHAPTER 11

The Two-Week Challenge:
Meal Planning and Simple Meals

IN THIS CHAPTER YOU WILL LEARN

- How to go two weeks without using seed oils.
- How to quickly assemble healthy ingredients into a meal, so you can free yourself from dependence on food bars, snacks, and junk food.
- How to clear your cupboard of seed-oil-soaked foods.
- What to eat to prevent pathologic hunger while improving energy and concentration.
- In the longer term, preventing pathologic hunger will cure metabolic sugar addictions and change your food cravings from unhealthy to healthy.
- By losing your fear of real food, you can free yourself from dependence on processed foods and the healthcare system.

I would like to invite you to take a Two-Week Challenge and go vegetable-oil-free to prove to yourself it can be done and to start detoxifying your body. In this chapter, I'll get you started with a meal plan of simple basic foods that you can easily make even if your kitchen confidence is low. I'll provide suggestions for easy breakfasts, lunches, and dinners, along with tips for healthy desserts.

In this short time, you will most likely notice more energy and less inflammation and belly bloating. If you test your blood sugar, you'll notice it improving as you start to reverse insulin resistance. If you choose to continue beyond two weeks, you will find that you can slow or even reverse the processes that degenerate and age us. By freeing yourself from dependence on processed foods, you'll be freeing yourself from dependence on the healthcare industry, too, while supporting the producers of real food who are more deserving of your hard-earned money.

Avoiding seed oils is not easy, and many people need to start small, by avoiding the worst of the worst and then gradually expanding their avoidance of seed oils over time. So there are degrees of seed-oil avoidance, and when I work with people I actually ask them to rate their current level of seed-oil avoidance on a scale from 1 to 10, with 1 meaning you don't avoid them and 10 meaning you never eat them. The goal of the Two-Week Challenge is to become a 10, for just a limited time. Hopefully you will feel so much better that you'll want to continue operating at a 10 for the rest of your life.

This is just to get you started. The breakfast and lunch examples are intended to show you how easily you can make meals fast using real-food ingredients, so that you can get in the habit of assembling your own dishes instead of opening boxes and packages. The dinner examples are intentionally basic. This is not a lesson in fancy cuisine, it's a lesson in strategizing for self-sufficiency. If you choose to continue you will need more variety, and I am confident that the concepts you've learned will help you better identify recipes from the billion available online.

Just to be clear, this Two-Week Challenge is going to help you eliminate the Hateful Eight toxic oils from your *diet*. They will still be present in your body fat, however. The body-fat detoxification process takes much longer, roughly two years for each forty or so pounds of fat on our bodies. That's the bad news. The good news is that it means you will continue to notice your body feeling better, and your mind functioning more efficiently on the job and at home, during the months and years to come.

"As a pilot I've always been health-conscious, but still my weight crept up, and so did my blood pressure. Your advice has been tremendously effective. I lost thirty pounds in five months. I have more energy. I feel much better to go work out. I've been saying to my wife, 'Let's get out of the house and do something,' and that's new because I didn't used to feel like it. Folks at the gym are asking what's changed, and I tell them they won't believe it—just cut out sugar and vegetable oil."

—Gerhard M.

FOR EVERYONE WHO GRAZES AND SNACKS

With more and more people snacking, fewer and fewer people are eating three square meals a day. One survey showed that at least 60 percent of people still do eat three meals, though, and most of them snack on top of their three meals. In my experience working with patients, one reason for snacking is simply being too busy to sit down and eat. This problem is easily solved by planning meals that you don't need to sit down to eat, and I've included several in this category, listed as "Meals on the Go" in the Two-Week Challenge section, after the listing for lunch.

Another common reason for snacking is being too busy to eat a meal at the intended time, and getting pathologic hunger as a result. This chapter will also help you to resolve that problem. It's far healthier to plan meals that prevent your hunger so you don't need to rely on snacks than it is to carry snacks. In the meal suggestions in this chapter, I have not included any healthy snacks because there really is no such thing. Plus, I'm hoping that you will experience for yourself the benefits of the energizing and satiety-inducing fats that you'll be eating. If you're snacking, you won't be able to notice any of that. Avoiding sugary beverages and alcohol will also go a long way toward helping you get the most out of this experiment.

"I want to thank you for changing my life. After I saw you on *Bill Maher* I immediately implemented the changes you recommend. After three weeks I had no more carb cravings. I have so much energy now [a year later] I've lost weight without any effort. I want to keep eating this way but now my doctor is worried about my cholesterol and I don't want to find a new doctor. I feel like my whole life, there was a secret out there, and this was the secret."

—Marrisa M.

HOW TO PREVENT PATHOLOGIC HUNGER

Once we fix pathologic hunger, we're starting our journey to total metabolic health. Fixing pathologic hunger comes down to choosing foods that take longer for our systems to digest, so they can sustain our energy for longer. This prevents blood sugar peaks, insulin spikes, and blood sugar dips and keeps your brain energy at an even keel. The meals in the breakfast, lunch, and dinner menu will prevent pathologic hunger. These are just a few examples, and you can make up your own following the same few simple principles:

1. Eat energizing fats at every meal (see the list of energizing fats in the Resources section). You should get 100 to 400 calories from these fats per *meal*.
2. Eat slow-digesting carbs at least twice a day, and limit sweets. To reverse insulin resistance, aim for 160 to 400 calories

from these foods per *day* (see chapter 10 and the list of slow-digesting carbs in the Resources section). For fastest results, limit sweet calories to less than 40 or so for the day. The *best* time to eat anything sweet is *after dinner*. During the day, you've emptied out your body's little carbohydrate storage suitcases, making space for blood sugar to flow right in. The worst time is at breakfast, though for the challenge I have included some naturally sweetened options for breakfast and lunch, because having something appealing matters more for these two weeks.

3. Eat real-food protein, not protein powders, hydrolysates, isolates, or fake-food protein. Find your daily needs using the protein calculator in Appendix A. It doesn't matter if you eat all your daily protein in one, two, or three meals.

4. Do not snack. The whole point of this strategy is learning to build meals that prevent pathologic hunger. If you eat or drink anything with calories between meals, you'll never know if it's working. If you do experience pathologic hunger after breakfast, lunch, or dinner, it means that tomorrow you need to modify that meal by adding either more fat or more carbohydrate. Drink only unflavored water, black coffee, or tea. (For a more detailed strategy, consult my previous book *The Fatburn Fix*.)

Tip: If you like healthy snack foods, try planning to eat some as a meal. This can include nuts, cheese cubes, kale chips, and the like.

How to Treat Between-Meal Hunger

It's okay to ignore hunger if your hunger is not pathologic. (Review Figure 4–1 if you're not sure.)

If your hunger is pathologic, then it's best to treat it, because it may not go away. Go ahead and eat something starchy that gets into your system fast, like a pretzel or two. Don't overdo it. Just two pretzels will break down quickly and bump your blood sugar for long enough to make it to your next meal. If it's hours away, then you should also support your energy levels with something more sustaining. A small handful of almonds or other nuts is a great choice.

For many people who are habitual snackers or grazers and who were not in the habit of eating meals, it can be very difficult to make the leap to less frequent eating. If this sounds like you, then focus first on avoiding seed oils and sugary, sweet foods for the first week while continuing to graze. In other words, follow the aforementioned Steps 1 through 3 for a week before you try to tackle Step 4.

YOUR TWO-WEEK CHALLENGE MEAL-PLANNING MENU

A Two-Week Challenge might sound—well—challenging, but really, it can be very simple. The number one goal is to prove to yourself that you and processed food are ready for a divorce: you don't need to live on food bars, take-out, boxed or frozen meals, snacks, or any other junk. The number two goal is to see how good you feel after you've ejected these toxic oils from your diet. In the first week you are most likely to notice improved digestive health and mental focus. If you continue, you will notice much, much more.

These are not recipes. They are meal concepts, and they are so simple they really don't require a recipe. They also have the advantage of being nonspecific, so that by their nature they are open to variation. For example, take avocado toast, which was a huge thing about ten years ago. You can very easily go online and find hundreds of great ways to make avocado toast delicious and fun to experiment with. Other meal concepts are more about giving you permission to eat foods that you probably know how to make but didn't realize were super healthy, such as burgers. If you follow these meal concepts during the Two-Week Challenge, you don't need to bother counting carbs or macros. It's built in.

To keep your shopping list short, pick no more than three from each meal category and buy enough to repeat that dish for the week. (If you want to shop just once for both weeks, that's great, but be sure to choose food items that will keep that long; fresh meats may need to be frozen.)

I've included a shopping list beneath each of the meal ideas. That may seem a little unnecessary given the simplicity of the meal, but if you're not used to making your own meals from scratch, you're probably not used to making shopping lists either. Making a shopping list is every bit as essential to success as being able to cook a few simple meals.

Remember, the goal is just getting through two weeks without seed oils so that you can get a taste of what's waiting for you once you become a full-time seed-oil avoider. We're not going for a complex meal plan or new cooking methods. If you are okay with eating the same thing for breakfast every day, then go for it. One patient I worked with who confessed to having zero cooking ability of any kind, and wanted to lose weight for a wedding, ended up doing nothing but almonds, pre-peeled hard-boiled eggs, and lots of milk for three months straight. He lost nearly sixty pounds. He felt fantastic—so good, that he started to learn a few skills. Eight years later, he'd developed quite a repertoire, including making family meals every other day and making his own bone broth from scratch (he also lost the other eighty pounds he wanted to shed).

Are you ready? Here are some of the most popular, easiest, fastest, and most healthy vegetable-oil-free options I recommend to get you started down the healing path.

Breakfast

EGGS

This meal consists of two to three eggs cooked any way you like. If you like hard-boiled eggs but want to skip cooking and peeling, most grocery stores now carry peeled hard-boiled eggs in bags. They taste amazing with melted butter and salt. Or, if you want to be fancy, try a splash of soy sauce. In England, a common meal is an egg with olives, relish, and other items mashed into it. This can also go on a slice of sprouted-grain toast.

Shopping List
- Eggs.
  - ○ *Optional:* Butter, olives, relish, and sprouted-grain bread (such as Ezekiel) or sourdough (or the healthiest type of bread you can find).

> **Tip:** Most grocery stores now carry peeled hard-boiled eggs—a real time saver!

AVOCADO TOAST

Use one or two slices of the healthiest bread you can find. Top with avocado slices and sprinkle with an "everything bagel" type of seasoning mix, or just with salt and pepper. Coconut flakes or cream also go well.

Shopping List
- Sprouted-grain bread, sourdough, or another healthy bread.
- Avocado.
  - ○ *Optional:* "Everything bagel" seasoning or coconut flakes.

> **Tip:** Sprouted-grain bread is sold in the freezer section.

CINNAMON BUTTER TOAST

Use one or two slices of the healthiest bread you can find. Top with 1–2 tablespoons each of butter and peanut butter (or almond butter), sprinkled with cinnamon if you like, and dotted with raisins or your favorite dried fruit.

Shopping List
- Bread.
- Peanut butter or almond butter.
  - *Optional:* Cinnamon, raisins, other dried fruit.

TYPE C TOAST

Use one or two slices of the healthiest bread you can find. Spread real cream cheese and top with smoked salmon. You can also use herbed cream cheese.

Shopping List
- Bread.
- Cream cheese.
- Smoked salmon.
  - *Note:* If you don't like smoked salmon, have it plain or buy herbed cream cheese.

YOGURT

Use one to one-and-a-half cups of plain whole-milk yogurt with one-quarter cup fresh melon or berries (optionally sweetened with jelly, honey, or dried fruits), and top with nuts.

Shopping List
- Yogurt (if regular is too sour for your taste, try Greek, but get the plain, whole-milk type).
- Fresh fruit, jelly, honey, or dried fruits.
- Nuts.

> **Tip:** Dried coconut, almonds, and vanilla extract make a great combination without the need for added sugar.

COTTAGE CHEESE

If you don't like yogurt, try full-fat cottage cheese, in the same amount as the yogurt (above) and with the same toppings.

Shopping List
- Cottage cheese, plus the toppings listed above.

TRAIL MIX

Make your own favorite blend of seed-oil-free nuts and dried fruits. Aim for three-quarters nuts and one-quarter or less fruits.

Shopping List
- One to three types of nuts (raw, sprouted, or roasted without seed oils).
- One or two types of dried fruits.

> **Tip:** Tropical fruits and apricots are less likely to be coated with vegetable oil than berries and raisins.

MILK SHAKE, UNSHAKEN

Add up to two ounces of cream to milk and flavor it with a few ounces of coffee, tea, or flavored stevia drops. If you don't normally have milk in the house, then, for this experimental week, just buy half-and-half and use a cup or so of that instead. (A cup of half and half has 285 calories and will keep you satisfied longer than that 300-calorie plain bagel.)

Shopping List
- Milk, cream, or half-and-half.
  - *Optional:* Flavoring (coffee, tea, or flavored stevia).

COFFEE

If you normally use a creamer with seed oils, instead use real dairy cream. Or try drinking it black. Remember, it's just two weeks!

No Breakfast Is Also an Option

If you're not accustomed to eating breakfast, there's no need to start. But if you've been skipping breakfast and snacking before lunch, that's actually just eating breakfast at a different time. So you'll need to have a seed-oil-free option. Hard-boiled eggs are easy to bring to work, as is the trail mix.

Lunch

SIMPLE DELI SANDWICH

Make a simple deli sandwich using the healthiest bread you can find (sprouted-grain or sourdough), plenty of slices of your favorite deli meat(s), and your favorite cheese(s), with avocado-oil or olive-oil mayonnaise and/or mustard and/or relish. The more meat and cheese, the more filling it will be. In fact, if you want to dabble with low carb, skip the bread and try the sliced meat and cheese rolled together. Popular combinations are ham and Swiss, roast turkey and Swiss, roast beef and provolone, or roast chicken and provolone.

Note: Deli meat gets a bad rap due to its high salt content. But, as we've seen, salt is not a problem. Another strike against it are the nitrites, which is a valid point. Nitrites are chemically more reactive and dangerous than nitrates. That's why I only recommend nitrite-free deli meat. Nitrite-free deli meat contains nitrates from natural sources like celery salt, which do not harm our health the way nitrites do.

Shopping List

- Sprouted-grain bread, sourdough, or another healthy bread.
- Nitrite-free deli slices (buy two pounds if you'll be eating this all week).

- Deli sliced cheese (or a block if you're okay with slicing it yourself).
- Avocado-oil or olive-oil mayonnaise.
- Mustard or relish for extra flavor.

> **Tip:** Roast beef, pastrami, and prosciutto are among the least mechanically processed options.

PEANUT BUTTER AND JELLY

Use healthy bread, plenty of peanut butter, plus jelly or fresh apple slices. A small carton of whole milk goes well with this lunch option.

Shopping List
- Sprouted-grain bread, sourdough, or another healthy bread.
- Peanut butter without added sugar or additional oils.
- Whole milk.

> **Tip:** The tastiest peanut butter is freshly ground in the store. It also does not separate. Almond and cashew butter are also great choices that usually don't contain added oils.

CELERY BOATS

Use two or three celery stalks generously filled with peanut butter or your favorite nut butter. Optional toppings could be sunflower seeds, raisins, or "everything bagel" seasoning.

Shopping List
- Celery.
- Peanut butter or other nut butter.
  - *Optional:* Toppings (sunflower seeds, raisins, or "everything bagel" seasoning).

PITA HUMMUS

Stuff a pita pocket with hummus and other ingredients to suit your taste, such as goat cheese, avocado, olives, baby greens or sprouts, shredded carrots, or chopped celery.

Shopping List

- Pita that is free of seed oils.
- Hummus made with olive oil.
- Goat cheese and/or olives, shredded carrots, chopped celery, greens, or other vegetables.

> **Tip:** You can find ingredients lists online for most products to save time reading them in the store. (The Instacart search works well for this even if you don't purchase through the app or website, for example. Company websites also usually include ingredients lists.)

FLAT TACO

Never heard of a flat taco? I made it up. It's a tostada that you don't have to toast (but if you'd like to, feel free to toast it, of course). I use a corn tortilla straight out of the bag, top it with cheddar or Monterey Jack cheese, melt the cheese in the microwave till just soft (thirty to forty seconds), then drizzle with red or green salsa.

Shopping List

- Yellow corn tortillas.
- At least one pound of cheese to last all week (it's cheaper to buy a block and slice it yourself).
- Red or green salsa.

> **Tip:** If you want to avoid added sugar, green salsa is a better option than red.

DECONSTRUCTED CORN DOG

This one is the same as a flat taco except that you add ham partway through the microwaving (just to warm it up). Instead of salsa, top it with mustard or sauerkraut.

Shopping List

- Yellow corn tortillas.
- At least one pound of cheese to last all week.
- At least one pound of nitrite-free ham.
- Mustard and/or sauerkraut.

> **Tip:** The best sauerkraut is fermented, and a nationally available brand is Bubbies.

Meals on the Go

KID'S LUNCH

Make a peanut-butter-and-jelly sandwich. Spread peanut butter on both pieces of bread to protect the bread from softening. Include a thermos of whole milk.

Shopping List

- Sprouted-grain bread, sourdough, or another healthy bread.
- No-stir natural peanut butter.
- Low-sugar jelly (the lowest number of grams of sugar per tablespoon that you can find). Or better yet, use fresh or frozen berries instead of jelly.
- Milk.

> **Tip:** You can buy eight-ounce packs of shelf-stable organic milk at Walmart and other stores. It's not as healthy as regular milk, but far healthier than a protein shake or soda.

MOBILE PICNIC
Pack a few ounces of cheese and meat cubes with a few nuts and maybe some grapes all together in a Tupperware container. Plop in an insulated bag with an ice pack. You can make your own insulated bag out of any cloth bag and a beach towel or two. Eat with toothpicks. Hard cheeses work well. As for the meat, for a taste of Spain try chorizo, and for an Italian option, choose prosciutto. Remember to choose nitrite-free whenever possible.

Shopping List
- Cheese: Manchego, mozzarella, Swiss, cheddar, Parmesan, Gouda, Edam, etc.
- Meat: salami, pepperoni, chorizo, prosciutto, or your favorite cured meat.
- White seedless grapes.
- Olives.
- Salted almonds.

DO-IT-YOURSELF DELI
Pack a deli sandwich into a Tupperware-type container or sandwich baggie. Plop it into an insulated bag with an ice pack (see above if you don't have an insulated bag). Add a nice dill pickle.

Shopping List
- Sprouted-grain bread, sourdough, or another healthy bread.
- Nitrite-free smoked turkey (or other deli sliced meat).
- Sliced Swiss cheese or other favorite cheese.
- Mustard and/or avocado-oil or olive-oil mayonnaise.
- Your favorite brand of dill pickles.

> **Tip:** The best pickles are naturally fermented, and a nationally available brand is Bubbies.

TRAIL MIX

Make your own healthy trail mix with a granola that's made using coconut oil or other non-seed-oil ingredients, or use popcorn in place of the granola. To a small ziplock bag, add one-third to one-half a cup of the granola (or popcorn), add an ounce or two of your favorite nuts, and maybe another ounce of shredded coconut or dried fruit. Bring along a thermos of milk.

Shopping List
- Healthy granola (such as Bob's Red Mill Granola).
- Nuts (raw, sprouted, or roasted without seed oils). Options include pistachios, macadamia nuts, almonds, walnuts, pecans, etc.
- Milk.
  ○ *Optional:* Use popcorn instead of granola.

HEALTHY SNACKS AS A MEAL

If you have a favorite snack that has all the nutrients you need to suppress pathologic hunger (see "How to Prevent Pathologic Hunger," above), just plan on eating that for a meal! A few popular examples include kale chips, nuts, including spiced nuts and hulled, salted pistachios, string cheese, Epic bars, and select flavors of Kind bars (read ingredients carefully to avoid the Hateful Eight).

Shopping List
- Your favorite healthy snack.

STORE-BOUGHT SUSHI

If you're near a grocery store and feeling hungry, one of the fastest, healthiest options is a pack of their premade sushi. Skip some of the rice to avoid some empty calories.

Shopping List

- Grocery store sushi.

> **Tip:** It's best not to buy sushi more than a day before you plan to eat it, so sushi is the exception to my recommendation to buy ahead.

Dinner

These dishes require no special skill, no special equipment, no exotic ingredients, and very little prep and cook time. If you are looking for more detailed recipes, I have shared a few of my favorites in the section "Select Recipes" at the end of the book, and you'll find many more on my website. Visit https://drcate.com/recipes.

If you've already got dinner nailed, and many people do, then there's nothing magical about these ideas except that they are super simple, fast, and great for beginning home cooks. Remember, the number one rule is avoiding seed oils. Number two is to make starchy carbs a side and not the star of the plate (if you eat them at all). Small amounts of pasta, rice, potatoes, and the like with a sauce, for example, are okay. All proteins, veggies, herbs, and spices are super-healthy.

When it comes to dinner planning, the biggest mistake I've seen people make is underestimating how tired they are at the end of the day, and not wanting to cook the more elaborate meals they may have planned. Another mistake is buying too many fresh vegetables, not using them, then throwing them out. These fast dinner protein and vegetable ideas are designed to be end-of-the-day fatigue proof.

HOW TO MAKE DINNER PROTEINS *FAST*

How much to cook? That depends on how much protein you need and what you've eaten earlier in the day. You can find formulas to calculate your protein needs, but I've found that some of them underestimate and others overestimate the amounts needed. I created a protein calculator for you based on what I think makes the most sense (see Appendix A).

You can get fancy and pick out a vegetable that's specially selected to pair well with the protein, or you can just make whatever you like from the list of veggie sides below.

ROTISSERIE CHICKEN

Most grocery stores sell rotisserie chickens near the deli. All the work is done for you. Be sure to check the ingredients list for seed oils before buying. If you're feeling like taking on more of a cooking project, save the bones to make bone stock.

Shopping List
• Rotisserie chicken.

> **Tip:** Since many of the flavored chickens will be coated with seed oil, the "original flavor" may be your best bet.

SHRIMP COCKTAIL

This meal is already made for you in the deli section of most grocery stores. Be sure to check the sauce for seed oils.

Shopping List
• Shrimp with cocktail sauce.

TUNA MELT

Mix together one can of tuna packed in olive oil (don't drain all the oil—it will save you expensive mayonnaise), a chopped small carrot, a chopped small celery stalk, one or two tablespoons of avocado-oil or olive-oil mayonnaise, and an eighth or quarter of a teaspoon each of onion powder, garlic powder, and salt. Melt a couple of ounces of cheddar or Monterey Jack cheese onto one of those six-inch yellow corn tortillas (thirty or forty seconds in the microwave), pile on the tuna, and enjoy.

Shopping List
- Canned tuna in olive oil.
- Carrot and/or celery.
- Garlic powder and/or onion powder.
- Avocado-oil or olive-oil mayonnaise.
- Cheddar or Monterey Jack cheese.
- Yellow corn tortillas.

> **Tip:** This would be a great place to try a Mexican spice blend. When purchased from the spice rack they are more likely to be free of fillers and contain just spices and salt.

STEAK
The secret to tasty steak is in the marinade. To make the simplest marinade ever, drizzle a few drops of Worcestershire sauce per steak per side and generously salt and pepper each side. Let it marinate in the fridge for between twenty minutes and twenty-four hours. The healthiest way to cook steak is rare.

Shopping List
- Steak.
- Worcestershire sauce.

CHEESEBURGERS AND LAMB BURGERS
The secret to quickly making burgers is to use 70 to 80 percent lean ground beef or ground lamb (which is naturally fatty). Avoid lean ground beef, which generally requires fussing with egg, oatmeal, or other binders to help it stay juicier and hold together. The secret to making burgers taste

more savory is adding a few drops of Worcestershire sauce, and plenty of salt. If you want to avoid the empty-calorie buns, toast some sourdough bread. Or just eat the burger without a bun, which is what I do. If you want burgers multiple days this week, for variety try experimenting with different cheeses or cheesy combinations.

Shopping List

- Ground beef (preferably grass-fed and 70–80 percent lean). If only leaner grass-fed beef is available, add one egg per pound to help prevent crumbling when flipping the burger.
- Worcestershire sauce.
  - *Note:* Lamb is always quite fatty. Also, it goes so well with rosemary, mixing it into the blend should be mandatory.

> **Tip:** If you can't find a grass-fed grind that's not super-lean, try mixing in a quarter to a third of a pound of ground pork per pound of ground beef.

FISH FILLET

Fish tastes great fried in generous amounts of butter, olive oil, or coconut oil. Just a few minutes on each side will cook most fish through, including salmon, halibut, and cod. Mahi-mahi and ahi tuna taste great rolled in sesame seeds; seared in sesame, peanut, or coconut oil; then sliced and dipped in soy sauce (this is popular at sushi restaurants). Or cook it any way you like. Be sure to add salt.

Shopping List

- Fish fillet, fresh or frozen.
- Butter or healthy cooking oil.
  - *Optional:* Soy sauce and sesame seeds.

> **Tip:** If you are shopping once for both weeks of the challenge, choose frozen fish, or freeze your fish if you're not using it soon.

FRIED CHICKEN HEARTS

This is the healthiest chicken meat you can buy in typical grocery stores (other than the liver). Chicken hearts are extremely cheap and surprisingly delicious. Melt one or two tablespoons of butter per half pound of hearts in a medium hot pan. Fry them for three or four minutes on each side, stirring often enough to cook all sides. Salt generously. If you are a fan of fennel (which tastes like black licorice) and sage, for the last three minutes of cooking add about half a teaspoon each of fresh ground fennel and sage. Season to taste.

Shopping List
- Chicken hearts.
- Butter.
  - *Optional:* Fennel, rubbed sage.

FRIED CHICKEN LIVERS

This is the simplest way to start liking liver and when you've perfected your technique it will taste better than chicken nuggets. Chicken livers are usually sold a pound at a time. Dredge all the little livers in plenty of flour, then let it soak in and press in some more flour. Load it up with flour, which is going to sizzle in the butter and taste great. Fry them in the butter for just a few minutes on each side until the livers firm up. Sprinkle generously with salt while cooking. They're done when slightly crumbly and barely pink in the middle. Add black pepper to taste.

Shopping List
- Chicken livers.
- Butter.

- All-purpose flour, or, for a lighter texture, try "00 flour" (a finely ground Italian flour).
- Black pepper.

HOW TO MAKE DINNER VEGETABLES *FAST*

If you've got too many vegetables in the fridge and you're worried about how to prepare them, fear not. Most veggies taste great together, whether steamed, sautéed, or roasted.

STEAMED VEGETABLES WITH MELTED BUTTER

Broccoli and the combination of carrots and red bell peppers are two of my favorites, but many veggies taste great steamed and drizzled with salt, butter, or garlic butter and sprinkled with spices or herbs. Try steaming them first, then pouring melted butter over the top and salting generously. A sprinkle of nutmeg tastes great on broccoli and Brussels sprouts. Curry powder goes well with cauliflower. For the best garlic butter, use fresh, minced garlic that you've heated in the melting butter.

Shopping List
- Fresh vegetables.
- Butter.
  - ○ *Optional:* Garlic bulb.

> **Tip:** If you're shopping for both weeks of the challenge, you might want to choose frozen vegetables for Week 2, as fresh vegetables are best consumed the week they are purchased. Refer to the instructions below for cooking frozen vegetables.

ROASTED VEGETABLES

Brussels sprouts and string beans are my two favorites for roasting, but beets, mushrooms, bell peppers, carrots, and other root vegetables also taste great when roasted, as do many other vegetable blends. Toss with olive oil (or any other healthy oil) and add a generous sprinkling of salt and pepper. Other fresh herb and spice blends can add pizazz. Set your oven to 425 degrees and roast for twenty or twenty-five minutes in a rimmed baking sheet or baking dish. Stir midway through cooking.

Shopping List
- Fresh vegetables.
- Healthy oil.
  - *Optional:* Fresh herbs or spices.

FROZEN VEGETABLES—FRIED IN BUTTER

Frozen vegetables are usually par-cooked and so all you really need to do is warm them up, making them even faster than steaming. Two of my favorite frozen veggies to cook this way are peas and lima beans. Just dump them in the pan, throw in a bunch of butter, heat until the butter is melted and the veggies are heated through and cooked to your taste, and salt them generously. Lima beans taste best when cooked for a while, but peas are just the opposite, so I don't recommend mixing these together. Spinach works, too, but tastes better if you use garlic butter, especially with fresh garlic. Frozen zucchini and summer squash are great when sautéed in butter and with fresh garlic added for the last few minutes. Salt these generously.

Shopping List
- Frozen vegetables.
- Butter.
  - *Optional:* Garlic.

SALAD

A side salad can be giant or tiny, depending on your mood. The hardest part for most people is the dressing, since most of your favorites from the store probably have seed oils. Using a quality olive oil whisked with vinegar and salt is a good way to start. Try adding granulated garlic or mustard for variety. Use two to three times as much oil as vinegar and salt to taste.

Shopping List
- Salad greens.
- Olive oil.
- Vinegar (balsamic or apple cider vinegar both taste great and are versatile).
  - Optional: Granulated garlic or mustard.

> **Tip:** Salad greens can go bad quickly, so try to find the packages with the best expiration dates.

COOKED GREENS

When I get too much spinach or baby kale to use in salad, I cook it down in a pan all by itself—a whole tub turns into about two servings. Then I add lots of garlic butter and salt.

Shopping List
- Spinach or baby kale.
- Butter.
  - Optional: Fresh garlic.

Dessert Recommendations

We all need dessert once in a while. These are my recommendations for simple, healthy desserts.

Note: Eating dessert within an hour after eating a mixed meal can minimize blood-sugar spikes.

POPCORN

Air pop or microwave dry kernels in a silicone popper (typical microwave popcorn is full of vegetable oils). Drizzle with melted butter, salt, and optional *furikake* seasoning or nutritional yeast. Furikake seasoning is a Japanese blend that uses seaweed, sesame seeds, and other ingredients (see the Shopping List link in the Resources section for seed-oil-free popcorn recommendations).

COCONUT MACAROONS

Coconut sustains our energy especially well, making macaroons an excellent choice for treating pathologic hunger in those (hopefully rare) instances where your meal plans didn't quite cut it. Buy the ones with the lowest sugar content you can find (see the Shopping List link in the Resources section).

ICE CREAM

Get ice cream with the shortest possible ingredients list that puts cream as high up in the list as possible (see the Shopping List link in the Resources section).

CREPE

See listing in "Select Recipes" section. Serve with cream or fruit.

PUTTING THE CHALLENGE INTO ACTION

The key to success is coordinating your shopping and your planning so that you only buy foods when you have a plan for what you are going to do with them. (For instance, two pounds of ground beef will become two nights of burgers for two people; two thirty-two-ounce tubs of yogurt and a small jar of blueberry jelly will be breakfast for the week for one person, and so on.) When you have a plan, you've already done the heavy mental lifting for when you come home tired, or need to rush out the door in the morning.

After you've gone through the suggested meals for breakfast, lunch, and dinner, circle the three or four from each category that you'll choose for both weeks of the Two-Week Challenge. Put together your initial shopping list. (You'll find many specific brand recommendations in the Resources section and at https://drcate.com/shopping-list.) You might shop once or several times during the challenge. If you want to shop once for both weeks, just plan to have more of the longer-lived goods on hand for Week 2, as the fresh meats and vegetables are best enjoyed the same week they are purchased. Of course, if you freeze your meat, do remember to thaw it out in the refrigerator a day or so ahead of when you'll need it.

Next, it's time to undergo the kitchen detox (if you haven't already!). Revisit the "Kitchen Detox Worksheet" in chapter 9. If you are ready to throw out, give away, or donate all the vegetable oils and vegetable-oil-containing foods in your kitchen, I applaud you. If you're not quite ready to get rid of the food, I understand where you're coming from. For the next two weeks, you might consider finding a box for the foods you ultimately want to get out of your kitchen. If the foods are in your fridge or freezer, you can stick them in their own box or bag there. Just do *something* to make the foods a little harder to access if you decide to keep them around during the challenge.

Go easy on yourself during these two weeks. As we discussed in chapter 4, if you are accustomed to snacking, making a switch to three square meals can be difficult; both your metabolism and your habits may be working against you. If you do find yourself experiencing the symptoms of pathologic hunger, it's more than reasonable for you to have a small snack—a couple of small pretzels or some nuts, as long as they contain no seed oils—to get you to the next meal.

You might also want to keep a log of how you are feeling each day (or even at various points each day). Make a note of any hunger pangs or cravings and your general mood and energy level. It's especially important to track when you experience pathologic hunger. If you do, that's your cue that there was something missing from your previous meal, so be sure to go back and revisit "How to Prevent Pathologic Hunger" on page 286. Also, check out the downloadable Free Reader's Tools for a pathological hunger tracker as well as tips on overcoming many of the common everyday challenges we face.

After working with thousands of patients and clients, I've consistently gotten feedback that most people start to feel more energized beginning on day one—literally within hours of getting started. When your breakfast includes healthy fats, you will probably notice that you have more energy all morning. Something as simple as eating good old scrambled eggs and toast can start your day out right.

At the end of the second week, it's time to take stock of how you feel. (I've found that paying close attention to how we feel is vital to long-term success. It's far more important than how fast we're losing weight.) If you're not sure that you are feeling more energy by then, it can help to revisit the list of inflammatory conditions to see if any of these other common issues have improved (see Figure 2–3).

Of course, if you still didn't notice anything, reassess, on a scale of 1–10, how well you did with avoiding seed oils. (Even if you give yourself a low score on the seed-oil-avoidance scale, you're still doing better than 99 percent of the population that has never heard about the dangers of these oils.) If you didn't do as well as you liked, take a few moments to answer the following questions:

- What challenges did I experience?
- How much can I commit to doing going forward?
- Do I need a partner to share stories with? (It doesn't even have to be someone avoiding seed oils, it can be anyone—especially if they are handy in the kitchen.)

Many people tell me that two weeks into it they are already feeling incredible—hence the Two-Week Challenge. But some people need to stick with it a little longer, so don't be discouraged. If you can commit to eating this way for three to six months, you will probably feel so much better that you can barely recognize yourself. And as you continue reducing your bodily burden of oxidative-stress-inducing oils over the coming years, you'll continue to notice improvements to your health, particularly when it comes to your brain.

As I went through this transformation myself, I started to realize just how many more "good" days I was having where I felt like myself—my moods were brighter, my concentration was sharp, and I could take joy from simple tasks that used to feel like drudgery. That transformation came from the enhanced performance I was getting from my own brain. It was like I got 30 percent more life every day for the small amount of additional time I spent focusing on buying and making healthier food.

The time you spend avoiding seed oils will pay itself back a thousandfold.

CONCLUSION

If something in this book has struck a chord with you, and you are ready to cut seed oils from your diet, know this: despite the challenges you may face, you are in good company. Growing numbers of chefs, nutritionists, naturopaths, osteopaths, dietitians, medical doctors, chiropractors, physical therapists, respiratory therapists, athletic trainers, athletes, social workers, biohackers, podcasters, journalists, educators, moms, and military personnel and other public servants are seeing the light. We all just want to eat real food that gives our bodies a chance to be energized, to feel healthy, and to allow us to do the things we want to do in this precious time we have on Earth. And we know that vegetable oil is not a part of that happy story.

If you do nothing more than make a conscious effort to get these oils out of your life, you are going to feel better. But you can go further. Our bodies are starving for a connection to the natural world. That connection is most powerfully created by eating intensely flavorful, fresh ingredients raised in healthy soil. When you celebrate good food, you are celebrating your body—believe this as if your life depended on it, because it does.

When you do make the change, and you start feeling better, I ask that you spread the word. If after cutting vegetable oil you've ditched medications, have more energy, and start to feel younger, try not to keep it a secret. Seed oils may be the missing piece in the puzzle for your friend, your neighbor, your office mate, your in-laws—and they might need to hear it from you, because they might not otherwise.

And remember also to enjoy and share real food, and honor where it comes from. Those whose daily labors create such quality foods—from the farmer to the chef to the home cook—are in short supply. The more we celebrate these people, the more we encourage our children to join their ranks, and the better life will be for all of us.

At the level of our governmental institutions and the biggest suppliers in our food supply chain, change might be a long time coming. But in your kitchen, change can start today.

One thing I've learned over the years is that the hardest part of making positive change is the part where you decide if you actually want to make the change or not. Obstacles, both in our vegetable-oil-saturated world and in our own minds and habits, can be a lot to overcome. But once you decide you really do want to make this change—when you're truly ready to commit—then you'll automatically start looking for ways you can do it.

And once you *believe* you can do this, you can become unstoppable.

Vegetable oil stole your health. Here's how we can take it back . . .

Feel Better Faster: Boost Your Health with These Seven Free Reader's Tools

- Use the **Protein Calculator** to confidently know you're getting enough
- Quickly identify and avoid bad fats with my **Good vs. Bad Fats Cheat Sheet**
- Use the **Kitchen Detox Assistant** to establish a roadmap for purging the bad fats
- Help loved ones boost their health with my **Metabolic Vicious Cycle 2 Pager**
- Leverage my **Carb Calculator** so you can assess amounts and easily find better carbs
- Cut planning hassle with my **One-Week Meal Planner and Shopping List**
- Detect metabolism issues and improve and track them using my **Pathologic Hunger Tracker**

Go here now to claim the resources you earned:
https://drcate.com/darkcaloriesdownloads/

SCAN ME

RESOURCES

THE SHOPPER'S GUIDE TO GOOD FATS AND BAD FATS

The lists on these pages are available for download on my website (see https://drcate.com/darkcaloriesdownloads), along with additional free resources. Be sure to also see Appendix A, which includes a protein calculator and the estimated protein content of different foods, and Appendix B, "Simply Counting Carbohydrates," which will help you select the best slow-digesting carbs.

These are the good fats you'll want to be sure to keep stocked. Start with at least one or two of them; most people only need three or four. Some you have to make yourself, like bacon fat, which is as easy as pouring it out of the pan. I like to keep butter along with olive, peanut, coconut, and sesame oil around at all times.

ASSESSING YOUR NEED FOR MINERALS

Contrary to some lab testing claims, there is no good blood test that can help you find out if you're getting enough minerals. The body regulates blood levels, and most can look normal even if your diet is deficient. The best way to find out if you are getting enough is to track your intake. My favorite free website for nutrient tracking is cronometer.com.

Good Fats—the Delightful Dozen (plus one!)

- Butter
- Extra virgin olive oil or unfiltered refined olive oil
- Unrefined peanut oil
- Unrefined coconut oil
- Unrefined avocado oil
- Ghee
- Sesame oil
- Unrefined palm oil
- Bacon fat
- Tallow
- Lard
- Chicken fat
- Unrefined tree nut oils (almond, hazelnut, pecan, etc.)

Take the two lists below with you to the grocery store too so that you can make quick choices as to which fats to buy and which to avoid. You can snap a picture of this page on your smartphone and take it with you. (You won't find many of the Delightful Dozen in processed foods.)

Okay but Not Great—Refined Fats and Oils

- Refined avocado oil
- Refined peanut oil
- Refined olive oil
- Refined coconut oil
- Refined palm oil
- Hydrogenated fats and oils (coconut oil, palm oil, or lard)

Bad Fats and Oils—the Hateful Eight and Others

- Corn oil
- Rapeseed oil
- Cottonseed oil
- Soybean oil
- Sunflower seed oil
- Safflower oil
- Grapeseed oil
- Rice bran oil
- Vegetable oil (catchall term for any of the above)
- Partially hydrogenated oils
- Vegetable lecithin
- Interesterified fats

ENERGIZING FATS

These two categories of foods provide saturated and monounsaturated fats that help prevent pathologic hunger.

These are examples of fats you can add to lower-fat foods to make them more sustaining:

- Avocado
- Bacon fat
- Butter
- Cream
- Cream cheese
- Coconut oil or cream
- Coconut flakes
- Dark chocolate
- Lard
- Macadamia nuts
- Olive oil
- Tallow

These are examples of high-fat foods that also contain enough protein to stand on their own:

- Bacon
- Full-fat cheese and 4 percent (or higher) cottage cheese
- Eggs
- Sausage and pepperoni
- Almonds and peanuts
- 70 percent lean ground beef

HOW TO FIND HOMA-IR TESTING

Few doctors know what HOMA-IR testing is, so you will need to go in armed with information that I provide on my webpage "Insulin Resistance and Metabolic Health Testing Using HOMA-IR," found at https://drcate .com/insulin-resistance-and-metabolic-health. Scroll to the bottom of that page for information on how to order a HOMA-IR blood test online.

RECOMMENDED SUPPLEMENTS AND FISH OIL FACTS

For recommended supplements to support your body's antioxidant enzymes, see my page at https://drcate.com/recommended-supplements. For more information on fish oil supplements, see https://drcate.com/should -i-take-fish-oil-supplements-benefits-and-harms.

WHERE TO GET A CONTINUOUS GLUCOMETER IF YOUR DOCTOR WON'T WRITE A PRESCRIPTION

For continuous glucometer (CGMs), see Levelshealth.com and Nutrisense .com.

GRASS-FINISHED STEAK

These sources will ship grass-finished steaks to your door, and their seasoned advice will help you to cook it.

- **Primal Pastures:** https://primalpastures.com/blogs/primal-blog /5-tips-for-cooking-grass-fed-beef

- **Butcher Box:** https://justcook.butcherbox.com/grass-fed-beef /how-to-cook
- **True Organic Beef:** https://truorganicbeef.com/blogs/beef -wiki/how-to-cook-grass-fed-steaks-the-right-way
- **Grassroots Foods:** https://grassrootsfoods.biz/cooking -instructions
- **Alderspring:** www.alderspring.com/faqs/cooking-grassfed -beef
- And my own article about how to cook grass-fed beef: https:// drcate.com/heres-how-to-cook-grass-fed-aka-pasture-raised -steak

OMEGA-3 SUPPLEMENTATION

Only choose products that mention controlling for oxidation in their marketing materials. For more details, visit https://drcate.com/should-i-take -fish-oil-supplements-benefits-and-harms.

INFANT FORMULA

For recipe guidance and more details on this topic, visit https://drcate.com /infant-formula-how-and-why-to-make-your-own.

TECH RESOURCES TO SUPPORT A SEED-OIL-FREE LIFESTYLE

Seed-Oil Scout: An app enabling the community of conscious diners to map out restaurants that care for their customers by cooking with healthy oils: www.seedoilscout.com.

Seedy: Find thousands of seed-oil-free products at your favorite stores with Seedy. Create shopping lists. Search by category, brand, and store—you can even search by voice chat: www.seedyapp.com (currently pending launch).

PEOPLE TO FOLLOW

Aseem Malhotra, MD: British cardiologist leading the charge in warning other MDs about the harms of statins and the fallacy of the cholesterol theory: https://doctoraseem.com.

Ken Berry, MD: Family medicine MD practicing in rural Tennessee who provides his Patreon supporters with an abundance of science-based advice on reversing diabetes: https://drberry.com.

Philip Ovadia, MD: Cardiologist in Rockford, Illinois, who wrote the book *Stay Off My Operating Table*. He also has a podcast.

Nadir Ali, MD: Houston-based cardiologist with many helpful YouTube videos about why not to worry about high cholesterol.

Uffe Ravnskov, MD, PhD: Danish family physician and scientist who first sounded the alarm on the fake science supporting the cholesterol theory decades ago. One of the last surviving experts to have witnessed firsthand the demonization of those who spoke out in defense of science, he runs THINCS.org, a website dedicated to "cholesterol skepticism."

David Diamond, PhD: University of South Florida neuroscientist with many helpful videos on how doctors are miseducated about statins and cholesterol.

Nina Teicholz:. New York City–based journalist and founder of the Nutrition Coalition, with many helpful and engaging videos explaining how the science supporting our current nutrition guidelines is flawed.

Tro Kalayjian, MD: New York City–based weight loss specialist who runs a nationwide telehealth practice using seed-oil avoidance and carbohydrate restriction to reverse diabetes.

GREAT RECIPES

- *Eat Smarter Family Cookbook* by Shawn Stevenson. This cookbook aligns with the fundamentals of my first book, *Deep Nutrition*, and takes a family- and kid-friendly approach to avoiding vegetable oils and processed foods in general.
- *Sunny Side Up: A 28-Day Breakfast Meal Plan for Busy Families* by Haley Scheich and Dr. Tarek Pacha.
- @CookWithChris (X, formerly known as Twitter) and website: https://cookingwithchris.crd.co.

I will be releasing a number of resources to help busy people make fast, easy meals, and if you would like to be notified, be sure to subscribe to drcate.com for updates!

REGENERATIVE AGRICULTURE

Here are just a few of the many organizations working to restore our ecology, the ultimate source of all nutrition.

The Carbon Underground: Their mission includes accelerating the adoption of regenerative agriculture at scale: https://thecarbon underground.org.

Permaculture Education Institute: Online resource for courses, masterclasses, free workshops, and more to help weave permaculture thinking and practice into your life—personally and professionally: https://permacultureeducationinstitute.org.

Groundswell: Hosts an annual conference focusing on no-till agriculture: https://groundswellag.com.

Polyface Farms: Founded by Joel Salatin, author of *Everything I Want to Do Is Illegal: War Stories from the Local Food Front.* He now trains budding farmers on his regenerative ranch in Virginia: https://polyfacefarms.com/education.

APPENDIX A

PROTEIN REQUIREMENTS "CALCULATOR"
Recommended intake, grams per day

WOMEN

Height	Pre-Menopausal	Post-Menopausal
Under 5'0"	55–80	50–70
5'0" to 5'4"	60–85	55–75
5'5" to 5'8"	65–90	60–80
5'10" to 6'0" +	70–95	65–85

MEN

Height	Age Under 60	Age Over 60
Under 5'4"	65–90	60–85
5'5" to 5'8"	70–95	65–90
5'9" to 6'0"	75–100	70–95
6'1" to 6'4"	80–120	80–110

Note: Weight and protein content are not the same. To estimate protein content, see next page.

Appendix A–1

ESTIMATING PROTEIN CONTENT

An ounce of uncooked lean meat or fish has about 6 grams (g) of protein.

Beef (weighed raw)
- Hamburger 80% lean, 4 oz, 28g
- Steak, 6 oz, 36g
- Most cuts of beef, 6g per oz

Chicken
- Chicken breast, 6 oz weighed raw, 36g
- Chicken thigh, 10g (for average size)
- Drumstick, 11g
- Wing, 6g
- Chicken meat, cooked, 4 oz, 35g

Fish
- Most fish fillets or steaks are about 22g for 3.5 oz (100g) of cooked fish, or 6g per oz
- Tuna, 5 oz can, 29g

Pork
- Pork chop, average, 22g
- Pork loin or tenderloin, 4 oz (weighed raw), 25g
- Ham, 3 oz serving, 18g
- Ground pork, 1 oz raw, 5g; 3 oz cooked, 22g
- Bacon, thin slice, 2g; thick cut, 5g
- Canadian-style bacon (back bacon), slice, 5–6g

Eggs and Dairy (full fat)
- Egg, large, 6g
- Milk, 1 cup, 8g
- Cottage cheese, ½ cup, 7g
- Yogurt, 1 cup, 8g; Greek, 9g
- Soft cheeses (Brie, Camembert), 6g per oz
- Medium cheeses (cheddar, Swiss, mozzarella), 7 or 8g per oz
- Hard cheeses (Parmesan), 10g per oz

Beans (including soy)
- Tofu, ½ cup, 20g
- Tofu, 1 oz, 2.3g
- Soy milk, 1 cup, 6–10g
- Most beans (black, pinto, lentils, etc) about 7–10g per half cup of cooked beans
- Soy beans, ½ cup cooked, 14g
- Split peas, ½ cup cooked, 8g

Nuts and Seeds
- Peanut butter, 2 tablespoons, 8g
- Almonds, ¼ cup, 8g
- Peanuts, ¼ cup, 9g
- Cashews, ¼ cup, 5g
- Pecans, ¼ cup, 2.5g
- Sunflower seeds, ¼ cup, 6g
- Pumpkin seeds, ¼ cup, 8g
- Flax seeds, ¼ cup, 8g

APPENDIX B

SIMPLY COUNTING CARBOHYDRATES

STARCHY FOODS: These foods contain about 15 grams of total carbohydrate per serving (measured after cooking). **Good sources of "slow-digesting" carb are indicated in bold.**

- ¼ large bagel OR large muffin
- ½ hamburger bun, hot-dog bun, pita bread, English muffin
- ½ flour tortilla (10-inch size)
- ½ to ¾ cup boxed cereal (label will tell you!)
- ⅓ cup white or brown rice, pasta, millet, couscous
- 1 oz slice of regular white or whole wheat flour bread
- 1 oz slice of **sourdough bread** including **Bavarian dark rye**
- 1 ½ slices **sprouted grain bread**
- 1 yellow corn tortilla (6-inch size)
- 6 saltine crackers or 3 graham squares
- ½ cup **steel cut oats, kasha, grits, bulgur, quinoa**
- ½ cup **wild rice**
- ½ cup **beans (i.e., pinto, kidney, garbanzo, lentils)**
- ½ cup starchy vegetable (potato, corn, sweet potato, yam)
- 3 cups **popped popcorn**

SEMI-STARCHY VEGETABLES: These vegetables contain about **15 grams of slow-digesting carb per serving** (measured chopped, if large, and measured cooked, unless stated otherwise).

- 1 artichoke, cooked whole
- 1.5 medium onions
- 1 cup beets, pumpkin (pureed), tomato puree or tomato sauce
- 1 cup green peas
- 2 cups Brussels sprouts, carrots, leeks, turnip puree

LOW-CARB VEGETABLES: These vegetables contain insignificant carbs in amounts normally consumed.

- asparagus
- baby greens
- bell peppers
- broccoli
- cabbage
- cauliflower
- celery
- eggplant
- jicama
- kohlrabi
- lettuce
- mushrooms
- okra
- pea pods (snow peas)
- spinach (also high protein)
- summer squashes (i.e., yellow squash, zucchini)
- tomato (raw)
- turnip (chopped)

SIMPLY COUNTING CARBOHYDRATES

NUTS and SEEDS
Most nuts and seeds contain about **5 grams of slow-digesting carb** per ounce (handful).

All foods below contain about **15 grams of carb per serving**. Good sources of **slow-digesting carb indicated in bold.**

MILK GROUP
The sugars in fermented dairy products have been modified by the fermenting organisms so that they do not spike our blood sugar, indicated in bold.
- 10 oz milk
- 1 cup soy milk
- 10 oz **cultured buttermilk**
- 10 oz **plain whole milk regular or Greek yogurt**
- 2 cups **cottage cheese**

FRUITS GROUP
The sugars in the fruits indicated in bold are also slowly released **due to the abundance of fiber.**

- ½ oz dried mango
- 1 date
- 3 prunes
- 1 oz raisins or dried, sweetened cranberries, cherries, or blueberries
- 7 dried apricot halves
- ½ average apple, peach, pear, or banana
- ½ grapefruit
- ½ cup unsweetened applesauce
- ½ cup orange juice, apple juice, or grapefruit juice
- 1 large kiwi

- 100g **unsweetened dark chocolate**
- 4 oz **unsweetened coconut flakes**
- ¾ cup fresh pineapple chunks, blueberries, blackberries, or grapes
- 1 cup cantaloupe, honeydew, or papaya
- 1 ¼ cups strawberries or watermelon
- 3 small **avocados**
- 80 **black olives**
- 100 **green olives**

SWEETS GROUP
- cookie 2 ½ inch
- ice cream ½ cup
- brownie 1 oz
- donut 1 oz

- milk chocolate or candy bar 1 oz
- dark chocolate (85%) 1 oz

SELECT RECIPES

Unlike the meal ideas in chapter 11, each of which stands for many different variations on basic ideas, these are detailed recipes. The first three are all-in-one dinner solutions, which I love because there is no need to plan a separate side dish. Everything goes into the same pot!

Some of these do take advantage of special kitchen equipment that I find super handy.

The trick to making these meals go smoothly and quickly is to prep—measure, peel, and chop—*before* you start cooking. Chefs call this *mise en place* (MEEZ ahn plahs), a French term meaning "put in place." Picture any cooking show where everything is all measured out and arranged on little plates that the chef dumps into their pots. It makes the cooking process look so easy. That's the beauty of the MEEZ.

Kale and Chorizo Instant Pot Soup

If you like chili, you will love this soup, which combines smoky chorizo with beef, beans, and greens for a deliciously satisfying meal-in-a-bowl. It freezes well, too. I can easily eat this for days on end.

Prep time: 10 minutes (not counting the bean-soaking process)

Cook time: 30 minutes

Serves 6 to 8

Ingredients

1 pound bulk chorizo sausage

1 pound ground beef

2 medium yellow onions, chopped

3 celery stalks, roughly chopped (with a few leafy tops)

4 garlic cloves, minced

4 cups chicken bone broth or stock

2 cups dried cannellini or garbanzo beans, soaked (see note)

1 teaspoon red pepper flakes

1 (28-ounce) can crushed tomatoes

1 small bunch kale, roughly chopped

1–2 teaspoons lemon juice

Salt and pepper to taste

Shredded cheddar or Monterey Jack cheese, for topping

Yellow corn tortillas, for topping (optional)

Instructions

Set an Instant Pot to sauté. Add the chorizo and ground beef and cook, breaking up the meat, until it begins to brown, about 5 minutes. Add the onion and celery and cook until they begin to soften, scraping up any browned bits stuck to the bottom of the pot with a wooden spoon, about 3–5 minutes. Add the garlic for the last minute or so of this portion (garlic burns easily so it shouldn't get too much heat at this point).

Add the stock, soaked beans, red pepper flakes, and tomatoes and stir to combine.

Place the lid on the Instant Pot and set to the "sealing" position. Set the timer for 12 minutes. The Instant Pot will warm up for about 10 minutes and then start cooking. After 12 minutes, quick-release the pressure by flipping the release valve to "venting." Remove the lid.

Add the kale and lemon juice. Stir to combine and season with salt and pepper to taste. Ladle the soup into bowls. Sprinkle with shredded cheese before serving. If you like, tear up a yellow corn tortilla to sprinkle over top.

Note: *To soak the beans, pour them into a bowl and cover with cool water. Let the beans sit 8–12 hours (or overnight). Before using them in your recipe, drain and rinse. Optionally, you can germinate the beans by allowing them to sit undisturbed and covered for an additional 12 to 24 hours.*

Sweet and Savory Pork with Cashews

You'll never need take-out again once you master the art of making your own East Asian–inspired sauces. This dish combines pork, colorful vegetables, and cashews with a sweet-savory sauce.

Prep time: 15 minutes

Cook time: 15 minutes

Serves 2

Ingredients

1–3 tablespoons coconut oil, divided*

1–3 tablespoons sesame oil, divided*

1–3 tablespoons peanut oil, divided*

12–16 ounces pork tenderloin or boneless pork chop, sliced into ½ to ¾ inch rounds or strips

1 small or medium onion, chopped

6–8 ounces white mushrooms, sliced

2 medium carrots, sliced

1–2 ribs celery, sliced

1 red bell pepper, diced

2 tablespoons soy sauce

2 tablespoons rice cooking wine

1 teaspoon malt vinegar

½ teaspoon fish sauce

1 (4-ounce) can sliced water chestnuts, drained

2 ounces cashews

*Note: Divided means that you add a portion of the total amount in different steps.

Instructions

Heat a large frying pan over medium-high heat. Melt ½ to 1 tablespoon of coconut oil for a few seconds, then add ½ to 1 tablespoon each of the sesame and peanut oils (melting the coconut oil first creates a platform that will protect the fragile, high-PUFA sesame oil). Tilt the pan or push the oil around with a flat-bottomed wooden spoon to evenly coat the pan.

Add the sliced pork, laying each slice separately. You may need to work in batches to not crowd the pan. When the meat begins to sizzle, reduce the heat to medium. (Overcooking will dry out the meat and make it less tender.) When the meat starts to release from the pan (lifts easily without sticking), usually after about 2 minutes, it's ready to flip. Flip each slice of meat one at a time, then cook till the meat just starts to firm up, usually about 2 minutes more. Remove from pan and set aside on clean plate when done.

Add some of the onion to the pan and cook until the onion starts to soften. The juices released from the onion will start to loosen those flavorful browned bits stuck to the pan; use a flat-edged wood turner to help release them.

Note: A flat-edged wooden turner or spatula is an essential tool for deglazing—the culinary word for releasing caramelized bits of food from the pan with a slightly acidic liquid (most often wine or broth). It also makes the later job of cleaning up much easier.

Melt another ½ to 1 tablespoon of the coconut oil, then add another ½ to 1 tablespoon each of the peanut oil and sesame oil. Add the remaining vegetables, except the water chestnuts.

Cook, stirring occasionally, until the veggies reach your desired doneness: if you like them still crispy, about 5 minutes; if you prefer them soft, about 10 minutes.

For the last 1–2 minutes of cooking, add the soy sauce, rice cooking wine, malt vinegar, and fish sauce and stir to coat.

Remove the pan from heat. Add the water chestnuts and stir in the pork to rewarm briefly. Serve topped with a small handful of cashews.

Mediterranean Seafood Medley in Tomato Cream Sauce

This scrumptious and versatile sauce takes advantage of a few delicious Mediterranean veggie preserves that I always have on hand because of their potent flavors and great shelf lives. If you don't have fresh herbs, substitute dried and add them earlier.

This recipe also works great with chicken instead of seafood. Simply swap in 1 to 1 ½ pounds boneless skinless chicken.

Prep time: 15 minutes

Cook time: 20 minutes

Serves 4

Ingredients

1–1 ½ tablespoons butter

1 tablespoon olive oil (to cover pan)

1–1 ½ pounds fresh scallops, raw peeled shrimp (or chicken breast, cut into pieces)

¼ cup white cooking wine or dry white wine

½ cup chicken stock

2 garlic cloves, minced

½-inch piece ginger, minced (this is optional)

1 large fresh tomato, or 1 cup of any tomato sliced into ½-inch pieces

1 teaspoon dried thyme

1 large red bell pepper, chopped

1 shallot or ¼ onion, sliced

3 sun-dried tomatoes, cut into pieces

3 artichoke hearts, cut into pieces

12 pitted kalamata olives, cut in half

1 ounce pine nuts

10 fresh basil leaves, chopped small

5 fresh flat-leaf (Italian) parsley leaves, chopped small

½ cup cream

Grated Parmesan, for topping

Salt to taste

Instructions

Heat olive oil in a large frying pan over medium high heat. When hot and shimmery, add the bell pepper and onion and sauté together for 3–4 minutes, stirring occasionally. Turn heat down to medium, add butter and when that starts to melt, stir in the garlic, ginger, tomato, and thyme, and let the ingredients sit over medium heat for 4–5 minutes, stirring occasionally.

Add the olives, sun-dried tomatoes, artichoke hearts, wine, and stock and use a flat wooden spoon to deglaze anything that sticks to the pan. When it comes back to simmering, turn down heat slightly to make sure it is just simmering (and not boiling), and allow the stock and wine to reduce down and the sauce to thicken slightly for 2–4 minutes.

Add scallops, shrimp, or chicken and cook through for about 4–5 minutes. Add cream and pine nuts, stir through, and heat for another 2 minutes. Add salt to taste.

Serve in a bowl with or without pasta (shell or bowtie pasta work better than spaghetti).

Top with parsley and Parmesan cheese.

Lowest-Carb Crepe

Most crepe recipes call for equal amounts flour and eggs by weight. This one makes three to four thin crepes and calls for just a tablespoon of flour per egg; once you get the hang of the recipe, you can make it work with ¾ tablespoon per egg. Each tablespoon of flour has just 6 grams of carbohydrate. To enjoy the crepes for dessert, try them with maple syrup, or fill with whipped cream and blueberries and roll up. For a savory crepe, you can roll sautéed minced shallots, sautéed mushrooms, lump crabmeat, or steamed spinach with the excess moisture squeezed out.

Prep time: 5 minutes
Cook time: 6–8 minutes
Serves 2

Ingredients
1 egg
1 tablespoon flour
1 tablespoon milk
Pinch of salt
2–3 tablespoons butter, divided

Instructions

In a bowl, whisk together the egg, flour, milk, and salt.

Heat a large frying pan over medium heat. Melt about a teaspoon of the butter and swirl to coat the pan. Pour a third or a fourth of the batter onto the pan toward the side (as opposed to in the middle). For a nice thin crepe, tilt the pan around so that the batter coats as much of the pan as possible. In less than 30 seconds, the crepe will have formed up and bubbled up away from the pan. Flip the crepe and cook for another 10 seconds; then, with a spatula, remove it to a plate. Repeat to make 2 to 3 more crepes.

Melt a little additional butter in the pan and pour it over the crepes. Enjoy hot with any fillings you like (see the headnote for ideas).

Crispy, Skin-on Salmon with Simple Mustard Sauce

Skin-on salmon is a real treat when cooked to crispy perfection. Please don't overcook it! The flesh of the fish should flake, but just barely. The simple accompanying sauce can be used for many other fish as well.

Prep time: 5 minutes

Cook time: 10 minutes

Serves 2

Ingredients

1 ½ pounds salmon fillet, skin on if possible

Salt

Olive oil

½ cup cream or ¾ cup half-and-half

1 tablespoon Dijon mustard

1 tablespoon chopped fresh dill or 1 teaspoon dried tarragon

Lemon slices, for serving

Instructions

Pat the salmon dry and season it liberally with salt. Cut the fillet in half if needed to accommodate the pan.

Heat a large frying pan on high. Pour in olive oil to a depth of about ⅛ inch and heat until shimmering. Add the fish, skin side down, and reduce the heat to medium. Cook the salmon until it's about 80 percent done (you can tell by the color—the side of the salmon will become opaque as it cooks), then flip and sear it on the other side for 10 seconds or until the flesh just barely flakes. Remove the salmon to a plate and let it rest while you make the sauce.

In another pan (or clean out the pan you used for the fish), warm the cream or half-and-half over low heat. Add the mustard and stir to combine. Continue stirring and heating a little longer to thicken if desired. Add the dill or tarragon, and stir.

Finish with a gentle flourish of fresh-cut dill and a slice of lemon on the side of the plate.

Check for doneness before serving. The flesh should flake apart but still be moist.

ACKNOWLEDGMENTS

I've been wanting to write a book like this since 2002, when I first learned of vegetable oils' toxicity and the backward world of medicine I'd been living in. But back then, the message would have been incomplete due to lack of available information—and, frankly, too radical-seeming. Times have changed. I want to begin by thanking the scientific heroes whose work helped me to complete the message, as well as the passionate influencers whose work collectively has facilitated the cultural changes that (I hope) primed the world to appreciate the messages of *Dark Calories.*

I am grateful for all the lipid scientists who fight the necessary battles to get funded and publish, particularly Dr. Eric Decker, Dr. Martin Grootveld, Dr. Glen D. Lawrence, and Dr. Frances Sladek, who all generously donated time to answering my questions—thank you. I am also indebted to the late Efraim Racker and Gerhard Spiteller, who both tried to warn the world about seed oils generations ago; their work greatly informed my understanding of oxidative stress and radically changed my worldview.

I also owe thanks to many others for inviting me to participate in podcasts, broadcasts, and other projects well before vegetable oil was a topic of interest, particularly Sean Croxton, Jeff Hayes, Mark Sisson, Brad Kearns, Ancestral Health Symposium organizers Kamal Patel and Katherine Morrison, Paleo FX organizers Michelle and Keith Norris, and chapter leaders of the Weston A. Price Foundation throughout the world. And to those who of you who have also now taken up the cause, especially Andrea Donsky, Ben Azadi, Cynthia Thurlow, Dr. Ken Berry, Dr. Phil Ovadia, Dr. David Perlmutter, Dr. Joe Mercola, Ben Greenfield, Dr. Paul

Saladino, Dr. Shawn Baker, Juliet and Kelly Starrett, Dave Asprey, Abel James, Dr. Daniel Pompa, Dr. Anthony Gustin, Dr. Michelle Gordon, Dr. Brian Kerley, David Gornowski, Dr. Drew Pinsky, Dr. Tro Kalajian, Dr. Brian Lenzkes, Dr. Jason Fung, Dr. Jeffrey Gerber, Vinnie Tortorich, Dixie Huey, and many more on X (formerly Twitter), Instagram, Facebook, and so on—there have been so many that I have lost track, and I apologize for this disservice to your support. Last, I need to acknowledge the readers of my other books who have reached out to share success stories and describe how they have become "insufferable converts" within their own communities. Awareness of vegetable oil as a health problem could always have begun only as a grassroots movement: you are collectively keeping that grass growing faster than it's mowed down.

I am extremely grateful to the scientists and practitioners who generously donated time to answer my technical questions and share their experiences within academia and industry, including Jennifer Hays, Mark Matlock, Matt Donovan, Candace Rassias, Dr. Klaus Schmidt-Rohr, Dr. Thomas Seyfried, Dr. Roy Baumeister, Dr. Chris Knobbe, Dr. Shebani Sethi, Dr. Georgia Ede, Dr. Dominic D'Agostino, and Dr. Phil Ovadia. And especially to Nina Teicholz, for uncovering the 1948 transaction that changed the course of medical history.

Much of the inspiration for Part Two of this book comes from seeing the financial burdens brought to bear on American employers and their employees by nutrition disinformation, along with the twisting of so-called preventive medicine in service of the healthcare industry. For that I thank the board of ABC Fine Wine and Spirits, particularly Charlie Bailes IV, who had the visionary idea of directly hiring a doctor.

I need to point out that this book would have never seen the light of day without the patience, support, guidance, and Earth-moving skills of my incredible agents at Folio, Dado Derviskadic and Steve Troha. I am forever grateful to Hachette, and especially my steadfast editor Lauren Marino. And for the absolute brilliance of Claire Schulz, the chess master of books, whose insights and masterful edits almost single-handedly kept this book alive.

Several members of my family deserve special mention. My brother, Dan Shanahan, whom I can always count on to create the exact perfect cartoon illustration; my sisters, who made writing breaks more fun; my mom, who passed on her dogged problem-solving skills; and my dad, who donated the all-important self-control gene. This book owes much to you.

NOTES

INTRODUCTION (PAGES IX THROUGH XVII)

Figure 0–1: Note that hydrogenated vegetable oils include both partially and fully hydrogenated oils, and since the trans-fat ban of 2018 in the United States, the majority of hydrogenated oils in the food supply are now fully hydrogenated—which has greatly increased the consumption of less stable, more toxic liquid oils. Sources used to create this figure include the following:

> For historical data from 1909 to 1999: Tanya L. Blasbalg, Joseph R. Hibbeln, Christopher E. Ramsden, Sharon F. Majchrzak, and Robert R. Rawlings, "Changes in Consumption of Omega-3 and Omega-6 Fatty Acids in the United States During the 20th Century," *American Journal of Clinical Nutrition* 93, no. 5 (2011): 950–962.

> For calorie availability and vegetable oil versus animal fat availability from 1909 to 2010: S. Gerrior, L. Bente, and H. Hiza, *Nutrient Content of the U.S. Food Supply, 1909–2010*, Home Economics Research Report Number 56, US Department of Agriculture, Center for Nutrition Policy and Promotion (CNPP), November 2004, https://grist.org/wp-content/uploads/2006/08/foodsupply1909-2000.pdf.

> For current calorie intake: Zhilei Shan, Colin D. Rehm, Gail Rogers, Mengyuan Ruan, Dong D. Wang, Frank B. Hu, Dariush Mozaffarian, Fang Fang Zhang, and Shilpa N. Bhupathiraju, "Trends in Dietary Carbohydrate, Protein, and Fat Intake and Diet Quality Among US Adults, 1999–2016," *JAMA* 322, no. 12 (2019): 1178–1187, https://doi.org/10.1001/jama.2019.13771.

> For consumption of each of the Hateful Eight oils in the United States between 2000 and 2020: Statistica.com. See, for example, "Soybean Oil Consumption in the United States from 2000 to 2022," Statistica, March 2023, www.statista.com/statistics/301037/soybean-oil-consumption-united-states.

1.   In the absence of published data on this topic, I reviewed the one hundred top sellers in the average US grocery store online and based the figure on this group of products. Based on shopping experience, the actual figure of food items by SKU is likely higher than 80 percent. See "List of 100 Top Selling Grocery Items 2023 & Tips," BusinessNES, January 2, 2023, https://businessnes.com/list-of-top-selling-grocery-items-and-tips.

2. Mary Enig, *Know Your Fats: The Complete Primer for Understanding the Nutrition of Fats, Oils and Cholesterol* (Bethesda, MD: Bethesda Press, 2000), 21.

CHAPTER 1 (PAGES 3 THROUGH 27)

1. P. F. Fox, T. Uniacke-Lowe, P. L. H. McSweeney, and J. A. O'Mahony, "Chemistry and Biochemistry of Fermented Milk Products," in *Dairy Chemistry and Biochemistry*, 2nd ed., 547–567 (Cham: Springer, 2015), https://doi.org/10.1007/978-3-319-14892-2_13.

2. Richard D. O'Brien, Lynn A. Jones, C. Clay King, Phillip J. Wakelyn, and Peter J. Wan, "Cottonseed Oil," in *Bailey's Industrial Oil and Fat Products*, vol. 2, *Edible Oil and Fat Products: Edible Oils*, 6th ed., ed. Fereidoon Shahidi, 173–280 (Hoboken, NJ: John Wiley and Sons, 2005).

3. Gary R. List and Michael A. Jackson, "Giants of the Past: The Battle over Hydrogenation (1903–1920)," *Inform* 18, no. 6 (2007): 403–405, www.ars.usda.gov/research/publications/publication/?seqNo115=210614.

4. Susan C. Pendleton, "Man's Most Important Food Is Fat: The Use of Persuasive Techniques in Procter & Gamble's Public Relations Campaign to Introduce Crisco, 1911–1913," *Public Relations Quarterly* 44, no. 1 (1999): 6–14.

5. N. K. Fairbank Company, "Cottolene, 'The New and Popular Health Food'" (advertising card), 1880 (date questionable), in Hagley Digital Archives, accessed September 4, 2023, https://digital.hagley.org/2270394#page/2/mode/2up.

6. William Shurtleff and Akiko Aoyagi, "History of Soy Oil Shortening—Part 2," SoyInfo Center, 2004, www.soyinfocenter.com/HSS/shortening2.php.

7. William Shurtleff and Akiko Aoyagi, "History of Soy Oil Shortening—Part 1," SoyInfo Center, 2004, www.soyinfocenter.com/HSS/shortening1.php.

8. Since there is no statistical data for total Hateful Eight, I've added up 2020 global annual revenue for each in US dollars as follows: cottonseed ($11 billion), canola ($26 billion), sunflower ($18.5 billion), soy ($47 billion), corn ($5 billion), rice bran ($1.3 billion), safflower ($7 billion). Each is expected to grow annually between 3 and 7 percent, except canola, which will stay flat or slightly decline. The projected 2027 value is based on an average increase of 5 percent. Data sources include the following:

Soybean oil: "Soybean Oil Market Size, Share & COVID-19 Impact Analysis, by Application (Cooking & Frying, Margarine & Shortening, Salad Dressings & Mayonnaise, Bakery Products, and Non-Food Applications), and Regional Forecast, 2021–2028," Fortune Business Insights, January 2022, www.fortunebusinessinsights.com/soybean-oil-market-106282.

Sunflower oil: "Sunflower Oil Market Size, Share & COVID-19 Impact Analysis, by Type (High-Oleic, Mid-Oleic, and Linoleic), End-Users (Household/Retail, Foodservice/HORECA, and Industrial) and Regional Forecast, 2021–2028," Fortune

Business Insights, January 2021, www.fortunebusinessinsights.com/industry-reports /sunflower-oil-market-101480.

Canola oil: Industry Research, "Canola Oil Market Size-Share Estimation 2022 Analysis by Industry Statistics, Covid-19 Impact, Global Trends Evaluation, Business Prospect, Geographical Segmentation, Revenue, Business Challenges and Investment Opportunities till 2027," Global Newswire, March 28, 2022, www.globenewswire.com /en/news-release/2022/03/28/2410651/0/en/Canola-Oil-Market-Size Share-Estimation -2022-Analysis-By-Industry-Statistics-Covid-19-Impact-Global-Trends-Evaluation -Business-Prospect-Geographical-Segmentation-Revenue-Business-C.html.

Cottonseed oil: "Mike," "Cotton Seed Price Index," BusinessAnalytiq, November 29, 2022, https://businessanalytiq.com/procurementanalytics/index/cotton-seed-price -index.

Corn oil: "Corn Oil Market Size, Share & COVID-19 Impact Analysis, by Type (Edible and Non-Edible), by Application (Food & Beverage, Pharmaceuticals, Cosmetics & Personal Care, Animal Feed, Industrial, and Biodiesel), and Regional Forecast, 2022– 2029," Fortune Business Insights, January 2023, www.fortunebusinessinsights.com /corn-oil-market-103810.

Rice bran oil: PRWireCenter News, "2023 Global Rice Bran Oil Market Growth: Key Players and Forecast 2030 | Industry Research Biz," Barchart, August 8, 2023, www .barchart.com/story/news/19169325/2023-global-rice-bran-oil-market-growth-key -players-and-forecast-2030-by-industry-research-biz#.

Safflower oil: "Safflower Oil," Tridge, accessed September 4, 2023, www.tridge.com /intelligences/safflower-oil.

Grapeseed oil: "Grape Seed Oil Market Size, Share & Trends Analysis Report by Application (Personal Care & Cosmetics, Food), by Extraction Process (Mechanically, Chemically), by Region, and Segment Forecasts, 2022–2026," Grand View Research, August 25, 2022, www.grandviewresearch.com/industry-analysis/grape-seed-oil-market.

9. Candace Rassias, Zoom interview with author, November 15, 2022.

10. Yacoob Bayat, "What's in Crude Vegetable Oil That Makes It Need to Be Refined So Extensively," American Oil Chemists' Society, December 12, 2022, www.informconnect.org /discussion/whats-in-crude-vegetable-oil-that-makes-it-need-to-be-refined-so-intensively.

11. Martin Grootveld, Victor Ruiz Rodado, and Christopher J. L. Silwood, "Detection, Monitoring, and Deleterious Health Effects of Lipid Oxidation," Inform 25, no. 10 (2014): 614–624, www.aocs.org/stay-informed/inform-magazine/featured-articles/detection -monitoring-and-deleterious-health-effects-of-lipid-oxidation-november/december-2014.

12. J. Bruce German, "Food Processing and Lipid Oxidation," in Impact of Processing on Food Safety: Advances in Experimental Medicine and Biology, vol. 459, ed. Lauren S. Jackson, Mark G. Knize, and Jeffrey N. Morgan (Boston: Springer, 1999), https://doi .org/10.1007/978-1-4615-4853-9_3; E. Choe and D. B. Min, "Chemistry of Deep-Fat

Frying Oils," *Journal of Food Science* 72, no. 5 (June/July 2007): R77–R86, https://doi.org/10.1111/j.1750-3841.2007.00352.x.

13. Haruki Okuyama, Sheriff Sultan, Naoki Ohara, Tomohito Hamazaki, Peter H. Langsjoen, Rokuro Hama, Yoichi Ogushi, et al., *Lipid Nutrition Guidelines: A Comprehensive Analysis* (Basel, Switzerland: MDPI, 2021), https://doi.org/10.3390/books978-3-03943-946-1.

14. Here I'm referring to the American Oil Chemists' Society Forum available to members online at www.informconnect.org/browse/allrecentposts.

15. Grootveld et al., "Detection, Monitoring, and Deleterious Health Effects."

16. Martin Grootveld, Benita C. Percival, Sarah Moumtaz, Miles Gibson, Katy Woodason, Azeem Akhtar, Michael Wawire, Mark Edgar, and Kerry L. Grootveld, "Commentary: Iconoclastic Reflections on the 'Safety' of Polyunsaturated Fatty Acid-Rich Culinary Frying Oils: Some Cautions Regarding the Laboratory Analysis and Dietary Ingestion of Lipid Oxidation Product Toxins," *Applied Sciences* 11, no. 5 (March 2021): 2351, https://doi.org/10.3390/app11052351; Martin Grootveld, Benita C. Percival, Justine Leenders, and Philippe B. Wilson, "Potential Adverse Public Health Effects Afforded by the Ingestion of Dietary Lipid Oxidation Product Toxins: Significance of Fried Food Sources," *Nutrients* 12, no. 4 (2020): 974, https://doi.org/10.3390/nu12040974; Sarah Moumtaz, Benita C. Percival, Devki Parmar, Kerry L. Grootveld, Pim Jansson, and Martin Grootveld, "Toxic Aldehyde Generation in and Food Uptake from Culinary Oils During Frying Practices: Peroxidative Resistance of a Monounsaturate-Rich Algae Oil," *Scientific Reports* 9 (2019): 4125, https://doi.org/10.1038/s41598-019-39767-1.

17. Martin Grootveld, "Evidence-Based Challenges to the Continued Recommendation and Use of Peroxidatively-Susceptible Polyunsaturated Fatty Acid-Rich Culinary Oils for High-Temperature Frying Practises: Experimental Revelations Focused on Toxic Aldehydic Lipid Oxidation Products," *Frontiers in Nutrition* 8 (2021): 711640, https://doi.org/10.3389/fnut.2021.711640.

18. Pierre Lambelet, André Grandgirard, Stéphane Gregoire, Pierre Juaneda, Jean-Louis Sebedio, and Constantin Bertoli, "Formation of Modified Fatty Acids and Oxyphytosterols During Refining of Low Erucic Acid Rapeseed Oil," *Journal of Agricultural and Food Chemistry* 51, no. 15 (July 2003): 4284–4290, https://doi.org/10.1021/jf030091u.

19. Martin Grootveld, Zoom interview with author, April 3, 2021.

20. Eric Decker, Zoom interview with author, July 8, 2022; "Why Does Lipid Oxidation in Foods Continue to Be Such a Challenge?," YouTube, posted by AOCS American Oil Chemists' Society, April 1, 2021, www.youtube.com/watch?v=B_U_9vvpDWo.

21. "Why Does Lipid Oxidation in Foods Continue to Be Such a Challenge?," YouTube.

22. Grootveld, Zoom interview with author.

23. Decker, Zoom interview with author.

24. "Aldehyde Generation in Cooking Oils; Professor Martin Grootveld," YouTube, posted by Zero Acre Farms, March 8, 2022, www.youtube.com/watch?v=HZV0nXYloh4, slide entitled "Estimating Human Dietary Intake of LOPs" at minute 40, and slide entitled "Aldehydes Are the Dominant Carcinogens in Cigarette Smoke" at minute 23. To support these, he cites multiple publications. See also Moumtaz et al., "Toxic Aldehyde Generation."

25. Telephone interview with the author. December 13, 2023.

26. Teicholz, *Big Fat Surprise*, 277–278.

27. Niamh Nic Daéid, Caroline Maguire, and Ailsa Walker, "An Investigation into the Causes of Laundry Fires—Spontaneous Combustion of Residual Fatty Acids," *Problems of Forensic Sciences* 46 (2001): 272–277, https://arch.ies.gov.pl/images/PDF/2001/vol_46/46_daeid4.pdf.

28. Chiung-Yu Peng, Cheng-Hang Lan, Pei-Chen Lin, and Yi-Chun Kuo, "Effects of Cooking Method, Cooking Oil, and Food Type on Aldehyde Emissions in Cooking Oil Fumes," *Journal of Hazardous Materials* 324, part B (February 2017): 160–167, https://doi.org/10.1016/j.jhazmat.2016.10.045; Ying-Chin Ko, Li Shu-Chuan Cheng, Chien-Hung Lee, Jhi-Jhu Huang, Ming-Shyan Huang, Eing-Long Kao, Hwei-Zu Wang, and Hsiang-Ju Lin, "Chinese Food Cooking and Lung Cancer in Women Nonsmokers," *American Journal of Epidemiology* 151, no. 2 (January 2000): 140–147, https://doi.org/10.1093/oxfordjournals.aje.a010181.

29. Sarah Moumtaz, Benita C. Percival, Devki Parmar, Kerry L. Grootveld, Pim Jansson, and Martin Grootveld, "Toxic Aldehyde Generation in and Food Uptake from Culinary Oils During Frying Practices: Peroxidative Resistance of a Monounsaturate-Rich Algae Oil," *Scientific Reports* 9 (2019): 4125, https:// doi.org/10.1038/s41598-019-39767-1.

CHAPTER 2 (PAGES 29 THROUGH 55)

1. Hippocrates, "The Oath," in *Hippocratic Writings*, ed. G. E. R. Lloyd, trans. J. Chadwick and W. N. Mann, Penguin Classics (New York: Penguin, 1983), and "The Sacred Disease" in the same work, 240.

2. C. Simon Herrington, ed., *Muir's Textbook of Pathology*, 15th ed. (Boca Raton, FL: CRC Press), 2014.

3. Ned Stafford, "Denham Harman," *BMJ* 350 (2015): h1092, https://doi.org/10.1136/bmj.h1092.

4. K. Kitani and G. O. Ivy, "'I Thought, Thought, Thought for Four Months in Vain and Suddenly the Idea Came': An Interview with Denham and Helen Harman," *Biogerontology* 4 (2003): 401–412, https://doi.org/10.1023/b:bgen.0000006561.15498.68.

5. Denham Harman, "Aging: A Theory Based on Free Radical and Radiation Chemistry," *Science of Aging Knowledge Environment* 2002, no. 37 (2002): cp14, https://doi.org/10.1126/sageke.2002.37.cp14.

6. John M. C. Gutteridge and B. Halliwell, "Invited Review. Free Radicals in Disease Processes: A Compilation of Cause and Consequence," *Free Radical Research Communications* i19, no. 3 (1993): 141–158, https://doi.org/10.3109/10715769309111598.

7. Tom O'Connor, "Dr. Denham Harman—Legendary Scientist—Dies at Age 98," University of Nebraska Medical Center, Newsroom, November 25, 2014, www.unmc.edu /newsroom/2014/11/25/dr-denham-harman-legendary-scientist-dies-at-age-98.

8. Josh Funk, "Denham Harman, Who Developed the 'Free-Radical Theory' of Aging, Dies at 98," *Washington Post*, November 29, 2014.

9. Margaret B. Wierman and Jeffrey S. Smith, "Yeast Sirtuins and the Regulation of Aging," *FEMS Yeast Research* 14, no. 1 (2014): 73–88, https://doi.org/10.1111/1567-1364.12115.

10. Rajindar S. Sohal and Michael J. Forster, "Caloric Restriction and the Aging Process: A Critique," *Free Radical Biology and Medicine* 73 (August 2014): 366–382, https://doi .org/10.1016/j.freeradbiomed.2014.05.015.

11. Etsuo Niki, "Role of Vitamin E as a Lipid-Soluble Peroxyl Radical Scavenger: In Vitro and In Vivo Evidence," *Free Radical Biology and Medicine* 66 (January 2014): 3–12, https://doi.org/10.1016/j.freeradbiomed.2013.03.022.

12. M. K. Horwitt, "Vitamin E and Lipid Metabolism in Man," *American Journal of Clinical Nutrition* 8, no. 4 (August 1960): 451–461, https://doi.org/10.1093/ajcn/8.4.451.

13. Maret G. Traber, "Vitamin E Inadequacy in Humans: Causes and Consequences," *Advances in Nutrition* 5, no. 5 (September 2014): 503–514, https://doi.org/10.3945 /an.114.006254; Daniel Raederstorff, Adrian Wyss, Philip C. Calder, Peter Weber, and Manfred Eggersdorfer, "Vitamin E Function and Requirements in Relation to PUFA," *British Journal of Nutrition* 114, no. 8 (2015): 1113–1122, https://doi.org/10.1017/S000711451500272X; Christopher Masterjohn, "AJCN Publishes a New PUFA Study That Should Make Us Long for the Old Days," Weston A. Price Foundation, May 17, 2012, www.westonaprice.org /ajcn-publishes-a-new-pufa-study-that-should-make-us-long-for-the-old-days.

14. Oxidized E was not measured, only normal E. "Used" vitamin E, called alpha-tocopherol quinone (or α-tocopherol quinone), is "a promising indicator of lipid peroxidation." See Desirée Bartolini, Rita Marinelli, Danilo Giusepponi, Roberta Galarini, Carolina Barola, Anna Maria Stabile, Bartolomeo Sebastiani, et al., "Alpha-Tocopherol Metabolites (The Vitamin E Metabolome) and Their Interindividual Variability During Supplementation," *Antioxidants (Basel)* 10, no. 2 (February 2021): 173, https://doi.org/10.3390 /antiox10020173.

15. Due to the oxidizability of omega-3, only omega-6 could be accurately analyzed, so his data reflects the most common omega-6 fatty acid found, called linoleic acid. We don't eat that much omega-3, so it probably would add only another 1 to 3 percentage points to the total PUFA. See Stephan J. Guyenet and Susan E. Carlson, "Increase in Adipose Tissue Linoleic Acid of US Adults in the Last Half Century," *Advances in Nutrition* 6, no. 6 (November 2015): 660–664, https://doi.org/10.3945/an.115.009944.

16. Data taken from the dataset used to create Figure 0-1, "Changes in Dietary Fat over 120 Years."

17. Stephan Guyenet, "Seed Oils and Body Fatness—A Problematic Revisit," Whole Health Source (blog), August 21, 2011, http://wholehealthsource.blogspot.com/2011/08 /seed-oils-and-body-fatness-problematic.html.

18. Masterjohn, "AJCN Publishes a New PUFA Study."

19. Taylor C. Wallace, Michael McBurney, and Victor L. Fulgoni III, "Multivitamin/ Mineral Supplement Contribution to Micronutrient Intakes in the United States, 2007– 2010," *Journal of the American College of Nutrition* 33, no. 2 (2014): 94–102, https://doi.org /10.1080/07315724.2013.846806; Victoria J. Drake, "Micronutrient Inadequacies in the US Population: An Overview," Oregon State University Linus Pauling Institute, March 2018, https://lpi.oregonstate.edu/mic/micronutrient-inadequacies/overview.

20. Michael T. Lin and M. Flint Beal, "The Oxidative Damage Theory of Aging," *Clinical Neuroscience Research* 2, no. 5–6 (January–February 2003): 305–315, http://dx.doi .org/10.1016/S1566-2772(03)00007-0.

21. Gerhard Spiteller, "The Relation of Lipid Peroxidation Processes with Atherogenesis: A New Theory on Atherogenesis," *Molecular Nutrition and Food Research* 49, no. 11 (November 2005): 999–1013, https://doi.org/10.1002/mnfr.200500055; Gözde Gürdeniz, Min Kim, Nicklas Brustad, Madeleine Ernst, Francesco Russo, Jakob Stokholm, Klaus Bønnelykke, et al., "Furan Fatty Acid Metabolite in Newborns Predicts Risk of Asthma," *Allergy* 78, no. 2 (February 2023): 429–438, https://doi.org/10.1111/all.15554.

22. Gerhard Spiteller and Mohammad Afzal, "The Action of Peroxyl Radicals, Powerful Deleterious Reagents, Explains Why Neither Cholesterol nor Saturated Fatty Acids Cause Atherogenesis and Age-Related Diseases," *Chemistry: A European Journal* 20 (2014): 14928–14945, https://doi.org/10.1002/chem.201404383.

23. Gerhard Spiteller, "Is Atherosclerosis a Multifactorial Disease or Is It Induced by a Sequence of Lipid Peroxidation Reactions?," *Annals of the New York Academy of Sciences* 1043, no. 1 (June 2005): 355–366, https://doi.org/10.1196/annals.1333.042; Gerhard Spiteller, "The Important Role of Lipid Peroxidation Processes in Aging and Age Dependent Diseases," *Molecular Biotechnology* 37 (2007): 5–12, https://doi.org/10.1007/s12033 -007-0057-6; Gerhard Spiteller, "Peroxyl Radicals Are Essential Reagents in the Oxidation Steps of the Maillard Reaction Leading to Generation of Advanced Glycation End Products," *Annals of the New York Academy of Sciences* 1126 (April 2008): 128–133, https://doi .org/10.1196/annals.1433.031.

24. Barry Halliwell and Martin Grootveld, "The Measurement of Free Radical Reactions in Humans: Some Thoughts for Future Experimentation," *FEBS Letters* 213, no. 1 (March 9, 1987): 9–14, https://doi.org/10.1016/0014-5793(87)81455-2.

25. Antonio Ceriello and Enrico Motz, "Is Oxidative Stress the Pathogenic Mechanism Underlying Insulin Resistance, Diabetes, and Cardiovascular Disease? The Common

Soil Hypothesis Revisited," *Arteriosclerosis, Thrombosis, and Vascular Biology* 24, no. 5 (May 2004): 816–823, https://doi.org/10.1161/01.ATV.0000122852.22604.78.

26. A. Koch, K. Zacharowski, O. Boehm, M. Stevens, P. Lipfert, H.-J. von Giesen, A. Wolf, and R. Freynhagen, "Nitric Oxide and Pro-inflammatory Cytokines Correlate with Pain Intensity in Chronic Pain Patients," *Inflammation Research* 56 (2007): 32–37, https://doi.org/10.1007/s00011-007-6088-4; Rebecca S. Y. Wong, "Inflammation in COVID-19: From Pathogenesis to Treatment," *International Journal of Clinical and Experimental Pathology* 14, no. 7 (2021): 831–844, www.ncbi.nlm.nih.gov/pmc/articles/PMC8339720.

27. Petra L. L. Goyens, Mary E. Spilker, Peter L. Zock, Martijn B. Katan, and Ronald P. Mensink, "Conversion of α-Linolenic Acid in Humans Is Influenced by the Absolute Amounts of α-Linolenic Acid and Linoleic Acid in the Diet and Not by Their Ratio," *American Journal of Clinical Nutrition* 84, no. 1 (July 2006): 44–53, https://doi.org/10.1093/ajcn/84.1.44.

28. Colin L. Masters and Dennis J. Selkoe, "Biochemistry of Amyloid β-Protein and Amyloid Deposits in Alzheimer Disease," *Cold Spring Harbor Perspectives in Medicine* 2, no. 6 (June 2012): a006262, https://doi.org/10.1101/cshperspect.a006262.

29. Akihiko Nunomura, George Perry, Gjumrakch Aliev, Keisuke Hirai, Atsushi Takeda, Elizabeth K. Balraj, Paul K. Jones, et al., "Oxidative Damage Is the Earliest Event in Alzheimer Disease," *Journal of Neuropathology and Experimental Neurology* 60, no. 8 (August 2001): 759–767, https://doi.org/10.1093/jnen/60.8.759; Akihiko Nunomura, Rudy J. Castellani, Xiongwei Zhu, Paula I. Moreira, George Perry, and Mark A. Smith, "Involvement of Oxidative Stress in Alzheimer Disease," *Journal of Neuropathology and Experimental Neurology* 65, no. 7 (July 2006): 631–641, https://doi.org/10.1097/01.jnen.0000228136.58062.bf.

30. Vivian W. Y. Leung, Sarah-Jeanne Pilon, Pierre O. Fiset, and Shaifali Sandal, "A Case Report on Lipofuscin Deposition in a Graft Biopsy Two Years After Kidney Transplantation: An Insignificant Bystander or a Pathogenic Benefactor?," *BMC Nephrology* 20 (2019): 376, https://doi.org/10.1186/s12882-019-1569-6; Joaquin Ponce-Zepeda, Wenchang Guo, Giorgioni Carmen, Daniel Moon Kim, Gregory C. Albers, Vishal Suresh Chandan, and Xiaodong Li, "Brown Bowel Syndrome Is a Rare and Commonly Missed Disease: A Case Report and Literature Review," *Case Reports in Gastrointestinal Medicine* 2021 (2021): 6684678, https://doi.org/10.1155/2021/6684678; Douglas A. Gray and John Woulfe, "Lipofuscin and Aging: A Matter of Toxic Waste," *Science of Aging Knowledge Environment* 2005, no. 5 (2005): re1, https://doi.org/10.1126/sageke.2005.5.re1.

31. A. Terman, "Garbage Catastrophe Theory of Aging: Imperfect Removal of Oxidative Damage?," *Redox Report* 6, no. 1 (2001): 15–26, https://doi.org/10.1179/135100001101535996.

32. R. Preston Mason, William J. Shoemaker, Lydia Shajenko, Timothy E. Chambers, and Leo G. Herbette, "Evidence for Changes in the Alzheimer's Disease Brain Cortical Membrane Structure Mediated by Cholesterol," *Neurobiology of Aging* 13, no. 3 (May–June 1992): 413–419, https://doi.org/10.1016/0197-4580(92)90116-F.

33. David M. Wilson and Lester I. Binder, "Free Fatty Acids Stimulate the Polymerization of Tau and Amyloid f Peptides: *In Vitro* Evidence for a Common Effector of

Pathogenesis in Alzheimer's Disease," *American Journal of Pathology* 150, no. 6 (June 1997): 2181–2195, www.ncbi.nlm.nih.gov/pmc/articles/PMC1858305.

34. L. Ebony Boulware, Spyridon Marinopoulos, Karran A. Phillips, Constance W. Hwang, Kenric Maynor, Dan Merenstein, Renee F. Wilson, et al., "Systematic Review: The Value of the Periodic Health Evaluation," *Annals of Internal Medicine* 146, no. 4 (February 2007): 289–300, https://doi.org/10.7326/0003-4819-146-4-200702200-00008; Lasse T. Krogsbøll, Karsten Juhl Jørgensen, Christian Grønøj Larsen, and Peter C. Gøtzsche, "General Health Checks in Adults for Reducing Morbidity and Mortality from Disease: Cochrane Systematic Review and Meta-Analysis," *BMJ* 345 (2012): e7191, https://doi.org/10.1136/bmj.e7191. The following articles provide a good overview and introduction to Dr. Welch, who has spent decades publishing in this area: Jennifer Durgin, "Are We Hunting Too Hard?," *Dartmouth Medicine* 29, no. 4 (Summer 2005): 40–47, https://dartmed.dartmouth.edu/summer05/pdf/hunting_too_hard.pdf; Ateev Mehrotra and Allan Prochazka, "Improving Value in Health Care—Against the Annual Physical," *New England Journal of Medicine* 373 (2015): 1485–1487, https://doi.org/10.1056/NEJMp1507485.

35. James F. Toole, M. René Malinow, Lloyd E. Chambless, J. David Spence, L. Creed Pettigrew, Virginia J. Howard, Elizabeth G. Sides, Chin-Hua Wang, and Meir Stampfer, "Lowering Homocysteine in Patients with Ischemic Stroke to Prevent Recurrent Stroke, Myocardial Infarction, and Death: The Vitamin Intervention for Stroke Prevention (VISP) Randomized Controlled Trial," *JAMA* 291, no. 5 (2004): 565–575, https://doi.org/10.1001/jama.291.5.565; J. L. Reay, M. A. Smith, and L. M. Riby, "B Vitamins and Cognitive Performance in Older Adults: Review," *International Scholarly Research Notices* 2013 (2013): 650983, https://doi.org/10.5402/2013/650983.

36. Roman N. Rodionov and Steven R. Lentz, "The Homocysteine Paradox," *Arteriosclerosis, Thrombosis, and Vascular Biology* 28 (2008): 1031–1033, https://doi.org/10.1161/ATVBAHA.108.164830.

CHAPTER 3 (PAGES 57 THROUGH 84)

Figure 3-1: Zhilei Shan, Colin D. Rehm, Gail Rogers, Mengyuan Ruan, Dong D. Wang, Frank B. Hu, Dariush Mozaffarian, Fang Fang Zhang, and Shilpa N. Bhupathiraju, "Trends in Dietary Carbohydrate, Protein, and Fat Intake and Diet Quality Among US Adults, 1999–2016," *JAMA* 322, no. 12 (2019): 1178–1187, https://doi.org/10.1001/jama.2019.13771; M. Shahbandeh, "Per Capita Consumption of Wheat Flour in the U.S., 2000–2023," Statista, May 15, 2023, www.statista.com/statistics/184084/per-capita-consumption-of-wheat-flour-in-the-us-since-2000; Gretchen Kuck and Gary Schnitkey, "An Overview of Meat Consumption in the United States," *Farmdoc Daily* 11, no. 76 (May 12, 2021), https://farmdocdaily.illinois.edu/2021/05/an-overview-of-meat-consumption-in-the-united-states.html; "How Much Sugar Do Americans Consume?," Sugar Association, accessed September 4, 2023, www.sugar.org/diet/intake; M. Shahbandeh, "Per Capita Consumption of High Fructose Corn Syrup in the U.S., 2000–2019," Statista, December 16, 2022, www.statista.com/statistics/328893/per-capita-consumption-of-high-fructose-corn-syrup-in-the-us.

Figure 3–2: Daniele Penzo, Chiara Tagliapietra, Raffaele Colonna, Valeria Petronilli, and Paolo Bernardi, "Effects of Fatty Acids on Mitochondria: Implications for Cell Death," *Biochimica et Biophysica Acta (BBA)—Bioenergetics* 1555, no. 1–3 (2002): 160–165, https://doi .org/10.1016/S0005-2728(02)00272-4.

Figure 3–4: Adapted from Louis Monnier, Claude Colette, Gareth J. Dunseath, and David R. Owens, "The Loss of Postprandial Glycemic Control Precedes Stepwise Deterioration of Fasting with Worsening Diabetes," *Diabetes Care* 30, no. 2 (2007): 263–269, https://doi .org/10.2337/dc06-1612; Daniel Cox, "A Paradigm Shift in the Management of Type 2 Diabetes: Glycemic Excursion Minimization (GEM)," VuMedi, August 4, 2023, www.vumedi .com/video/a-paradigm-shift-in-the-management-of-type-2-diabetes-glycemic-excursion -minimization-gem.

1. Hayley Wall, "Scientists Don't Agree on What Causes Obesity, but They Know What Doesn't," *New York Times*, November 21, 2022, www.nytimes.com/2022/11/21 /opinion/obesity-cause.html.

2. Weston A. Price, *Nutrition and Physical Degeneration* (Lemon Grove, CA: Price-Pottenger Nutrition Foundation, 2009); Catherine Shanahan, *Deep Nutrition: Why Your Genes Need Traditional Food* (New York: Flatiron Books, 2017).

3. Chris Knobbe, email communication with author, January 16, 2023.

4. Tanya L. Blasbalg, Joseph R. Hibbeln, Christopher E. Ramsden, Sharon F. Majchrzak, and Robert R. Rawlings, "Changes in Consumption of Omega-3 and Omega-6 Fatty Acids in the United States During the 20th Century," *American Journal of Clinical Nutrition* 93, no. 5 (2011): 950–962, https://doi.org/10.3945/ajcn.110.006643.

5. This is known as the LA VA study; participants in this study and the Elgin Project maintained a normal weight in spite of their high-PUFA diet, likely because their meals were portioned to maintain a healthy weight during the study and they had no access to snacks or outside food. See Seymour Dayton, Morton Lee Pearce, Sam Hashimoto, Wilfrid J. Dixon, and Uwamie Tomiyasu, "A Controlled Clinical Trial of a Diet High in Unsaturated Fat in Preventing Complications of Atherosclerosis," *Circulation* 40, no. 1s2 (1969), https:// doi.org/10.1161/01.CIR.40.1S2.II-1.

6. John Yudkin, *The Penguin Encyclopaedia of Nutrition* (New York: Penguin, 1986), 55.

7. G. Cohen, Y. Riahi, and S. Sasson, "Lipid Peroxidation of Poly-Unsaturated Fatty Acids in Normal and Obese Adipose Tissues," *Archives of Physiology and Biochemistry* 117, no. 3 (July 2011): 131–139, https://doi.org/10.3109/13813455.2011.557387; Giuseppe Murdolo, Desirée Bartolini, Cristina Tortoioli, Marta Piroddi, Luigi Iuliano, and Francesco Galli, "Lipokines and Oxysterols: Novel Adipose-Derived Lipid Hormones Linking Adipose Dysfunction and Insulin Resistance," *Free Radical Biology and Medicine* 65 (2013): 811–820, https://doi.org/10.1016/j.freeradbiomed.2013.08.007.

8. Charalambos Antoniades and Cheerag Shirodaria, "Detecting Coronary Inflammation with Perivascular Fat Attenuation Imaging: Making Sense from Perivascular

Attenuation Maps," *JACC: Cardiovascular Imaging* 12, no. 10 (October 2019): 2011–2014, https://doi.org/10.1016/j.jcmg.2018.12.024.

9. V. Van Harmelin, S. Reynisdottir, P. Eriksson, A. Thörne, J. Hoffstedt, F. Lönnqvist, and P. Arner, "Leptin Secretion from Subcutaneous and Visceral Adipose Tissue in Women," *Diabetes* 47, no. 6 (June 1998): 913–917, https://doi.org/10.2337/diabetes.47.6.913.

10. Jacek Karczewski, Aleksandra Zielínska, Rafał Staszewski, Piotr Eder, and Agnieszka Dobrowolska, "Metabolic Link Between Obesity and Autoimmune Diseases," *European Cytokine Network* 32, no. 4 (2021): 64–72, https://doi.org/10.1684/ecn.2021.0474; Victoria R. Kwiat, Gisienne Reis, Isela C. Valera, Kislay Parvatiyar, and Michelle S. Parvatiyar, "Autoimmunity as a Sequela to Obesity and Systemic Inflammation," *Frontiers in Physiology* 13 (2022), https://doi.org/10.3389/fphys.2022.887702; Giuseppina Rosaria Umano, Carmelo Pistone, Enrico Tondina, Alice Moiraghi, Daria Lauretta, Emanuele Miraglia Del Giudice, and Ilaria Brambilla, "Pediatric Obesity and the Immune System," *Frontiers in Pediatrics* 7 (2019), https://doi.org/10.3389/fped.2019.00487.

11. Jan Frohlich, George N. Chaldakov, and Manlio Vinciguerra, "Cardio- and Neurometabolic Adipobiology: Consequences and Implications for Therapy," *International Journal of Molecular Sciences* 22, no. 8 (April 2021): 4137, https://doi.org/10.3390/ijms22084137.

12. Philip B. Maffetone, Ivan Rivera-Dominguez, and Paul B. Laursen, "Overfat Adults and Children in Developed Countries: The Public Health Importance of Identifying Excess Body Fat," *Frontiers in Public Health* 5 (2017), https://doi.org/10.3389/fpubh.2017.00190.

13. Maffetone et al., "Overfat Adults and Children in Developed Countries."

14. Kenneth F. Kiple and Kriemhild Coneè Ornelas, eds., *The Cambridge World History of Food* (Cambridge: Cambridge University Press, 2000).

15. Chris A. Knobbe and Suzanne Alexander, *The Ancestral Diet Revolution: How Vegetable Oils and Processed Foods Destroy Our Health—and How to Recover!* (Boulder, CO: Ancestral Health Foundation, 2023).

16. Jules Hirsch, John W. Farquhar, E. H. Ahrens Jr., M. L. Peterson, and Wilhelm Stoffel, "Studies of Adipose Tissue in Man: A Microtechnic for Sampling and Analysis," *American Journal of Clinical Nutrition* 8, no. 4 (August 1960): 499–511, https://doi.org/10.1093/ajcn/8.4.499.

17. Dominique Langan, "In and Out: Adipose Tissue Lipid Turnover in Obesity and Dyslipidemia," *Cell Metabolism* 14, no. 5 (November 2011): 569–570; S. Bernard and K. L. Spalding, "Implication of Lipid Turnover for the Control of Energy Balance," *Philosophical Transactions of the Royal Society B* 378, no. 1888 (October 2023), https://doi/10.1098/rstb.2022.0202.

18. J. Luo, H. Yang, and B. L. Song, "Mechanisms and Regulation of Cholesterol Homeostasis," *Nature Reviews Molecular Cell Biology* 21 (2020): 225–245, https://doi.org/10.1038/s41580-019-0190-7.

Notes

19. Mitochondria contain a highly energized form of oxygen called superoxide, which is capable of initiating a free radical cascade within the mitochondrial phospholipid bilayer, polymerizing, stiffening, and destroying it.

20. Daniele Penzo, Chiara Tagliapietra, Raffaele Colonna, Valeria Petronilli, and Paolo Bernardi, "Effects of Fatty Acids on Mitochondria: Implications for Cell Death," *Biochimica et Biophysica Acta (BBA)—Bioenergetics* 1555, no. 1–3 (2002): 160–165, https://doi.org/10.1016/S0005-2728(02)00272-4.

21. Berton C. Pressman and Henry A. Lardy, "Effect of Surface Active Agents on the Latent ATPASE of Mitochondria," *Biochimica et Biophysica Acta* 21, no. 3 (September 1956): 458–466, https://doi.org/10.1016/0006-3002(56)90182-2; P. Borst, J. A. Loos, E. J. Christ, and E. C. Slater, "Uncoupling Activity of Long-Chain Fatty Acids," *Biochimica et Biophysica Acta* 62, no. 3 (August 1962): 509–518, https://doi.org/10.1016/0006-3002(62)90232-9.

22. Efraim Racker, "Editorial: Calories Don't Count—If You Don't Use Them," *American Journal of Medicine* 35, no. 2 (August 1963): 133–134.

23. Racker, "Editorial: Calories Don't Count."

24. Paweł Kowalczyk, D. Sulejczak, P. Kleczkowska, I. Bukowska-Ośko, M. Kucia, M. Popiel, E. Wietrak, K. Kramkowski, K. Wrzosek, and K. Kaczyńska, "Mitochondrial Oxidative Stress—A Causative Factor and Therapeutic Target in Many Diseases," *International Journal of Molecular Sciences* 22, no. 24 (2021): 13384, https://doi.org/10.3390/ijms222413384.

25. This article supports the idea that cells have trouble burning body fat. The authors write, "This process originates with the impaired or incomplete mitochondrial catabolism of intracellular lipid in insulin-resistant skeletal muscle." However, the authors are unaware that our body fat is high PUFA, so cannot draw the correct conclusions about some aspects of the process. See Nishanth E. Sunny, E. J. Parks, J. D. Browning, and S. C. Burgess, "Excessive Hepatic Mitochondrial TCA Cycle and Gluconeogenesis in Humans with Nonalcoholic Fatty Liver Disease," *Cell Metabolism* 14, no. 6 (December 2021): 804–810, https://doi.org/10.1016/j.cmet.2011.11.004.

26. Mitchell Roslin, "Obesity as a Mitochondrial Disease of Aging," keynote address, Australian New Zealand Metabolic and Obesity Society, October 2022.

27. This article is in contrast to studies comparing the effect of PUFAs versus saturated fats on substrate oxidation immediately after eating. In this case, PUFA promotes greater fat oxidation than saturated fat, probably because in the presence of insulin these oily, wiggly fatty acids get into cells so fast that they can then slip into the mitochondria without the proper mitochondrial controls. See Peter J. H. Jones and Dale A. Schoeller, "Polyunsaturated: Saturated Ratio of Diet Fat Influences Energy Substrate Utilization in the Human," *Metabolism* 37, no. 2 (February 1988): 145–151, https://doi.org/10.1016/S0026-0495(98)90009-9.

28. Melania Manco, Menotti Calvani, and Geltrude Mingrone, "Effects of Dietary Fatty Acids on Insulin Sensitivity and Secretion," *Diabetes, Obesity and Metabolism* 6, no.

6 (2004): 402–413, https://doi.org/10.1111/j.1462-8902.2004.00356.x; Meghana D. Gadgil, Lawrence J. Appel, Edwina Yeung, Cheryl A. M. Anderson, Frank M. Sacks, and Edgar R. Miller III, "The Effects of Carbohydrate, Unsaturated Fat, and Protein Intake on Measures of Insulin Sensitivity: Results from the OmniHeart Trial," *Diabetes Care* 36, no. 5 (May 2013): 1132–1137, https://doi.org/10.2337/dc12-0869.

29. C. Xiao, A. Giacca, A. Carpentier, and G. F. Lewis, "Differential Effects of Mono-unsaturated, Polyunsaturated and Saturated Fat Ingestion on Glucose-Stimulated Insulin Secretion, Sensitivity and Clearance in Overweight and Obese, Non-diabetic Humans," *Diabetologia* 49 (2006): 1371–1379, https://doi.org/10.1007/s00125-006-0211-x.

30. Nora D. Volkow, Gene-Jack Wang, Ehsan Shokri Kojori, Joanna S. Fowler, Helene Benveniste, and Dardo Tomasi, "Alcohol Decreases Baseline Brain Glucose Metabolism More in Heavy Drinkers Than Controls but Has No Effect on Stimulation-Induced Metabolic Increases," *Journal of Neuroscience* 35, no. 7 (2015): 3248–3255, https://doi.org/10.1523/jneurosci.4877-14.2015. The fact that when brain cells metabolize acetate they reduce their sugar use is generally taken as evidence that acetate is "preferred" by our cells.

31. "Understanding Insulin Resistance," American Diabetes Association, accessed September 7, 2023, https://diabetes.org/healthy-living/medication-treatments/insulin-resistance.

32. R. Firth, P. Bell, and R. Rizza, "Insulin Action in Non-Insulin-Dependent Diabetes Mellitus: The Relationship Between Hepatic and Extrahepatic Insulin Resistance and Obesity," *Metabolism, Clinical and Experimental* 36, no. 11 (November 1987): 1091–1095, https://doi.org/10.1016/0026-0495(87)90031-X.

33. R. Reynolds, B. R. Walker, H. E. Syddall, C. B. Whorwood, P. J. Wood, and D. I. Phillips, "Elevated Plasma Cortisol in Glucose-Intolerant Men: Differences in Responses to Glucose and Habituation to Venepuncture," *Journal of Clinical Endocrinology and Metabolism* 86, no. 3 (March 2001): 1149–1153, Figs. 1, 2, and 3. "Obesity (p = 0.033) and insulin resistance (p = 0.009) were associated with elevated glucagon levels": Martin Lundqvist, Kristina Almby, Urban Wiklund, Niclas Abrahamsson, Prasad Kamble, Maria Pereira, and Jan Eriksson, "Altered Hormonal and Autonomic Nerve Responses to Hypo- and Hyperglycaemia Are Found in Overweight and Insulin-Resistant Individuals and May Contribute to the Development of Type 2 Diabetes," *Diabetologia* 64, no. 3 (March 2021): 641–655.

34. Glucose intolerance is the earliest recognized stage of insulin resistance. See Robert C. Andrews, Olive Herlihy, Dawn E. W. Livingstone, Ruth Andrew, and Brian R. Walker, "Abnormal Cortisol Metabolism and Tissue Sensitivity to Cortisol in Patients with Glucose Intolerance," *Journal of Clinical Endocrinology and Metabolism* 87, no. 12 (December 2002): 5587–5593, https://doi.org/10.1210/jc.2002-020048. "Glucagon increases HGP by acutely stimulating glycogenolysis and chronically promoting gluconeogenesis": Dominic Santoleri and Paul M. Titchenell, "Resolving the Paradox of Hepatic Insulin Resistance," *Cellular and Molecular Gastroenterology and Hepatology* 7, no. 2 (2019): 447–456, https://doi.org/10.1016/j.jcmgh.2018.10.016.

35. Carine Beaupere, Alexandrine Liboz, Bruno Fève, Bertrand Blondeau, and Ghislaine Guillemain, "Molecular Mechanisms of Glucocorticoid-Induced Insulin Resistance," *International Journal of Molecular Sciences* 22, no. 2 (2021): 623, https://doi.org/10.3390/ijms22020623.

36. "Initially, there is a compensatory increase in insulin secretion which maintains glucose levels in normal range": Rajeev Goyal, Minhthao Nguyen, and Ishwarlal Jialal, "Glucose Intolerance," Stat Pearls, January 2023, www.ncbi.nlm.nih.gov/books/NBK499910.

37. Sunny et al., "Excessive Hepatic Mitochondrial TCA Cycle"; Santoleri and Titchenell, "Resolving the Paradox of Hepatic Insulin Resistance"; Ralph A. DeFronzo, "Pathogenesis of Type 2 Diabetes Mellitus," *Medical Clinics* 88, no. 4 (July 2024): 787–835, https://doi.org/10.1016/j.mcna.2004.04.013.

38. Evan D. Muse, Tony K. T. Lam, Philipp E. Scherer, and Luciano Rossetti, "Hypothalamic Resistin Induces Hepatic Insulin Resistance," *Journal of Clinical Investigation* 117, no. 6 (2007): 1670–1678, https://doi.org/10.1172/JCI30440.

39. Nal Ae Yoon and Sabrina Diano, "Hypothalamic Glucose-Sensing Mechanisms," *Diabetologia* 64, no. 5 (2021): 985–993, https://doi.org/10.1007/s00125-021-05395-6.

40. Noël Cano, "Bench-to-Bedside Review: Glucose Production from the Kidney," *Critical Care* 6, no. 4 (2002): 317, https://doi.org/10.1186/cc1517.

41. Samantha Hurrle and Walter H. Hsu, "The Etiology of Oxidative Stress in Insulin Resistance," *Biomedical Journal* 40, no. 5 (October 2017): 257–262, https://doi.org/10.1016/j.bj.2017.06.007.

42. "Insulin Resistance and Diabetes," Centers for Disease Control and Prevention, last reviewed June 20, 2022, www.cdc.gov/diabetes/basics/insulin-resistance.html.

43. Poonamjot Deol, Jane R. Evans, Joseph Dhahbi, Karthikeyani Chellappa, Diana S. Han, Stephen Spindler, and Frances M. Sladek, "Soybean Oil Is More Obesogenic and Diabetogenic Than Coconut Oil and Fructose in Mouse: Potential Role for the Liver," *PLOS One* 10, no. 7 (July 2015): e0132672, https://doi.org/10.1371/journal.pone.0132672.

44. Frances Sladek, telephone interview with the author, February 24, 2015.

45. "Dr Frances M. Sladek: Turning the Tables on 'Healthy' Fats," Scientia, February 18, 2017, www.scientia.global/dr-frances-m-sladek-turning-tables-healthy-fats.

46. Jean A Welsh, Andrea J. Sharma, Lisa Grellinger, and Miriam B. Vos, "Consumption of Added Sugars Is Decreasing in the United States," *American Journal of Clinical Nutrition* 94, no. 3 (September 2011): 726–734; Kelsey A. Vercammen, Alyssa J. Moran, Mark J. Soto, Lee Kennedy-Shaffer, and Sara N. Bleich, "Decreasing Trends in Heavy Sugar-Sweetened Beverage Consumption in the United States, 2003 to 2016," Academy of Nutrition and Dietetics, 2020, https://doi.org/10.1016/j.jand.2020.07.012.

47. Joana Araújo, Jianwen Cai, and June Stevens, "Prevalence of Optimal Metabolic Health in American Adults: National Health and Nutrition Examination Survey, 2009–2016,"

Metabolic Syndrome and Related Disorders 17, no. 1 (February 2019): 46–52, https://doi .org/10.1089/met.2018.0105; "Only 12 Percent of American Adults Are Metabolically Healthy, Carolina Study Finds," UNC Gillings School of Global Public Health, November 28, 2018, https://sph.unc.edu/sph-news/only-12-percent-of-american-adults-are-metabolically -healthy-study-finds.

48. One study (Matli et al.) suggests 1.0–1.1 as the lower limit of normal, and some of the data in this article suggests it could be lower than that. Other research (Kar) suggests 3.8 as one possible "normal" score. See Bassel Matli, Andreas Schulz, Thomas Koeck, Tanja Falter, Johannes Lotz, Heidi Rossmann, and Norbert Pfeiffer, et al., "Distribution of HOMA-IR in a Population-Based Cohort and Proposal for Reference Intervals," *Clinical Chemistry and Laboratory Medicine* 59, no. 11 (August 2021): 1844–1851, https://doi.org/10.1515 /cclm-2021-0643; S. Kar, "Metabolic Risks of the Lean PCOS Woman," *Fertility and Sterility* 100, no. 3 (September 2013): S359, https://doi.org/10.1016/j.fertnstert.2013.07.848.

49. Reference ranges for glucose are now 70 to 100 mg/dL. Back when I was in medical school, a normal range for fasting blood sugar was 65 to 85 mg/dL.

50. D. R. Matthews, J. R. Hosker, A. S. Rudenski, B. A. Naylor, D. F. Treacher, and R. C. Turner, "Homeostasis Model Assessment: Insulin Resistance and β-Cell Function from Fasting Plasma Glucose and Insulin Concentrations in Man," *Diabetologia* 28 (1985): 412–419; Catherine Marin DeUgarte, Alfred A. Bartolucci, and Ricardo Azziz, "Prevalence of Insulin Resistance in the Polycystic Ovary Syndrome Using the Homeostasis Model Assessment," *Fertility and Sterility* 83, no. 5 (May 2005): 1454–1460, https://doi .org/10.1016/j.fertnstert.2004.11.070.

51. Vibhu Parcha, Brittain Heindl, Rajat Kalra, Peng Li, Barbara Gower, Garima Arora, Pankaj Arora, "Insulin Resistance and Cardiometabolic Risk Profile Among Nondiabetic American Young Adults: Insights From NHANES," *Journal of Clinical Endocrinology and Metabolism* 107, no. 1 (January 2022): e25–e37, https://doi.org/10.1210/clinem/dgab645.

52. "Type 2 Diabetes Can Be Stopped in Childhood," Diabetes in Control, June 29, 2009, www.diabetesincontrol.com/type-2-diabetes-can-be-stopped-in-childhood; Brian Bennett, D. Enette Larson-Meyer, Eric Ravussin, Julia Volaufova, Arlette Soros, William T. Cefalu, Stuart Chalew, et al., "Impaired Insulin Sensitivity and Elevated Ectopic Fat in Healthy Obese vs. Nonobese Prepubertal Children," *Obesity* 20, no. 2 (February 2012): 371–375, https://doi.org/10.1038/oby.2011.264.

53. Bennett et al., "Impaired Insulin Sensitivity and Elevated Ectopic Fat."

54. Anton Holmgren, Aimon Niklasson, Andreas F. M. Nierop, Lars Gelander, A. Stefan Aronson, Agneta Sjöberg, Lauren Lissner, and Kerstin Albertsson-Wikland, "Pubertal Height Gain Is Inversely Related to Peak BMI in Childhood," *Pediatric Research* 81 (2017): 448–454, https://doi.org/10.1038/pr.2016.253.

55. Ottavio Vitelli, Alessandra Tabarrini, Silvia Miano, Jole Rabasco, Nicoletta Pietropaoli, Martina Forlani, Pasquale Parisi, and Maria Pia Villa, "Impact of Obesity on

Cognitive Outcome in Children with Sleep-Disordered Breathing," *Sleep Medicine* 16, no. 5 (May 2015): 625–630, https://doi.org/10.1016/j.sleep.2014.12.015.

56. Ida Gillberg Andersen, Jens-Christian Holm, and Preben Homøe, "Obstructive Sleep Apnea in Obese Children and Adolescents, Treatment Methods and Outcome of Treatment—A Systematic Review," *International Journal of Pediatric Otorhinolaryngology* 87 (August 2016): 190–197, https://doi.org/10.1016/j.ijporl.2016.06.017.

57. Coleen A. Boyle, Sheree Boulet, Laura A. Schieve, Robin A. Cohen, Stephen J. Blumberg, Marshalyn Yeargin-Allsopp, Susanna Visser, and Michael D. Kogan, "Trends in the Prevalence of Developmental Disabilities in US Children, 1997–2008," *Pediatrics* 127, no. 6 (2011): 1034–1042, https://doi.org/10.1542/peds.2010-2989.

58. "Childhood Cancer Fact Library," Coalition Against Childhood Cancer, updated 2022, https://cac2.org/interest-groups/awareness/childhood-cancer-fact-library.

59. Max D. Gehrman and Louis C. Grandizio, "Elbow Ulnar Collateral Ligament Injuries in Throwing Athletes: Diagnosis and Management," *Journal of Hand Surgery* 47, no. 3 (March 2022): 266–273, https://doi.org/10.1016/j.jhsa.2021.11.026; Chris G. Koutures, Andrew J. M. Gregory, and the Council on Sports Medicine and Fitness, "Injuries in Youth Soccer," *Pediatrics* 125, no. 2 (2010): 410–414, https://doi.org/10.1542/peds.2009-3009.

60. Moody's Analytics, "The Economic Consequences of Millennial Health," Blue Cross Blue Shield, November 6, 2019, www.bcbs.com/the-health-of-america/reports/how-millennials-current-and-future-health-could-affect-our-economy.

61. Hagai Levine, Niels Jørgensen, Anderson Martino-Andrade, Jaime Mendiola, Dan Weksler-Derri, Maya Jolles, Rachel Pinotti, and Shanna H. Swan, "Temporal Trends in Sperm Count: A Systematic Review and Meta-Regression Analysis of Samples Collected Globally in the 20th and 21st Centuries," *Human Reproduction Update* 29, no. 2 (March–April 2023): 157–176, https://doi.org/10.1093/humupd/dmac035.

CHAPTER 4 (PAGES 85 THROUGH 116)

1. Hana Kahleova, Jan Irene Lloren, Andrew Mashchak, Martin Hill, and Gary E. Fraser, "Meal Frequency and Timing Are Associated with Changes in Body Mass Index in Adventist Health Study 2," *Journal of Nutrition* 147, no. 9 (September 2017): 1722–1728, https://doi.org/10.3945/jn.116.244749; Physicians Committee for Responsible Medicine, "How to Optimize Your Diet to Boost Metabolism," VuMedi, March 24, 2022, www.vumedi.com/video/how-to-optimize-your-diet-to-boost-metabolism; Hana Kahleova, Lenka Belinova, Hana Malinska, Olena Oliyarnyk, Jaroslava Trnovska, Vojtech Skop, Ludmila Kazdova, et al., "Eating Two Larger Meals a Day (Breakfast and Lunch) Is More Effective Than Six Smaller Meals in a Reduced-Energy Regimen for Patients with Type 2 Diabetes: A Randomised Crossover Study," *Diabetologia* 57, no. 8 (2014): 1552–1560, https://doi.org/10.1007/s00125-014-3253-5.

2. Someone who is insulin resistant can produce ketones, but they are more likely to come from muscle than fat, which is not the normal process of brain fueling and doesn't work as well. We will discuss this in more detail in chapter 8. See Philip Felig, John Wahren, Robert Sherwin, and George Palaiologos, "Amino Acid and Protein Metabolism in Diabetes Mellitus," *Archives of Internal Medicine* 137, no. 4 (1977): 507–513, https://doi .org/10.1001/archinte.1977.03630160069014; Weimin Yu, Tomiko Kuhara, Yoshito Inoue, Isamu Matsumoto, Ryoji Iwasaki, and Shinpei Morimoto, "Increased Urinary Excretion of β-Hydroxyisovaleric Acid in Ketotic and Nonketotic Type II Diabetes Mellitus," *Clinica Chimica Acta* 188, no. 2 (April 1990): 161–168, https://doi.org/10.1016/0009-8981 (90)90160-T; Kohsuke Hayamizu, "Amino Acids and Energy Metabolism: An Overview," in *Sustained Energy for Enhanced Human Functions and Activity*, ed. Debasis Bagchi, 339–349 (London: Academic Press, 2017).

3. "A single cell uses about 10 million ATP molecules per second, and recycles all of its ATP molecules about every 20–30 seconds": "2.9: Glucose and ATP," in *Biology*, LibreTexts.org, accessed September 8, 2023, https://k12.libretexts.org/Bookshelves /Science_and_Technology/Biology/02%3A_Cell_Biology/2.09%3A_Glucose_and_ATP.

4. Benedetta Russo, Marika Menduni, Patrizia Borboni, Fabiana Picconi, and Simona Frontoni, "Autonomic Nervous System in Obesity and Insulin-Resistance—The Complex Interplay Between Leptin and Central Nervous System," *International Journal of Molecular Sciences* 22, no. 10 (2021): 5187, https://doi.org/10.3390/ijms22105187.

5. Michael M. Smith and Christopher T. Minson, "Obesity and Adipokines: Effects on Sympathetic Overactivity," *Journal of Physiology* 590, no. 8 (April 2012): 1787–1801, https://doi.org/10.1113/jphysiol.2011.221036.

6. Iltan Aklan, Nilufer Sayar Atasoy, Yavuz Yavuz, Tayfun Ates, Ilknur Coban, Fulya Koksalar, Gizem Filiz, et al., "NTS Catecholamine Neurons Mediate Hypoglycemic Hunger via Medial Hypothalamic Feeding Pathways," *Cell Metabolism* 31, no. 2 (February 4, 2020): 313–326, https://doi.org/10.1016/j.cmet.2019.11.016.

7. On the normal GLP-1 level between meals ~10 pmol/L, see M. A. Nauck, I. Vardarli, C. F. Deacon, J. J. Holst, and J. J. Meier, "Secretion of Glucagon-Like Peptide-1 (GLP-1) in Type 2 Diabetes: What Is Up, What Is Down?," *Diabetologia* 54 (2011): 10–18, https://doi.org/10.1007/s00125-010-1896-4. Comparing to the previous reference requires using the molar weight of Ozempic (4,133 daltons) as the conversion factor and adjusting units: Tine A. Baekdal, Mette Thomsen, Viera Kupčová, Cilie W. Hansen, and Thomas W. Anderson, "Pharmacokinetics, Safety, and Tolerability of Oral Semaglutide in Subjects with Hepatic Impairment," *Journal of Clinical Pharmacology* 58, no. 10 (October 2018): 1314–1323, https://doi.org/10.1002/jcph.1131.

8. University of Guelph, "Link Between Hunger and Mood Explained," Science Daily, September 25, 2018, www.sciencedaily.com/releases/2018/09/180925115218.htm; Thomas Horman, Maria Fernanda Fernandes, Yan Zhou, Benjamin Fuller, Melissa Tigert, and

Francesco Leri, "An Exploration of the Aversive Properties of 2-Deoxy-D-Glucose in Rats," *Psychopharmacology* 235 (2018): 3055–3063, https://doi.org/10.1007/s00213-018-4998-1.

9. University of Guelph, "Link Between Hunger and Mood Explained."

10. Thomas Horman, "An Exploration of the Aversive Properties of 2-Deoxy-D-Glucose in the Context of Metabolic Dysfunction and Mood Disorders" (master's thesis, University of Guelph, 2017).

11. Viren Swami, Samantha Hochstöger, Erik Kargl, and Stefan Stieger, "Hangry in the Field: An Experience Sampling Study on the Impact of Hunger on Anger, Irritability, and Affect," *PLOS One* (July 6, 2022), https://doi.org/10.1371/journal.pone.0269629.

12. Roy F. Baumeister and Joseph M. Boden, "Aggression and the Self: High Self-Esteem, Low Self-Control, and Ego Threat," in *Human Aggression: Theories, Research, and Implications for Social Policy* (Cambridge, MA: Academic Press, 1998), 111–137, https://doi.org/10.1016/B978-012278805-5/50006-7.

13. "Roy Baumeister—Willpower: Self-Control, Decision Fatigue, and Energy Depletion," YouTube, posted by TheIMHC (Institute for Human and Machine Cognition), November 7, 2012, www.youtube.com/watch?v=KfnUicHDNM8.

14. "Roy Baumeister—Willpower: Self-Control, Decision Fatigue, and Energy Depletion," YouTube; "Self-Control, Willpower, and Ego Depletion: Gradual Emergence of a Theory," YouTube, posted by Wydział Psychologii i Kognitywistyki UAM, June 13, 2022, www.youtube.com/watch?v=aa9AjpJnZJA.

15. "Roy Baumeister—Willpower: Self-Control, Decision Fatigue, and Energy Depletion," YouTube; "Self-Control, Willpower, and Ego Depletion: Gradual Emergence of a Theory," YouTube.

16. Thomas F. Denson, William von Hippel, Richard I. Kemp, and Lydia S. Teo, "Glucose Consumption Decreases Impulsive Aggression in Response to Provocation in Aggressive Individuals," *Journal of Experimental Social Psychology* 46, no. 6 (November 2010): 1023–1028, https://doi.org/10.1016/j.jesp.2010.05.023.

17. C. Nathan DeWall, Timothy Deckman, Matthew T. Gailliot, and Brad J. Bushman, "Sweetened Blood Cools Hot Tempers: Physiological Self-Control and Aggression," *Aggressive Behavior* 37, no. 1 (January–February 2011): 73–80, https://doi.org/10.1002/ab.20366.

18. Leigh M. Riby, Anna S. Law, Jennifer Mclaughlin, and Jennifer Murray, "Preliminary Evidence That Glucose Ingestion Facilitates Prospective Memory Performance," *Nutrition Research* 31 (2011): 370–377, https://doi.org/10.1016/j.nutres.2011.04.003.

19. Christine Gagnon, Carol E. Greenwood, and Louis Bherer, "The Acute Effects of Glucose Ingestion on Attentional Control in Fasting Healthy Older Adults," *Psychopharmacology (Berlin)* 211, no. 3 (2010): 337–346, https://doi.org/10.1007/s00213-010-1905-9.

20. D. O. Kennedy and A. B. Scholey, "Glucose Administration, Heart Rate and Cognitive Performance: Effects of Increasing Mental Effort," *Psychopharmacology* 149 (2000): 63–71, https://doi.org/10.1007/s002139900335; Michael A. Smith, Leigh M. Riby, J. Anke

M. van Eekelen, Jonathan K. Foste, "Glucose Enhancement of Human Memory: A Comprehensive Research Review of the Glucose Memory Facilitation Effect," *Neuroscience and Biobehavioral Reviews* 35 (2011): 770–783, https://doi.org/10.1016/j.neubiorev.2010.09.008.

21. Cheryl D. Fryar, Jeffery P. Hughes, Kirsten A. Herrick, and Namanjeet Ahluwalia, "Fast Food Consumption Among Adults in the United States, 2013–2016," NCHS Data Brief No. 322, October 2018, www.cdc.gov/nchs/data/databriefs/db322-h.pdf.

22. Danielle Wiener-Bronner, "How America Turned into a Nation of Snackers," KCRA, September 5, 2022, www.kcra.com/article/snacking-habits-americans/41082220.

23. "Roy Baumeister—Willpower: Self-Control, Decision Fatigue, and Energy Depletion," YouTube.

24. Brad Bushman, personal interview with author, May 3, 2023.

25. Brad J. Bushman, C. Nathan DeWall, Richard S. Pond Jr., and Michael D. Hanus, "Low Glucose Relates to Greater Aggression in Married Couples," ed. Roy Baumeister, *PNAS* 111, no. 17 (April 2014): 6254–6257, https://doi.org/10.1073/pnas.1400619111.

26. "Don't Get Hangry: Feed Your Brain Healthy Food | Brad Bushman | TEDx-Columbus," YouTube, posted by TEDx Talks, November 26, 2014, www.youtube.com/watch?v=UOn3zOp8JPE.

27. Gisela Telis, "Unhappy Marriages Due to Low Blood Sugar? Study Suggests Low Levels of Glucose in the Blood Spur Spouses to Fight," *Science*, April 14, 2014, www.science.org/content/article/unhappy-marriages-due-low-blood-sugar.

28. Morgana Mongraw-Chaffin, Daniel P. Beavers, and Donald A. McClain, "Hypoglycemic Symptoms in the Absence of Diabetes: Pilot Evidence of Clinical Hypoglycemia in Young Women," *Journal of Clinical and Translational Endocrinology* 18 (December 2019): 100202, https://doi.org/10.1016/j.jcte.2019.100202.

29. Mongraw-Chaffin et al., "Hypoglycemic Symptoms in the Absence of Diabetes"; "Erratum Regarding Missing Declaration of Competing Interest Statements in Previously Published Articles," *Journal of Clinical and Translational Endocrinology* 23 (December 2020): 100242, https://doi.org/10.1016/j.jcte.2020.100242.

30. Seok Joon Won, Byung Hoon Yoo, Tiina M. Kauppinen, Bo Young Choi, Jin Hee Kim, Bong Geom Jang, Min Woo Lee, et al., "Recurrent/Moderate Hypoglycemia Induces Hippocampal Dendritic Injury, Microglial Activation, and Cognitive Impairment in Diabetic Rats," *Journal of Neuroinflammation* 9 (2012): 182, https://doi.org/10.1186/1742-2094-9-182.

31. Ashish K. Rehni and Kunjan R. Dave, "Impact of Hypoglycemia on Brain Metabolism During Diabetes," *Molecular Neurobiology* 55 (2018): 9075–9088, https://doi.org/10.1007%2Fs12035-018-1044-6.

32. Joel Yager and Roy T. Young, "Non-Hypoglycemia Is an Epidemic Condition," *New England Journal of Medicine* 291 (October 24, 1974): 907–908, https://doi.org/10.1056/nejm197410242911713; Marianna Hall, Magdalena Walicka, Mariusz Panczyk, and Iwona

Traczyk, "Metabolic Parameters in Patients with Suspected Reactive Hypoglycemia," *Journal of Personalized Medicine* 11, no. 4 (April 2021): 276, https://doi.org/10.3390/jpm11040276; Michael T. McDermott, ed., *Management of Patients with Pseudo-Endocrine Disorders: A Case-Based Pocket Guide* (Berlin: Springer, 2019).

33. Mongraw-Chaffin et al., "Hypoglycemic Symptoms in the Absence of Diabetes."

34. Mongraw-Chaffin et al., "Hypoglycemic Symptoms in the Absence of Diabetes."

35. Ichiro Kishimoto and Akio Ohashi, "Subclinical Reactive Hypoglycemia Is Associated with Higher Eating and Snacking Frequencies in Obese or Overweight Men Without Diabetes," *Endocrines* 3, no. 3 (2022): 530–537, https://doi.org/10.3390/endocrines3030043.

36. Kishimoto and Ohashi, "Subclinical Reactive Hypoglycemia."

CHAPTER 5 (PAGES 119 THROUGH 138)

1. Jennifer Shike, "Most People Think They Eat Healthier Than They Do," Dairy Herd Management, June 22, 2022, www.dairyherd.com/news/education/most-people -think-they-eat-healthier-they-do; Jessica Thomson, Alicia Landry, and Tameka Walls, "Can United States Adults Accurately Assess Their Diet Quality?," *Current Developments in Nutrition* 6, no. Supplement 1 (June 2022): 952, https://doi.org/10.1093/cdn/nzac067.072.

2. Maria Luz Fernandez and Ana Gabriela Murillo, "Is There a Correlation Between Dietary and Blood Cholesterol? Evidence from Epidemiological Data and Clinical Interventions," *Nutrients* 14, no. 10 (May 2014): 2168, https://doi.org/10.3390/nu14102168.

3. "Angelo Scanu, MD," *University of Chicago: Medicine on the Midway*, May 15, 2018, 41.

4. Marc S. Penn and Guy M. Chisolm, "Oxidized Lipoproteins, Altered Cell Function and Atherosclerosis," *Atherosclerosis* 108, Supplement (August 1994): S21–S29, https:// doi.org/10.1016/0021-9150(94)90150-3; Dayuan Li and Jawahar L. Mehta, "Oxidized LDL, a Critical Factor in Atherogenesis," *Cardiovascular Research* 68, no. 3 (December 2005): 353–354, https://doi.org/10.1016/j.cardiores.2005.09.009.

5. Fumiaki Ito and Tomoyuki Ito, "High-Density Lipoprotein (HDL) Triglyceride and Oxidized HDL: New Lipid Biomarkers of Lipoprotein-Related Atherosclerotic Cardiovascular Disease," *Antioxidants* 9, no. 5 (2020): 362, https://doi.org/10.3390/antiox9050362.

6. "A new national study has shown that nearly 75 percent of patients hospitalized for a heart attack had cholesterol levels that would indicate they were not at high risk for a cardiovascular event, based on current national cholesterol guidelines": Amit Sachdeva, Christopher P. Cannon, Prakash C. Deedwania, Kenneth A. LaBresh, Sidney C. Smith Jr., David Dai, Adrian Hernandez, and Gregg C. Fonarow, on behalf of the GWTG [Get with the Guidelines] Steering Committee and Hospitals, "Lipid Levels in Patients Hospitalized with Coronary Artery Disease: An Analysis of 136,905 Hospitalizations in Get with the Guidelines," *American Heart Journal* 157, no. 1 (January 2009): 11–17, https://doi.org/10.1016/j .ahj.2008.08.010.

7. Sachdeva et al., "Lipid Levels in Patients Hospitalized with Coronary Artery Disease."

8. Nicholas A. Marston, Robert P. Giugliano, Jeong-Gun Park, Andrea Ruzza, Peter S. Sever, Anthony C. Keech, and Marc S. Sabatine, "Cardiovascular Benefit of Lowering Low-Density Lipoprotein Cholesterol Below 40 mg/dL," *Circulation* 144 (2021): 1732–1734, https://doi.org/10.1161/CIRCULATIONAHA.121.056536.

9. The value was 189 mg/dL in the 2013–2014 period. See Margaret D. Carroll, David A. Lacher, and Paul D. Sorlie, "Trends in Serum Lipids and Lipoproteins of Adults, 1960–2002," *JAMA* 294, no. 14 (2005): 1773–1781, https://doi.org/10.1001/jama.294.14.1773; Asher Rosinger, Margaret D. Carroll, David Lacher, and Cynthia Ogden, "Trends in Total Cholesterol, Triglycerides, and Low-Density Lipoprotein in US Adults, 1999–2014," *JAMA Cardiology* 2, no. 3 (2017): 339–341, https://doi.org/10.1001/jamacardio.2016.4396.

10. Ancel Keys, Joseph T. Anderson, and Francisco Grande, "Serum Cholesterol Response to Changes in the Diet: IV: Particular Saturated Fatty Acids in the Diet," *Metabolism* 14, no. 7 (1965): 776–787, https://doi.org/10.1016/0026-0495(65)90004-1.

11. Ivan D. Frantz Jr., Emily A. Dawson, Patricia L. Ashman, Laël C. Gatewood, Glenn E. Bartsch, Kanta Kuba, and Elizabeth R. Brewer, "Test of Effect of Lipid Lowering by Diet on Cardiovascular Risk: The Minnesota Coronary Survey," *Arteriosclerosis* 9, no. 1 (January–February 1989): 129–135, https://doi.org/10.1161/01.ATV.9.1.129.

12. Christopher E. Ramsden, Daisy Zamora, Sharon Majchrzak-Hong, Keturah R. Faurot, Steven K. Broste, Robert P. Frantz, John M. Davis, Amit Ringel, Chirayath M. Suchindran, and Joseph R. Hibbeln, "Re-evaluation of the Traditional Diet-Heart Hypothesis: Analysis of Recovered Data from Minnesota Coronary Experiment (1968–73)," *BMJ* (2016): 353, https://doi.org/10.1136/bmj.i1246.

13. Ramsden et al., "Re-evaluation of the Traditional Diet-Heart Hypothesis."

14. Staff, "Research Review: Old Data on Dietary Fats in Context with Current Recommendations," Harvard T.H. Chan School of Public Health, April 13, 2016, www.hsph .harvard.edu/nutritionsource/2016/04/13/diet-heart-ramsden-mce-bmj-comments.

15. U. Ravnskov, K. S. McCully, and P. J. Rosch, "The Statin-Low Cholesterol-Cancer Conundrum," *QJM: An International Journal of Medicine* 105, no. 4 (April 2012): 383–388, https://doi.org/10.1093/qjmed/hcr243.

16. Janice Hopkins Tanne, "Meta-Analysis Says Low LDL Cholesterol May Be Associated with Greater Risk of Cancer," *BMJ* 335, no. 7612 (July 28, 2007): 177, https://doi .org/10.1136/bmj.39287.415347.DB.

17. Naoki Nago, Shizukiyo Ishikawa, Tadao Goto, and Kazunori Kayaba, "Low Cholesterol Is Associated with Mortality from Stroke, Heart Disease, and Cancer: The Jichi Medical School Cohort Study," *Journal of Epidemiology* 21, no. 1 (2011): 67–74, https://doi .org/10.2188/jea.JE20100065.

18. Christopher E. Ramsden, Daisy Zamora, Boonseng Leelarthaepin, Sharon F. Majchrzak-Hong, Keturah R. Faurot, Chirayath M. Suchindran, Amit Ringel, John M.

Davis, and Joseph R. Hibbeln, "Use of Dietary Linoleic Acid for Secondary Prevention of Coronary Heart Disease and Death: Evaluation of Recovered Data from the Sydney Diet Heart Study and Updated Meta-Analysis," *BMJ* 346 (2013), https://doi.org/10.1136/bmj .e8707.

19. Y.-B. Lv, Z. X. Yin, C.-L. Chei, M. S. Brasher, J. Zhang, V. B. Kraus, F. Qian, Xiaoming Shi, D. B. Matchar, and Y. Zeng, "Serum Cholesterol Levels Within the High Normal Range Are Associated with Better Cognitive Performance Among Chinese Elderly," *Journal of Nutrition, Health and Aging* 20, no. 3 (2016): 280–287, https://doi.org/10.1007/s12603-016-0701-6.

20. Kenneth R. Feingold and Carl Grunfeld, "The Effect of Inflammation and Infection on Lipids and Lipoproteins," in *Endotext*, ed. Kenneth R. Feingold, Bradley Anawalt, Marc R. Blackman, Alison Boyce, George Chrousos, Emiliano Corpas, and Wouter W. de Herder, et al. (South Dartmouth, MA: MDText.com, 2000); Álvaro Aparisi, Carolina Iglesias-Echeverría, Cristina Ybarra-Falcón, Iván Cusácovich, Aitor Uribarri, Mario García-Gómez, Raquel Ladrón, et al., "Low-Density Lipoprotein Cholesterol Levels Are Associated with Poor Clinical Outcomes in COVID-19," *Nutrition, Metabolism and Cardiovascular Diseases* 31, no. 9 (August 2021): 2619–2627, https://doi.org/10.1016/j.numecd.2021.06.016; Mengmeng Zhao, Zhen Luo, Hua He, Bo Shen, Jinjun Liang, Jishou Zhang, Jing Ye, et al., "Decreased Low-Density Lipoprotein Cholesterol Level Indicates Poor Prognosis of Severe and Critical COVID-19 Patients: A Retrospective, Single-Center Study," *Frontiers in Medicine* 8 (2021): 585851, https://doi.org/10.3389/fmed.2021.585851; Angelo Zinellu, Panagiotis Paliogiannis, Alessandro G. Fois, Paolo Solidoro, Ciriaco Carru, and Arduino A. Mangoni, "Cholesterol and Triglyceride Concentrations, COVID-19 Severity, and Mortality: A Systematic Review and Meta-Analysis with Meta-Regression," *Frontiers in Public Health* (August 18, 2021), https://doi.org/10.3389/fpubh.2021.705916; Daniel A. Hofmaenner, Anna Kleyman, Adrian Press, Michael Bauer, and Mervyn Singer, "The Many Roles of Cholesterol in Sepsis: A Review," *American Journal of Respiratory and Critical Care Medicine* 205, no. 4 (February 2022): 388–396, https://doi.org/10.1164/rccm.202105-1197TR.

21. Lauriane Sèdes, Laura Thirouard, Salwan Maqdasy, Manon Garcia, Françoise Caira, Jean-Marc A. Lobaccaro, Claude Beaudoin, and David H. Volle, "Cholesterol: A Gatekeeper of Male Fertility?," *Frontiers in Endocrinology (Lausanne)* 9 (2018): 369, https://doi.org/10.3389/fendo.2018.00369.

22. There are numerous case reports. This is just one of them. See Erik A. H. Knauff, Hendrika E. Westerveld, Angelique J. Goverde, Marinus J. Eijkemans, Olivier Valkenburg, Evert J. P. van Santbrink, Bart Fauser, and Yvonne T. van der Schouw, "Lipid Profile of Women with Premature Ovarian Failure," *Menopause* 15, no. 5 (July 2008): 919–923, https://doi.org/10.1097/gme.0b013e31816b4509.

23. Feingold and Grunfeld, "The Effect of Inflammation and Infection on Lipids and Lipoproteins."

24. Lise Bathum, René Depont Christensen, Lars Engers Pedersen, Palle Lyngsie Pedersen, John Larsen, and Jørgen Nexøe, "Association of Lipoprotein Levels with Mortality in

Subjects Aged 50 + Without Previous Diabetes or Cardiovascular Disease: A Population-Based Register Study," *Scandinavian Journal of Primary Health Care* 31, no. 3 (2013), https://doi.org/10.3109/02813432.2013.824157.

25. Marcos Aparecido Sarria Cabrera, Selma Maffei de Andrade, and Renata Maciulis Dip, "Lipids and All-Cause Mortality Among Older Adults: A 12-Year Follow-Up Study," *Scientific World Journal* 2012 (2012): 930139, https://doi.org/10.1100/2012/930139.

26. Ya Liu, Liwen Zhang, Junxian Li, Wenjuan Kang, Mingli Cao, Fangfang Song, and Fengju Song, "Association Between Low Density Lipoprotein Cholesterol and All-Cause Mortality: Results from the NHANES 1999–2014," *Scientific Reports* 11 (2021): 22111, https://doi.org/10.1038/s41598-021-01738-w.

27. Glen D. Lawrence, "Perspective: The Saturated Fat–Unsaturated Oil Dilemma: Relations of Dietary Fatty Acids and Serum Cholesterol, Atherosclerosis, Inflammation, Cancer, and All-Cause Mortality," *Advances in Nutrition* 12, no. 3 (May 2021): 647–656, https://doi.org/10.1093/advances/nmab013.

28. Martha A. Belury, Emilio Ros, and Penny M. Kris-Etherton, "Weighing Evidence of the Role of Saturated and Unsaturated Fats and Human Health," *Advances in Nutrition* 13, no. 2 (March 2022): 686–688, https://doi.org/10.1093/advances/nmab160; Jeff M. Moore, "The Dietary Guidelines Are Correct: Saturated Fat Should Be Limited and Replaced with the Proposed Alternatives to Reduce Morbidity and Mortality," *Advances in Nutrition* 13, no. 2 (March 2022): 688–690, https://doi.org/10.1093/advances/nmab159.

29. Robyn M. Lucas and Rachael M. Rodney Harris, "On the Nature of Evidence and 'Proving' Causality: Smoking and Lung Cancer vs. Sun Exposure, Vitamin D and Multiple Sclerosis," *International Journal of Environmental Research and Public Health* 15, no. 8 (August 2018): 1726, https://doi.org/10.3390/ijerph15081726.

30. Carlos Zaragoza, Carmen Gomez-Guerrero, Jose Luis Martin-Ventura, Luis Blanco-Colio, Begoña Lavin, Beñat Mallavia, Carlos Tarin, Sebastian Mas, Alberto Ortiz, and Jesus Egido, "Animal Models of Cardiovascular Diseases," *Journal of Biomedicine and Biotechnology* 2011 (2011): 497841, https://doi.org/10.1155/2011/497841.

31. Zaragoza et al., "Animal Models of Cardiovascular Diseases."

32. Normal rodent chow contains 4 percent fat by weight. Atherogenic chow contains 23.5 percent fat by weight. And given that the average human eats about 1.5 Kg per day, doing the math, 1.5 percent is 22,500 mg of cholesterol. A stick of butter has 243 mg cholesterol. See source: Ross G. Gerrity, Herbert K. Naito, Mary Richardson, and Colin J. Schwartz, "Dietary Induced Atherogenesis in Swine," *American Journal of Pathology* 95 (1979): 775–793, www.ncbi.nlm.nih.gov/pmc/articles/PMC2042303.

33. Ilona Staprans, Xian-Mang Pan, Joseph H. Rapp, and Kenneth R. Feingold, "The Role of Dietary Oxidized Cholesterol and Oxidized Fatty Acids in the Development of Atherosclerosis," *Molecular Nutrition and Food Research* 49, no. 11 (November 2005): 1075–1082, https://doi.org/10.1002/mnfr.200500063.

34. S. Won Park and P. B. Addis, "HPLC Determination of C-7 Oxidized Cholesterol Derivatives in Foods," *Food Science* 50, no. 5 (September 1985): 1437–1441, https://doi.org /10.1111/j.1365-2621.1985.tb10494.x.

CHAPTER 6 (PAGES 139 THROUGH 164)

Figure 6–1: The data used to make this chart come from the following sources:

Saturated fat: S. Gerrior, L. Bente, and H. Hiza, *Nutrient Content of the U.S. Food Supply, 1909–2010*, Home Economics Research Report Number 56, US Department of Agriculture, Center for Nutrition Policy and Promotion (CNPP), November 2004, https://grist.org/wp-content/uploads/2006/08/foodsupply1909-2000.pdf.

Heart disease: James E. Dalen, Joseph S. Alpert, Robert J. Goldberg, and Ronald S. Weinstein, "The Epidemic of the 20th Century: Coronary Heart Disease," *American Journal of Medicine* 127, no. 9 (September 2014): 807–812, https://doi.org/10.1016/j .amjmed.2014.04.015; Stephen Sidney, Catherine Lee, Jennifer Liu, Sadiya S. Khan, Donald M. Lloyd-Jones, and Jamal S. Rana, "Age-Adjusted Mortality Rates and Age and Risk–Associated Contributions to Change in Heart Disease and Stroke Mortality, 2011–2019 and 2019–2020," *JAMA Network Open* 5, no. 3 (2022): e223872, https://doi .org/10.1001/jamanetworkopen.2022.3872; Farida B. Ahmad, Jodi A. Cisewski, Jiaquan Xu, and Robert N. Anderson, "Provisional Mortality Data—United States, 2022," *Morbidity and Mortality Weekly Report* 72, no. 18 (May 5, 2023): 488–492.

Rate of smoking: Richard J. Bonnie, Kathleen Stratton, and Robert B. Wallace, eds., *Ending the Tobacco Problem: A Blueprint for the Nation* (Washington, DC: National Academies Press, 2007), https://doi.org/10.17226/11795.

1. Ancel Keys, "Atherosclerosis: A Problem in Newer Public Health," *Journal of the Mount Sinai Hospital, New York* 20, no. 2 (July–August 1953): 119–139, text available from University of Minnesota School of Public Health, www.epi.umn.edu/cvdepi/wp-content /uploads/2014/03/Keys-Atherosclerosis-A-Problem-in-Newer-Public-Health.pdf.

2. J. Yerushalmy and Herman E. Hilleboe, "Fat in the Diet and Mortality from Heart Disease: A Methodologic Note," *New York State Journal of Medicine* 57, no. 14 (1957): 2343–2354, text available from CrossFit, https://library.crossfit.com/free/pdf/1957 _Yerushalmy_Hilleboe_Fat_Diet_Mortality_Heart_Disease.pdf; Zoë Harcombe, "Keys Six Countries Graph," Dr. Zoë Harcombe, PhD (blog), February 20, 2017, www.zoeharcombe .com/2017/02/keys-six-countries-graph.

3. Harcombe, "Keys Six Countries Graph"; Ancel Keys, "Epidemiologic Aspects of Coronary Artery Disease," *Journal of Chronic Disease* 6, no. 5 (1957): 552–559, https://doi .org/10.1016/0021-9681(57)90043-7.

4. Nina Teicholz, *The Big Fat Surprise: Why Butter, Meat and Cheese Belong in a Healthy Diet* (New York: Simon and Schuster, 2014).

5. Teicholz, *Big Fat Surprise*, 45–46.

6. Zoë Harcombe, Julien S. Baker, Stephen Mark Cooper, Bruce Davies, Nicholas Sculthorpe, James J. DiNicolantonio, and Fergal Grace, "Evidence from Randomised Controlled Trials Did Not Support the Introduction of Dietary Fat Guidelines in 1977 and 1983: A Systematic Review and Meta-Analysis," *Open Heart* 2 (2015): e000196, https://doi.org/10.1136/openhrt-2014-000196.

7. Keys, "Atherosclerosis: A Problem in Newer Public Health."

8. "Medicine: The Fat of the Land," *Time*, January 13, 1961, https://content.time.com/time/subscriber/article/0,33009,828721-1,00.html.

9. "Medicine: The Fat of the Land."

10. Ancel Keys and Flaminio Fidanza, "Serum Cholesterol and Relative Body Weight of Coronary Patients in Different Populations," *Circulation* 22, no. 6 (December 1960): 1091–1106, https://doi.org/10.1161/01.CIR.22.6.1091 and www.ahajournals.org/doi/epdf/10.1161/01.CIR.22.6.1091. (No other articles were found that represented his data prior to 1962.)

11. Ancel Keys, Alessandro Menotti, Christ Aravanis, Henry Blackburn, Bozidar S. Djordevič, Ratko Buzina, and A. S. Dontas, et al., "The Seven Countries Study: 2,289 Deaths in 15 Years," *Preventive Medicine* 13, no. 2 (March 1984): 141–154, https://doi.org/10.1016/0091-7435(84)90047-1.

12. Sally Fallon and Mary G. Enig, "The Oiling of America," Weston A. Price Foundation, January 17, 2019, www.westonaprice.org/health-topics/the-oiling-of-america.

13. "Our Lifesaving History," American Heart Association, accessed September 10, 2023, www.heart.org/en/about-us/history-of-the-american-heart-association and www.heart.org/-/media/Files/About-Us/History/History-of-the-American-Heart-Association.pdf; "Research Accomplishments," American Heart Association, accessed September 10, 2023, https://professional.heart.org/en/research-programs/aha-research-accomplishments.

14. Richard Doll and A. Bradford Hill, "The Mortality of Doctors in Relation to Their Smoking Habits," *British Medical Journal* 1 (1954): 1451, https://doi.org/10.1136/bmj.1.4877.1451.

15. David Kritchevsky, "History of Recommendations to the Public About Dietary Fat," *Journal of Nutrition* 128, no. 2 (February 1998): 449S–452S, https://doi.org/10.1093/jn/128.2.449S.

16. Irvine H. Page, Edgar V. Allen, Francis L. Chamberlain, Ancel Keys, Jeremiah Stamler, Fredrick J. Stare, and the Central Committee for Medical and Community Program of the American Heart Association and Ad Hoc Committee on Dietary Fat and Atherosclerosis, "Dietary Fat and Its Relation to Heart Attacks and Strokes," *Circulation* 23 (1961): 133–136, https://doi.org/10.1161/01.CIR.23.1.133 and www.ahajournals.org/doi/pdf/10.1161/01.cir.23.1.133.

17. Daan Kromhout, Alessandro Menotti, and Henry Blackburn, eds., *The Seven Countries Study, A Scientific Adventure in Cardiovascular Disease Epidemiology* (Bilthoven, Netherlands: Studio RIVM, 1984).

18. Ancel Keys, Henry Longstreet Taylor, Henry Blackburn, Josef Brozek, Joseph T. Anderson, and Ernst Simonson, "Coronary Heart Disease Among Minnesota Business and Professional Men Followed Fifteen Years," *Circulation* 23 (September 1963): 381–395, https://doi.org/10.1161/01.CIR.28.3.381.

19. *The Search*, 1953, produced by CBS News, hosted at University of Minnesota School of Public Health, www.epi.umn.edu/cvdepi/video/the-search-1953.

20. F. E. Kendall, W. Meyer, and M. Bevans, "Effect of Intravenous Injection of Oxidized Cholesterol Upon the Production of Atherosclerosis in Rabbits," *Federation Proceedings* 7, no. 1, part 1 (1948): 273.

21. Henry E. Armstrong, "Carbonic Oxide in Tobacco Smoke," *British Medical Journal* 1, no. 3208 (1922): 992.

22. Nutrition Coalition, "The Largest Promoters of High-Carb Diets Are Funded by Corporate Interests," January 19, 2018, www.nutritioncoalition.us/news/2018/1/19/the-largest-promoters-of-high-carb-diets-are-funded-by-corporate-interests.

23. AHA Financial Information from the American Heart Association. https://www.heart.org/en/about-us/aha-financial-information.

24. "Advocacy," American Heart Association, accessed September 10, 2023, www.heart.org/en/get-involved/advocate.

25. Harcombe et al., "Evidence from Randomised Controlled Trials Did Not Support the Introduction of Dietary Fat Guidelines in 1977 and 1983"; Nina Teicholz, "A Short History of Saturated Fat: The Making and Unmaking of a Scientific Consensus," *Current Opinions in Endocrinology, Diabetes and Obesity* 30, no. 1 (February 1, 2023): 65–71, https://doi.org/10.1097/med.0000000000000791; Zoë Harcombe, "Dietary Fat Guidelines Have No Evidence Base: Where Next for Public Health Nutritional Advice?," *British Journal of Sports Medicine* 51 (2017): 769–774, https://doi.org/10.1136/bjsports-2016-096734.

26. "Research Programs," American Heart Association Professional Heart Daily, accessed August 1, 2023, https://professional.heart.org/en/research-programs.

27. Frances Sladek, telephone interview with author, February 24, 2015.

28. W. Bruce Fye, "A History of the American Heart Association's Council on Clinical Cardiology," *Circulation* 87 (1993): 1057–1063, https://doi.org/10.1161/01.CIR.87.3.1057.

29. Fye, "A History of the American Heart Association's Council on Clinical Cardiology."

30. Fye, "A History of the American Heart Association's Council on Clinical Cardiology."

31. Fye, "A History of the American Heart Association's Council on Clinical Cardiology."

32. Minutes of the American Heart Association Meetings, 1948.

33. Teicholz, *Big Fat Surprise*, 47; Teicholz, "The Questionable Link Between Saturated Fat and Heart Disease," *Wall Street Journal*, May 6, 2014, www.wsj.com/articles /the-questionable-link-between-saturated-fat-and-heart-disease-1399070926.

34. Fye, "A History of the American Heart Association's Council on Clinical Cardiology."

35. Edward L. Bernays, *The Engineering of Consent* (Norman: University of Oklahoma Press, 1969).

36. "Water Fluoridation Data & Statistics," Centers for Disease Control and Prevention, reviewed June 9, 2023, www.cdc.gov/fluoridation/statistics/index.htm.

37. Edward L. Bernays, *Propaganda* (Brooklyn, NY: Ig Publishing, 2005).

38. Christopher Bryson, *The Fluoride Deception* (New York: Seven Stories Press, 2004), 159.

39. Bryson, *Fluoride Deception*, 159.

40. Larry Tye, *The Father of Spin: Edward L. Bernays and the Birth of Public Relations* (New York: Picador, 2002), 74.

41. Bernays, *Propaganda*, 37.

42. United States Department of Agriculture, *Yearbooks of the United States Department of Agriculture* (Washington, DC: Government Printing Office, 1904), available from https://archive.org/details/yoa1903/page/n1/mode/2up.

43. Bryson, *Fluoride Deception*, 159.

44. The program is still in place as of this writing. A business can get a license to use the "Heart Healthy" checkmark for an "administrative fee" of thousands of dollars per SKU per year as long as you meet their criteria, which include saturated fat limits on all products but no PUFA limits for many products. See "Heart-Check Food Certification Program Fee Structure," American Heart Association, www.heart.org/-/media/files /healthy-living/company-collaboration/heart-check-certification/hc-pricing-sheet.pdf; "Heart-Check Food Certification Program Nutrition Requirements," American Heart Association, www.heart.org/en/healthy-living/company-collaboration/heart-check-certification /heart-check-in-the-grocery-store/heart-check-food-certification-program-nutrition -requirements.

CHAPTER 7 (PAGES 165 THROUGH 182)

Figure 7–1: Uffe Ravinskov, *The Cholesterol Myths: Exposing the Fallacy That Saturated Fat and Cholesterol Cause Heart Disease* (White Plains, MD: NewTrends Publishing, 2000), 209.

1. In the United States, total cesareans run around 33–36 percent of all births. While there is currently a lot of publicity around unnecessary cesareans, in my own experience the majority are done for pregnancy complications such as amniotic fluid abnormalities and preeclampsia; issues that come up during delivery, like fetal malpresentation or distress; or

previous cesarean. According to the World Health Organization, "necessary" cesarean rates run between 10 and 15 percent. But this figure is based on decades-old data that fails to account for increased obesity, and obesity increases the need for cesareans.

2.   K. M. Venkat Narayan, James P. Boyle, Theodore J. Thompson, Stephen W. Sorensen, and David F. Williamson, "Lifetime Risk for Diabetes Mellitus in the United States," *JAMA* 290, no. 14 (2003): 1884–1890, https://doi.org/10.1001/jama.290.14.1884.

3.   Dr. Klish was later criticized for basing his comments on personal experience as a pediatrician rather than research data. Nevertheless, his statement was influential and widely cited in *JAMA* and other medical journals. It played a vital role in ending the complacency about our nation's overall health.

4.   Dariush Mozaffarian, Renata Micha, and Sarah Wallace, "Effects on Coronary Heart Disease of Increasing Polyunsaturated Fat in Place of Saturated Fat: A Systematic Review and Meta-Analysis of Randomized Controlled Trials," *PLOS Medicine* 7, no. 3 (2010): e1000252, https://doi.org/10.1371/journal.pmed.1000252.

5.   Suzanne White Junod, "Statins: A Success Story Involving FDA, Academia and Industry," *Update*, March–April 2017, www.fda.gov/media/110452/download.

6.   "WHO Cooperative Trial on Primary Prevention of Ischaemic Heart Disease with Clofibrate to Lower Serum Cholesterol: Final Mortality Follow-up: Report of the Committee of Principal Investigators," *Lancet* 2, no. 8403 (September 15, 1984): 600–604, https://pubmed.ncbi.nlm.nih.gov/6147641.

7.   Marco Studer, Matthias Briel, Bernd Leimenstoll, Tracy R. Glass, and Heiner C. Bucher, "Effect of Different Antilipidemic Agents and Diets on Mortality: A Systematic Review," *Archives of Internal Medicine* 165, no. 7 (2005): 725–730, https://doi.org/10.1001/archinte.165.7.725.

8.   Stephen J. Nicholls and Kristen Bubb, "The Mystery of Evacetrapib—Why Are CETP Inhibitors Failing?," *Expert Review of Cardiovascular Therapy* 18, no. 3 (2020), https://doi.org/10.1080/14779072.2020.1745633.

9.   Nicholls and Bubb, "The Mystery of Evacetrapib."

10.   Robert duBroff, "Cholesterol Paradox: A Correlate Does Not a Surrogate Make," *BMJ Evidence-Based Medicine* 22, no. 1 (2017): 15–19, http://dx.doi.org/10.1136/ebmed-2016-110602.

11.   Ihab Suliman, Abdulaziz Batarfi, Hassan Almohammadi, Hisham Aljeraisi, Hassan Alnaserallah, and Ali Alghamdi, "Prevalence of Self-Reported Muscle Pain Among Statin Users from National Guard Hospital, Riyadh," *Cureus* 14, no. 3 (March 2022): e23463, https://doi.org/10.7759/cureus.23463.

12.   Sarah Zhang, "America's Most Popular Drug Has a Puzzling Side Effect. We Finally Know Why," *Atlantic*, June 27, 2023, www.theatlantic.com/health/archive/2023/06/the-gene-that-explains-statins-most-puzzling-side-effect/674542.

13. Zhang, "America's Most Popular Drug Has a Puzzling Side Effect."

14. Peter H. Langsjoen, Jens O. Langsjoen, Alena M. Langsjoen, and Franklin Rosenfeldt, "Statin-Associated Cardiomyopathy Responds to Statin Withdrawal and Administration of Coenzyme Q10," *Permanente Journal* 23 (2019): 18–257, https://doi.org/10.7812/TPP /18.257.

15. Langsjoen et al., "Statin-Associated Cardiomyopathy Responds to Statin Withdrawal and Administration of Coenzyme Q10."

16. "Acute treatment of wild-type hippocampal slices with an inhibitor of the mevalonate pathway (a statin) also impairs LTP," meaning you can create the same memory-impairing nerve abnormalities with statins that you can by genetically modifying mice to give them dementia. Tiina J. Kotti, Denise M.O. Ramirez, Brad E. Pfeiffer, and David W. Russell, "Brain Cholesterol Turnover Required for Geranylgeraniol Production and Learning in Mice," *PNAS* 103, no. 10 (March 2006): 3869–3874, https://doi.org/10.1073/pnas .0600316103.

17. Anamaria Jurcau and Aurel Simion, "Cognition, Statins, and Cholesterol in Elderly Ischemic Stroke Patients: A Neurologist's Perspective," *Medicina (Kaunas)* 57, no. 6 (June 13, 2021): 616, https://doi.org/10.3390/medicina57060616.

18. Fan Nils Yang, Macdonell Stanford, and Xiong Jiang, "Low Cholesterol Level Linked to Reduced Semantic Fluency Performance and Reduced Gray Matter Volume in the Medial Temporal Lobe," *Frontiers in Aging Neuroscience* (March 31, 2020), https://doi .org/10.3389/fnagi.2020.00057.

19. Beatrice Alexandra Golomb, Michael H. Criqui, Halbert White, and Joel E. Dimsdale, "Conceptual Foundations of the UCSD Statin Study," *Archives of Internal Medicine* 164, no. 2 (2004): 153–162, https://doi.org/10.1001/archinte.164.2.153.

20. "How Statins Made Me Stupid | EpicReviewGuys in 4k CC," YouTube, posted by EpicReviewGuys, October 31, 2014, www.youtube.com/watch?v=MKYBp5aukQA.

21. "Psychiatric Side Effects of Statins | An Interview with Beatrice Golomb," YouTube, posted by Witt-Doering Psychiatry, June 28, 2023, www.youtube.com/watch?v= F7NizS-piiI; Golomb et al., "Conceptual Foundations of the UCSD Statin Study."

22. "Psychiatric Side Effects of Statins," YouTube.

23. Samaneh Asgari, Hengameh Abdi, Alireza Mahdavi Hezaveh, Alireza Moghisi, Koorosh Etemad, Hassan Riahi Beni, and Davood Khalili, "The Burden of Statin Therapy Based on ACC/AHA and NCEP ATP-III Guidelines: An Iranian Survey of Non-Communicable Diseases Risk Factors," *Scientific Reports* 8 (2018): 4928, https://doi .org/10.1038/s41598-018-23364-9; Martin Bødtker Mortensen and Børge Grønne Nordestgaard, "Comparison of Five Major Guidelines for Statin Use in Primary Prevention in a Contemporary General Population," *Annals of Internal Medicine* 168, no. 2 (January 16, 2018): 85–92, https://doi.org/10.7326/M17-0681.

24. Peter Ueda, Thomas Wai-Chun Lung, Philip Clarke, and Goodarz Danaei, "Application of the 2014 NICE Cholesterol Guidelines in the English Population: A Cross-Sectional Analysis," *British Journal of General Practice* 67, no. 662 (September 2017): e598–e608, https://doi.org/10.3399/bjgp17x692141. (The 2023 guidelines are largely unchanged.)

25. Andrew Paul DeFilippis, Rebekah Young, John W. McEvoy, Erin D. Michos, Veit Sandfort, Richard A. Kronmal, Robyn L. McClelland, and Michael J. Blah, "Risk Score Overestimation: The Impact of Individual Cardiovascular Risk Factors and Preventive Therapies on the Performance of the American Heart Association–American College of Cardiology-Atherosclerotic Cardiovascular Disease Risk Score in a Modern Multi-Ethnic Cohort," *European Heart Journal* 38, no. 8 (February 21, 2017): 598–608, https://doi.org/10.1093/eurheartj/ehw301.

26. Jacqui Wise, "Long Term Study Backs Statins for Patients with High LDL and No Other Risk Factors," *BMJ* 358 (2017), https://doi.org/10.1136/bmj.j4171.

27. David M. Diamond, "Misleading Communication of Benefits of Long-Term Statin Treatment," *BMJ* 358 (2017): j4171, https://doi.org/10.1136/bmj.j4171.

28. "Dr. Aseem Malhotra—'Evidence Based Medicine Has Been Hijacked,'" YouTube, posted by Low Carb Down Under, August 20, 2022, https://youtu.be/qwovXFzUvfg?si=zryK-7o21scLNW3A&t=1560; M. L. Kristensen, P. M. Christensen, J. Hallas, "The Effect of Statins on Average Survival in Randomised Trials, an Analysis of End Point Postponement," *BMJ Open* 5 (2015): e007118, https://doi.org/10.1136/bmjopen-2014-007118.

29. "Healthcare Spending in the United States Remains High," Peter G. Peterson Foundation, April 5, 2023, www.pgpf.org/blog/2023/04/healthcare-spending-in-the-united-states-remains-high; Steven Zahniser and Kathleen Kassel, "What Is Agriculture's Share of the Overall US Economy?," US Department of Agriculture Economic Research Service, updated January 6, 2023, www.ers.usda.gov/data-products/chart-gallery/gallery/chart-detail/?chartId=58270; "The United States Spends More on Defense Than the Next 10 Countries Combined," Peter G. Peterson Foundation, April 24, 2023, www.pgpf.org/blog/2023/04/the-united-states-spends-more-on-defense-than-the-next-10-countries-combined; Statista Research Department, "Tech GDP as a Percent of Total GDP in the U.S. 2017–2022," Statista, July 11, 2023, www.statista.com/statistics/1239480/united-states-leading-states-by-tech-contribution-to-gross-product.

30. "Food Prices and Spending," US Department of Agriculture, Economic Research Service, updated September 26, 2023, www.ers.usda.gov/data-products/ag-and-food-statistics-charting-the-essentials/food-prices-and-spending; "Healthcare Spending Will Be One-Fifth of the Economy Within a Decade," Peter G. Peterson Foundation, July 27, 2023, www.pgpf.org/blog/2023/07/healthcare-spending-will-be-one-fifth-of-the-economy-within-a-decade.

31. John Abramson, *Overdosed America: The Broken Promise of American Medicine* (New York: Harper Perennial, 2008).

32. John Abramson, *Sickening: How Big Pharma Broke American Health Care and How We Can Repair It* (New York: Mariner Books, 2022).

33. Abramson, *Overdosed America*.

34. Matti Marklund, Jason H. Y. Wu, Fumiaki Imamura, Liana C. Del Gobbo, Amanda Fretts, Janette de Goede, Peilin Shi, et al., "Biomarkers of Dietary Omega-6 Fatty Acids and Incident Cardiovascular Disease and Mortality," *Circulation* 139, no. 21 (May 21, 2019): 2422–2436, https://doi.org/10.1161/CIRCULATIONAHA.118.038908; Jason H. Y. Wu, Matti Marklund, Fumiaki Imamura, Nathan Tintle, Andres V. Ardisson Korat, Janette de Goede, Xia Zhou, et al., "Omega-6 Fatty Acid Biomarkers and Incident Type 2 Diabetes: Pooled Analysis of Individual-Level Data for 39 740 Adults from 20 Prospective Cohort Studies," *Lancet Diabetes and Endocrinology* 5, no. 12 (2017): 965–974, http://doi.org/10.1016/S2213-8587(17)30307-8.

35. Q. Qi, A. Y. Chu, J. H. Kang, J. Huang, L. M. Rose, M. K. Jensen, et al. "Fried Food Consumption, Genetic Risk, and Body Mass Index: Gene-Diet Interaction Analysis in Three US Cohort Studies." *BMJ* 348 (2014): g1610, doi:10.1136/bmj.g1610.

CHAPTER 8 (PAGES 183 THROUGH 212)

1. Kana Miyahara, Naoharu Takano, Yumiko Yamada, Hiromi Kazama, Mayumi Tokuhisa, Hirotsugu Hino, Koji Fujita, et al., "BRCA1 Degradation in Response to Mitochondrial Damage in Breast Cancer Cells," *Scientific Reports* 11 (2021): 8735, https://doi.org/10.1038/s41598-021-87698-7; Minsoo Kim, Mahnoor Mahmood, Ed Reznik, and Payam A. Gammage, "Mitochondrial DNA Is a Major Source of Driver Mutations in Cancer," *Trends in Cancer* 8, no. 12 (December 2022): 1046–1059, https://doi.org/10.1016/j.trecan.2022.08.001.

2. "Compared with nuclear DNA, the mitochondrial DNA (mtDNA) is more prone to be affected by DNA damaging agents, and accumulated DNA damages may cause mitochondrial dysfunction and drive the pathogenesis of a variety of human diseases, including neurodegenerative disorders and cancer": Ziye Rong, Peipei Tu, Peiqi Xu, Yan Sun, Fangfang Yu, Na Tu, Lixia Guo, and Yanan Yang, "The Mitochondrial Response to DNA Damage," *Frontiers in Cell and Developmental Biology*, Sec. Cell Death and Survival 9 (May 2021), https://doi.org/10.3389/fcell.2021.669379.

3. Takako Yoshida, Shinji Goto, Miho Kawakatsu, Yoshishige Urata, and Tao-sheng Li, "Mitochondrial Dysfunction, a Probable Cause of Persistent Oxidative Stress After Exposure to Ionizing Radiation," *Free Radical Research* 46, no. 2 (2012): 147–153, https://doi.org/10.3109/10715762.2011.645207.

4. "Clonal Evolution in Cancer," Mission Bio, accessed September 9, 2023, https://missionbio.com/resources/learning-center/clonal-evolution-in-cancer.

5. Lawrence A. Loeb, Keith R. Loeb, and Jon P. Anderson, "Multiple Mutations and Cancer," *PNAS* 100, no. 3 (February 2003): 776–781, https://doi.org/10.1073/pnas.0334858100.

6. Douglas E. Brash, "Melanoma: Accelerating Cancer Without Mutations," *Cancer Biology* (March 21, 2019), https://doi.org/10.7554/eLife.45809.

7. Thomas Seyfried, Zoom interview with author, December 1, 2022.

8. Purna Mukherjee, Zachary M. Augur, Mingyi Li, Collin Hill, Bennett Greenwood, Marek A. Domin, Gramoz Kondakci, et al., "Therapeutic Benefit of Combining Calorie-Restricted Ketogenic Diet and Glutamine Targeting in Late-Stage Experimental Glioblastoma," *Communications Biology* 2 (2019): 200, https://doi.org/10.1038/s42003-019-0455-x.

9. "Top Cancer Expert: This Is the WORST Food to Feed Cancer" (interview with Dr. Thomas Seyfried conducted by Dr. Anthony Chaffee), YouTube, posted by Anthony Chaffee, MD, July 22, 2022, www.youtube.com/watch?v=1ebPZP9hBPA.

10. Seyfried, Zoom interview with author.

11. Seyfried, Zoom interview with author.

12. Terence A. Ketter, Tim A. Kimbrell, Mark S. George, Robert T. Dunn, Andrew M. Speer, Brenda E. Benson, Mark W. Willis, et al., "Effects of Mood and Subtype on Cerebral Glucose Metabolism in Treatment-Resistant Bipolar Disorder," *Biological Psychiatry* 49, no. 2 (January 2001): 97–109, https://doi.org/10.1016/s0006-3223(00)00975-6.

13. Ling Shao, Maureen V. Martin, Stanley J. Watson, Alan Schatzberg, Huda Akil, Richard M. Myers, Edward G. Jones, William E. Bunney, and Marquis P. Vawter, "Mitochondrial Involvement in Psychiatric Disorders," *Annals of Medicine* 40, no. 4 (2008): 281–295, https://doi.org/10.1080/07853890801923753.

14. Benjamin Ang, Mark Horowitz, and Joanna Moncrieff, "Is the Chemical Imbalance an 'Urban Legend'? An Exploration of the Status of the Serotonin Theory of Depression in the Scientific Literature," *SSM—Mental Health* 2 (December 2022): 100098, https://doi.org/10.1016/j.ssmmh.2022.100098.

15. Albert Danan, Eric C. Westman, Laura R. Saslow, and Georgia Ede, "The Ketogenic Diet for Refractory Mental Illness: A Retrospective Analysis of 31 Inpatients," *Frontiers in Psychiatry*, Sec. Public Mental Health 13 (July 6, 2022), https://doi.org/10.3389/fpsyt.2022.951376.

16. Georgia Ede, Zoom interview with author, November 29, 2022.

17. James W. Wheless, "History of the Ketogenic Diet," *Epilepsia* 49, no. s8 (November 2008): 3–5, https://doi.org/10.1111/j.1528-1167.2008.01821.x.

18. Emanuele Bartolini, Anna Rita Ferrari, Simona Fiori, and Stefania Della Vecchia, "Glycaemic Imbalances in Seizures and Epilepsy of Paediatric Age: A Literature Review," *Journal of Clinical Medicine* 12, no. 7 (2023): 2580, https://doi.org/10.3390/jcm12072580.

19. Prathama Guha, Piyanku Mazumder, Malay Ghosal, Indranil Chakraborty, and Prabir Burman, "Assessment of Insulin Resistance and Metabolic Syndrome in Drug Naive Patients of Bipolar Disorder," *Indian Journal of Clinical Biochemistry* 29 (2014): 51–56, https://doi.org/10.1007/s12291-012-0292-x.

20. US Department of Health and Human Services, "More Americans Have Epilepsy Than Ever Before," CDC.gov, August 10, 2017, www.cdc.gov/media/releases/2017/p0810-epilepsy-prevalence.html; Laura Blakeslee, Megan Rabe, Zoe Caplan, and Andrew Roberts, "An Aging U.S. Population with Fewer Children in 2020," Census.gov, May 25, 2023, www.census.gov/library/stories/2023/05/aging-united-states-population-fewer-children-in-2020.html; Stella U. Ogunwole, Megan A. Rabe, Andrew W. Roberts, and Zoe Caplan, "Population Under Age 18 Declined Last Decade," United States Census Bureau, August 12, 2021, www.census.gov/library/stories/2021/08/united-states-adult-population-grew-faster-than-nations-total-population-from-2010-to-2020.html.

21. J. Peplies, D. Jiménez-Pavón, S. C. Savva, C. Buck, K. Günther, A. Fraterman, and P. Russo, "Percentiles of Fasting Serum Insulin, Glucose, HbA1c and HOMA-IR in Prepubertal Normal Weight European Children from the IDEFICS Cohort," *International Journal of Obesity* 38 (2014): S39–S47, https://doi.org/10.1038/ijo.2014.134.

22. Ameer Y. Taha, "Role and Metabolism of Omega-6 Linoleic Acid in the Brain," *Clinical Neurophysiology* 130, no. 8 (August 2019): e117–e118, https://doi.org/10.1016/j.clinph.2019.03.020; Christopher E. Ramsden, Marie Hennebelle, Susanne Schuster, Gregory S. Keyes, Casey D. Johnson, Irina A. Kirpich, Jeff E. Dahlen, et al., "Effects of Diets Enriched in Linoleic Acid and Its Peroxidation Products on Brain Fatty Acids, Oxylipins, and Aldehydes in Mice," *Biochimica et Biophysica Acta (BBA)—Molecular and Cell Biology of Lipids* 1863, no. 10 (October 2018): 1206–1213, https://doi.org/10.1016/j.bbalip.2018.07.007; Ameer Y. Taha, "Linoleic Acid—Good or Bad for the Brain?," *npj Science of Food* 4, no. 1 (2020): 1, https://doi.org/10.1038/s41538-019-0061-9; Zhichao Zhang, Shiva Emami, Marie Hennebelle, Rhianna K. Morgan, Larry A. Lerno, Carolyn M. Slupsky, Pamela J. Lein, and Ameer Y. Taha, "Linoleic Acid–Derived 13-Hydroxyoctadecadienoic Acid Is Absorbed and Incorporated into Rat Tissues," *Biochimica et Biophysica Acta (BBA)—Molecular and Cell Biology of Lipids* 1866, no. 3 (March 2021): 158870, https://doi.org/10.1016/j.bbalip.2020.158870.

23. "What Can I Eat?," American Diabetes Association, July 18, 2019, https://diabetes.org/blog/what-can-i-eat.

24. "It is the position of the American Diabetes Association (ADA) that there is not a 'one-size-fits-all' eating pattern for individuals with diabetes": Alison B. Evert, Jackie L. Boucher, Marjorie Cypress, Stephanie A. Dunbar, Marion J. Franz, Elizabeth J. Mayer-Davis, Joshua J. Neumiller, et al., "Nutrition Therapy Recommendations for the Management of Adults with Diabetes," *Diabetes Care* 37, Supplement 1 (2014): S120–S143, https://doi.org/10.2337/dc14-S120.

25. Neal D. Barnard, Joshua Cohen, David J. A. Jenkins, Gabrielle Turner-McGrievy, Lise Gloede, Amber Green, and Hope Ferdowsian, "A Low-Fat Vegan Diet and a Conventional Diabetes Diet in the Treatment of Type 2 Diabetes: A Randomized, Controlled, 74-wk Clinical Trial," *American Journal of Clinical Nutrition* 89, no. 5 (2009): 1588S–1596S, https://doi.org/10.3945/ajcn.2009.26736H; Gunadhar Panigrahi, Sally M. Goodwin, Kara

Livingston Staffier, and Micaela Karlsen, "Remission of Type 2 Diabetes After Treatment with a High-Fiber, Low-Fat, Plant-Predominant Diet Intervention: A Case Series," *American Journal of Lifestyle Medicine* (June 15, 2023), https://doi.org/10.1177/155982762311 81574.

26. Irene Roncero-Ramos, Francisco M. Gutierrez-Mariscal, Francisco Gomez-Delgado, Alejandro Villasanta-Gonzalez, Jose D. Torres-Peña, Silvia De La Cruz-Ares, Oriol A. Rangel-Zuñiga, et al., "Beta Cell Functionality and Hepatic Insulin Resistance Are Major Contributors to Type 2 Diabetes Remission and Starting Pharmacological Therapy: From CORDIOPREV Randomized Controlled Trial," *Translational Research* 238 (December 2021): 12–24, https://doi.org/10.1016/j.trsl.2021.07.001.

27. Sarah Hallberg, "A Comprehensive List of Low Carb Research," Virta Health, January 31, 2018, www.virtahealth.com/blog/low-carb-research-comprehensive-list. This list includes five studies showing that low-carb diets are not superior to higher-carb MyPlate-style diets.

28. Hallberg, "Comprehensive List of Low Carb Research"; Matthew J. Landry, Anthony Crimarco, Dalia Perelman, Lindsay R. Durand, Christina Petlura, Lucia Aronica, Jennifer L. Robinson, Sun H. Kim, and Christopher D. Gardner, "Adherence to Ketogenic and Mediterranean Study Diets in a Crossover Trial: The Keto–Med Randomized Trial," *Nutrients* 13, no. 3 (2021): 967, https://doi.org/10.3390/nu13030967.

29. Megan Molteni, "The Struggles of a $40 Million Nutrition Science Crusade," *Wired*, June 18, 2018, www.wired.com/story/how-a-dollar40-million-nutrition-science-crusade-fell -apart.

30. Kohsuke Hayamizu, "Amino Acids and Energy Metabolism: An Overview," in *Sustained Energy for Enhanced Human Functions and Activity*, ed. Debasis Bagchi, 339–349 (London: Academic Press, 2017).

31. W. R. Beisel, "Alterations in Hormone Production and Utilization During Infection," in *Infection: The Physiologic and Metabolic Responses of the Host*, ed. M. C. Powanda and P. G. Canonico, 147–172 (Amsterdam: Elsevier North Holland Biomedical Press, 1981).

32. Brian S. Fuehrlein, Michael S. Rutenberg, Jared N. Silver, Matthew W. Warren, Douglas W. Theriaque, Glen E. Duncan, Peter W. Stacpoole, and Mark L. Brantly, "Differential Metabolic Effects of Saturated Versus Polyunsaturated Fats in Ketogenic Diets," *Journal of Clinical Endocrinology and Metabolism* 89, no. 4 (2004): 1641–1645, https://doi .org/10.1210/jc.2003-031796.

33. For a figure showing ketone production at fourteen weeks 50 percent higher on soy than coconut oil, see Poonamjot Deol, Jane R. Evans, Joseph Dhahbi, Karthikeyani Chellappa, Diana S. Han, Stephen Spindler, and Frances M. Sladek, "Soybean Oil Is More Obesogenic and Diabetogenic Than Coconut Oil and Fructose in Mouse: Potential Role for the Liver," *PLOS One* (July 22, 2015), https://doi.org/10.1371/journal.pone.0132672.

34. Gerald Grandl, Leon Straub, Carla Rudigier, Myrtha Arnold, Stephan Wueest, Daniel Konrad, and Christian Wolfrum, "Short-Term Feeding of a Ketogenic Diet Induces More Severe Hepatic Insulin Resistance Than an Obesogenic High-Fat Diet," *Journal of Physiology* 596, no. 19 (2018): 4597–4609, https://doi.org/10.1113/JP275173.

35. Tanya J. W. McDonald and Mackenzie C. Cervenka, "Lessons Learned from Recent Clinical Trials of Ketogenic Diet Therapies in Adults," *Current Opinion in Clinical Nutrition and Metabolic Care* 22, no. 6 (November 2019): 418–424, https://doi.org/10.1097 /MCO.0000000000000596.

36. André Lefèvre, Howard Adler, and Charles S. Lieber, "Effect of Ethanol on Ketone Metabolism," *Journal of Clinical Investigation* 49, no. 10 (October 1970): 1775–1782, https:// doi.org/10.1172/jci106395.

37. Y. Kashiwaya, K. Sato, N. Tsuchiya, S. Thomas, D. A. Fell, R. L. Veech, and J. V. Passonneau, "Control of Glucose Utilization in Working Perfused Rat Heart," *Journal of Biological Chemistry* 269, no. 41 (1994): 25502–25514; email communication between Dr. Kashiwaya and the author, December 3, 2012.

38. Bret H. Goodpaster and Lauren M. Sparks, "Metabolic Flexibility in Health and Disease," *Cell Metabolism* 25, no. 5 (May 2, 2017): 1027–1036, http://doi.org/10.1016/j .cmet.2017.04.015.

39. Kevin D. Hall, Thomas Bemis, Robert Brychta, Kong Y. Chen, Amber Courville, Emma J. Crayner, Stephanie Goodwin, et al., "Calorie for Calorie, Dietary Fat Restriction Results in More Body Fat Loss Than Carbohydrate Restriction in People with Obesity," *Cell Metabolism* 22, no. 3 (2015): 427–436, https://doi.org/10.1016/j.cmet.2015.07.021; Kevin D. Hall, Kong Y. Chen, Juen Guo, Yan Y. Lam, Rudolph L. Leibel, Laurel E. S. Mayer, Marc L. Reitman, et al., "Energy Expenditure and Body Composition Changes After an Isocaloric Ketogenic Diet in Overweight and Obese Men," *American Journal of Clinical Nutrition* 104, no. 2 (2016): 324–333, https://doi.org/10.3945/ajcn.116.133561; Kevin D. Hall, Juen Guo, Amber B. Courville, James Boring, Robert Brychta, Kong Y. Chen, Valerie Darcey, et al., "Effect of a Plant-Based, Low-Fat Diet Versus an Animal-Based, Ketogenic Diet on Ad Libitum Energy Intake," *Nature Medicine* 27, no. 2 (2021): 344–353, https://doi.org/10.1038 /s41591-020-01209-1.

40. Philip Felig, John Wahren, Robert Sherwin, and George Palaiologos, "Amino Acid and Protein Metabolism in Diabetes Mellitus," *Archives of Internal Medicine* 137 (1977): 507–513, https://doi.org/ 10.1001/archinte.1977.03630160069014; Weimin Yu, Tomiko Kuhara, Yoshito Inoue, Isamu Matsumoto, Ryoji Iwasaki, and Shinpei Morimoto, "Increased Urinary Excretion of β-Hydroxyisovaleric Acid in Ketotic and Nonketotic Type II Diabetes Mellitus," *Clinica Chimica Acta* 188, no. 2 (April 1990): 161–168, https://doi.org/10.1016/0009 -8981(90)90160-T; Kohsuke Hayamizu, "Amino Acids and Energy Metabolism."

41. Christopher D. Gardner, Matthew J. Landry, Dalia Perelman, Christina Petlura, Lindsay R. Durand, Lucia Aronica, Anthony Crimarco, et al., "Effect of a Ketogenic Diet Versus Mediterranean Diet on Glycated Hemoglobin in Individuals with Prediabetes and

Type 2 Diabetes Mellitus: The Interventional Keto-Med Randomized Crossover Trial," *American Journal of Clinical Nutrition* 116, no. 3 (September 2022): 640–652, https://doi .org/10.1093/ajcn/nqac154.

42. This study lacked a "washout" period that would have allowed participants to return to their baseline state, which critics point out deviated from normal. However, this gives us a unique opportunity to assess the effect of "preparing" for keto.

CHAPTER 9 (PAGES 215 THROUGH 250)

Figure 9–1: My calculations are as follows:

Based on trends since the year 1800 (Walrabenstein et al.), the average person eats 2,500 calories a day. (Note: The numbers below don't add up, and amounts of added fats are lower than in other sources, while the added sugar is high; Walrabenstein and colleagues seem to have a low-carb agenda):

Flour and cereal (aka refined grain): 600

Added sugar: 350

Added fats: 350

Meat, eggs, and nuts: 530 (includes fat from these foods)

Dairy: 250

Vegetables: 130

Fruit: 80

Based on data below, the total calories available are 3,540 per person per day (per UN News). Note that this figure reflects per capita annual *availability*, but the media always reports it as *consumption*:

Calories per Person per Day from Flours and Sugars:

Corn flour: 35.5 pounds per person per year at 1,729 calories per pound = 168 calories per person per day.

Wheat flour: 129.3 pounds per person per year at 1,651 calories per pound = 583 calories per person per day.

Other flour: 5.2 pounds per person per year (use wheat calories) = 24 calories per day.

Total caloric sweeteners: 127.3 pounds per person per year (use sugar calories) at 1,775 calories per pound = 619 calories per day.

Calories per Person per Day from Fats and Oils:

Seed oils consumed: 62 pounds per person per day at 4,002 calories per pound = 679 calories per day.

Unrefined fats: Total = 107 calories per person per day based on figures below.

Butter: 6.3 pounds per person per year at 3,258 calories per pound = 56 calories per person per day.

Olive oil: 1 liter per person per year (2 pounds at 4,000 calories per pound) = 22 calories per person per day.

Tallow: 1 pound per person per year = 11 calories per person per day.

Lard: 1.5 pounds per person per year = 18 calories per person per day.

Calories per Person per Day from Other Sources:

Fresh food: Total = 695 calories per person per day (Note: this includes nuts and probably also includes nut butters and almond milk—i.e., not fresh).

Fruit = 81 calories per person per day.

Vegetables = 126 calories per person per day.

Nuts = 72 calories per person per day.

Meat/poultry/fish = 416 calories per person per day.

Dairy = 234 calories per person per day.

Eggs = 37 calories per person per day.

Sources: US Department of Agriculture (USDA), "Food Availability (Per Capita) Data System," updated April 14, 2023, www.ers.usda.gov/data-products/food-availability-per-capita -data-system; Wendy Walrabenstein, Catharina S. de Jonge, Anna M. Kretova, Marieke van de Put, Carlijn A. Wagenaar, Franktien Turkstra, Hana Kahleova, Simon J. Hill, and Dirkjan van Schaardenburg, "Commentary: United States Dietary Trends Since 1800: Lack of Association Between Saturated Fatty Acid Consumption and Non-communicable Diseases," *Frontiers in Nutrition* 9 (April 28, 2022), https://doi.org/10.3389/fnut.2022.891792; UN News, "Once Again, US and Europe Way Ahead on Daily Calorie Intake," United Nations, December 12, 2022, https://news.un.org/en/story/2022/12/1131637; S. Gerrior, L. Bente, and H. Hiza, *Nutrient Content of the U.S. Food Supply, 1909–2010*, Home Economics Research Report Number 56, US Department of Agriculture, Center for Nutrition Policy and Promotion (CNPP), November 2004, https://grist.org/wp-content/uploads/2006/08/foodsupply1909 -2000.pdf; Tanya L. Blasbalg, Joseph R. Hibbeln, Christopher E. Ramsden, Sharon F. Majchrzak, and Robert R. Rawlings, "Changes in Consumption of Omega-3 and Omega-6 Fatty Acids in the United States During the 20th Century," *American Journal of Clinical Nutrition* 93, no. 5 (2011): 950–962, https://doi.org/10.3945/ajcn.110.006643; Andrzej Blazejczyk and Linda Kantor, "Food Availability and Consumption," US Department of Agriculture Economic Research Service, updated May 5, 2023, www.ers.usda.gov/data-products/ag-and -food-statistics-charting-the-essentials/food-availability-and-consumption; M. Shahbandeh, "Corn Oil Consumption in the U.S., 2004/05–2022/23," Statista, August 24, 2023, www .statista.com/statistics/1022603/corn-oil-consumption-in-the-us; Nils-Gerrit Wunsch, "U.S. Canola Oil Consumption, 2000–2022," Statista, June 13, 2023, www.statista.com /statistics/301036/canola-oil-consumption-united-states; Nils-Gerrit Wunsch, "U.S. Soybean

Oil Consumption, 2000–2022," Statista, June 13, 2023, www.statista.com/statistics/301037 /soybean-oil-consumption-united-states; Nils-Gerrit Wunsch, "U.S. Palm Oil Consumption, 2000–2022," Statista, June 13, 2023, www.statista.com/statistics/301032/palm-oil -consumption-united-states; Nils-Gerrit Wunsch, "U.S. Sunflowerseed Oil Consumption, 2000–2022," Statista, June 13, 2023, www.statista.com/statistics/301040/sunflowerseed-oil -consumption-united-states; M. Shahbandeh, "Per Capita Consumption of Butter in the U.S., 2000–2021," Statista, November 16, 2022, www.statista.com/statistics/184011/per -capita-consumption-of-butter-in-the-us-since-2000; "Olive Oil Consumption," North American Olive Oil Association, accessed September 10, 2023, www.aboutoliveoil.org /olive-oil-consumption; Statista Research Department, "Per Capita Consumption of Edible Beef Tallow in the U.S., 2000–2009," Statista, September 30, 2011, www.statista.com/statistics /184042/per-capita-consumption-of-edible-beef-tallow-in-the-us-since-2000; Statista Research Department, "Per Capita Consumption of Lard in the U.S., 2000–2009," Statista, September 30, 2011, www.statista.com/statistics/184032/per-capita-consumption-of-lard-in -the-us-since-2000; Sarah Rehkamp, "A Look at Calorie Sources in the American Diet," US Department of Agriculture Economic Research Department, December 5, 2016, www.ers .usda.gov/amber-waves/2016/december/a-look-at-calorie-sources-in-the-american-diet. See also sources for Figure 0–1 in introduction.

1. Hilary S. Green and Selina C. Wang, "Purity and Quality of Private Labelled Avo-cado Oil," *Food Control* 152 (October 2023): 109837, https://doi.org/10.1016/j.foodcont .2023.109837.

2. "Why EVERYONE Should Learn to Fry at Home (…and How to Do It Easily)," You-Tube, posted by Pasta Grammar, July 30, 2023, www.youtube.com/watch?v=wzExs5wHYs4.

3. From a recording of a conversation for a documentary called *The Real Skinny on Fat* that took place November 4, 2017, in Manhattan. Jeff Hays Films, hosted by Naomi Whittel, released on March 15, 2018. Used with permission.

4. Zhifei Chen, Fabian Leinisch, Ines Greco, Wei Zhang, Nan Shu, Christine Y. Chuang, Marianne N. Lund, and Michael J. Davies, "Characterisation and Quantification of Protein Oxidative Modifications and Amino Acid Racemisation in Powdered Infant Milk Formula," *Free Radical Research* 53, no. 1 (2019): 68–81, https://doi.org/10.1080/10715762 .2018.1554250.

5. Hong-xin Jia, Wen-Liang Chen, Xiao-Yan Qi, and Mi-Ya Su, "The Stability of Milk-Based Infant Formulas During Accelerated Storage," *CyTA—Journal of Food* 17, no. 1 (2019): 96–104, https://doi.org/10.1080/19476337.2018.1561519.

6. "Proteins present in infant formulas are modified by oxidation and glycation during processing": Zhifei Chen, Alina Kondrashina, Ines Greco, Luke F. Gamon, Mari-anne N. Lund, Linda Giblin, and Michael J. Davies, "Effects of Protein-Derived Amino Acid Modification Products Present in Infant Formula on Metabolic Function, Oxidative Stress, and Intestinal Permeability in Cell Models," *Journal of Agricultural and Food Chemistry* 67, no. 19 (May 15, 2019): 5634–5646, https://doi.org/10.1021/acs.jafc.9b01324.

7. Cheryl Rothwell, "AAP's Relationship with Formula Companies," United States Lactation Consultant Association, August 14, 2019, https://uslca.org/clinical-pearl/aap-and-formula-companies.

8. K. Naidoo, R. Naidoo, and V. Bangalee, "Understanding the Amino Acid Profile of Whey Protein Products," *Global Journal of Health Science* 10, no. 9 (2018), https://doi.org/10.5539/gjhs.v10n9p45.

9. Naidoo et al., "Understanding the Amino Acid Profile of Whey Protein Products."

10. "Defining the Quality of Plant-Based Proteins: Challenges and Opportunities for Pulses," YouTube, posted by AOCS American Oil Chemists' Society, April 28, 2019, www.youtube.com/watch?v=GPHnOTBVRQY.

11. "U.S. Protein Supplements Market Size, Share & COVID-19 Impact Analysis, by Product (Protein Powder, RTD, Protein Bars, and Others), by Source (Plant-Based and Animal-Based), by Distribution Channel (Specialty Retailers, Online Stores, and Others), and Country Forecast, 2022–2029," Fortune Business Insights, Food Supplements, US Protein Supplements Market, February 2023, www.fortunebusinessinsights.com/u-s-protein-supplements-market-107171.

12. Aaron O'Neill, "Average Prices for Soybean Oil Worldwide from 2014 to 2024," Statista, August 3, 2023, www.statista.com/statistics/675815/average-prices-soybean-oil-worldwide.

13. Linda Giblin, A. Süha Yalçın, Gökhan Biçim, Anna C. Krämer, Zhifei Chen, Michael J. Callanan, Elena Arranz, and Michael J. Davies, "Whey Proteins: Targets of Oxidation, or Mediators of Redox Protection," *Free Radical Research* 53, Sup. 1 (2019): 1136–1152, https://doi.org/10.1080/10715762.2019.1632445.

14. Megyn Kelly, "Brutal Inflation, 1/6 Manipulation, and Motherhood, w/ Eric Bolling, Michael Knowles, & Christina P.," YouTube, posted by Megyn Kelly, June 10, 2022, https://youtu.be/tv4GzFsvl1M?t=3343.

CHAPTER 10 (PAGES 251 THROUGH 282)

1. This idea is well supported by Dan Buettner's book *The Blue Zones: Lessons for Living Longer from the People Who've Lived the Longest* (Washington, DC: National Geographic Society, 2008). The author visited four villages around the world where people were healthy into their late seventies and early eighties and interviewed some of the elders he met in each village. Unfortunately, his expenses were paid in part by the Seventh-Day Adventist Church, which has a fixed set of beliefs about what constitutes a healthy diet, specifically that it should be plant based. Although his observations included seeing people in the villages being heavily reliant on animal products (such as weekly purchases of "two-liter plastic bottles to fill with liquefied lard"), the book's highlights and conclusions seem heavily influenced by the project benefactor's agenda.

2. Maria Luz Fernandez and Ana Gabriela Murillo, "Is There a Correlation Between Dietary and Blood Cholesterol? Evidence from Epidemiological Data and Clinical Interventions," *Nutrients* 14, no. 10 (May 2014): 2168, https://doi.org/10.3390/nu14102168.

3. Thomas M. Devlin, ed., *Textbook of Biochemistry* (Hoboken, NJ: Wiley-Liss, 2002), 722.

4. Y. Kashiwaya, K. Sato, N. Tsuchiya, S. Thomas, D. A. Fell, R. L. Veech, and J. V. Passonneau, "Control of Glucose Utilization in Working Perfused Rat Heart," *Journal of Biological Chemistry* 269, no. 41 (1994): 25502–25514.

5. Stephanie M. Fanelli, Owen J. Kelly, Jessica L. Krok-Schoen, and Christopher A. Taylor, "Low Protein Intakes and Poor Diet Quality Associate with Functional Limitations in US Adults with Diabetes: A 2005–2016 NHANES Analysis," *Nutrients* 13, no. 8 (July 2021): 2582, https://doi.org/10.3390/nu13082582.

6. P. Grasgruber, M. Sebera, E. Hrazdíra, J. Cacek, and T. Kalina, "Major Correlates of Male Height: A Study of 105 Countries," *Economics and Human Biology* 21 (May 2016): 172–195, https://doi.org/10.1016/j.ehb.2016.01.005.

7. Takuya Yamaoko, Atsushi Araki, Yoshiaki Tamura, Shiro Tanaka, Kazuya Fujihara, Chika Horikawa, Rei Aida, et al., "Association Between Low Protein Intake and Mortality in Patients with Type 2 Diabetes," *Nutrients* 12, no. 6 (2020): 1629, https://doi.org/10.3390/nu12061629.

8. Rajavel Elango, Mohammad A. Humayun, Ronald O. Ball, and Paul B. Pencharz, "Evidence That Protein Requirements Have Been Significantly Underestimated," *Current Opinion in Clinical Nutrition and Metabolic Care* 13, no. 1 (January 2010): 52–57, https://doi.org/10.1097/mco.0b013e328332f9b7.

9. See Bobby Gill, "Soil Carbon Sequestration with Holistic Planned Grazing: A Map of Published Rates," Savory, March 8, 2023, https://savory.global/soil-carbon-sequestration-with-holistic-planned-grazing-a-map-of-published-rates.

10. "Cancer: Carcinogenicity of the Consumption of Red Meat and Processed Meat," World Health Organization, October 26, 2015, www.who.int/news-room/questions-and-answers/item/cancer-carcinogenicity-of-the-consumption-of-red-meat-and-processed-meat.

11. IARC Working Group on the Evaluation of Carcinogenic Risks to Humans, *Red Meat and Processed Meats*, vol. 114, IARC Monographs on the Evaluation of Carcinogenic Risks to Humans (Lyon, France: International Agency for Research on Cancer, 2015), 385.

12. IARC Working Group, *Red Meat and Processed Meats*, 388–393.

13. "Chemicals in Meat Cooked at High Temperatures and Cancer Risk," National Cancer Institute, reviewed July 11, 2017, www.cancer.gov/about-cancer/causes-prevention/risk/diet/cooked-meats-fact-sheet; David Forman, "Meat and Cancer: A Relation in Search of a Mechanism," *Lancet* 353, no. 9154 (February 27, 1999): 686–687, https://doi.org/10.1016/S0140-6736(98)00377-8.

14. "RR for every 50 g/day increase in processed meat was 1.18" (50 grams is roughly the amount of one hot dog): Doris S. M. Chan, Rosa Lau, Dagfinn Aune, Rui Vieira, Darren C. Greenwood, Ellen Kampman, and Teresa Norat, "Red and Processed Meat and Colorectal Cancer Incidence: Meta-Analysis of Prospective Studies," *PLOS One* 6, no. 6 (2011): e20456, https://doi.org/10.1371/journal.pone.0020456.

15. Loïc Le Marchand, Jean H. Hankin, Lisa M. Pierce, Rashmi Sinha, Pratibha V. Nerurkar, Adrian A. Franke, and Lynne R. Wilkens, et al., "Well-Done Red Meat, Metabolic Phenotypes and Colorectal Cancer in Hawaii," *Mutation Research / Fundamental and Molecular Mechanisms of Mutagenesis* 506–507 (September 30, 2002): 205–214, https://doi.org/10.1016/S0027-5107(02)00167-7.

16. Naomi Fliss-Isakov, Shira Zelber-Sagi, Dana Ivancovsky-Wajcman, Oren Shibolet, and Revital Kariv, "Ultra-Processed Food Intake and Smoking Interact in Relation with Colorectal Adenomas," *Nutrients* 12, no. 11 (November 2020): 3507, https://doi.org/10.3390/nu12113507.

17. H.-K. Biesalski, "Meat as a Component of a Healthy Diet—Are There Any Risks or Benefits If Meat Is Avoided in the Diet?," *Meat Science* 70, no. 3 (July 2005): 509–524, https://doi.org/10.1016/j.meatsci.2004.07.017; Keli M. Hawthorne, Jill Castle, and Sharon M. Donovan, "Meat Helps Make Every Bite Count: An Ideal First Food for Infants," *Nutrition Today* 51, no. 1 (January/February 2022): 8–13, https://doi.org/10.1097/NT.0000000000000523.

18. Hawthorne et al., "Meat Helps Make Every Bite Count."

19. Audra Boscoe, Clark Paramore, and Joseph G. Verbalis, "Cost of Illness of Hyponatremia in the United States," *Cost Effectiveness and Research Allocation* 4 (2006): 10, https://doi.org/10.1186/1478-7547-4-10.

20. Alyssa J. Moran, Maricelle Ramirez, and Jason P. Block, "Consumer Underestimation of Sodium in Fast Food Restaurant Meals: Results from a Cross-Sectional Observational Study," *Appetite* 113 (June 2017): 155–161, https://doi.org/10.1016/j.appet.2017.02.028.

21. China Salt Substitute Study Collaborative Group, "Salt Substitution: A Low-Cost Strategy for Blood Pressure Control Among Rural Chinese. A Randomized, Controlled Trial," *Journal of Hypertension* 25, no. 10 (October 2007): 2011–2018, https://doi.org/10.1097/hjh.0b013e3282b9714b; Li Che, Wei Song, Ying Zhang, Yan Lu, Yunpeng Cheng, Yinong Jiang, "A Randomized, Double-Blind Clinical Trial to Evaluate the Blood Pressure Lowing Effect of Low-Sodium Salt Substitution on Middle-Aged and Elderly Hypertensive Patients with Different Plasma Renin Concentrations," *Journal of Clinical Hypertension (Greenwich)* 24, no. 2 (February 2022): 140–147, https://doi.org/10.1111/jch.14396.

INDEX

Vegetable oil stole your health. Here's how we can take it back . . .

Feel Better Faster: Boost Your Health with These Seven Free Reader's Tools

- Use the **Protein Calculator** to confidently know you're getting enough
- Quickly identify and avoid bad fats with my **Good vs. Bad Fats Cheat Sheet**
- Use the **Kitchen Detox Assistant** to establish a roadmap for purging the bad fats
- Help loved ones boost their health with my **Metabolic Vicious Cycle 2 Pager**
- Leverage my **Carb Calculator** so you can assess amounts and easily find better carbs
- Cut planning hassle with my **One-Week Meal Planner and Shopping List**
- Detect metabolism issues and improve and track them using my **Pathologic Hunger Tracker**

Go here now to claim the resources you earned:
https://drcate.com/darkcaloriesdownloads/

SCAN ME